Nuclear Medicine Self-Study Program III: NUCLEAR MEDICINE CARDIOLOGY

Topic 5: Myocardial Perfusion Scintigraphy—Technical Aspects

Series Editor

Elias H. Botvinick, MD
University of California at San Francisco, California

Contributors

Elias H. Botvinick, MD
Neil Ratzlaff, MS, CNMT
University of California at San Francisco, California
J.I.E. Hoffman, MD
University of California at San Francisco, California
Jamshid Maddahi, MD
University of California at Los Angeles, California
Ernest Garcia, MD, PhD
Emory Medical Center, Atlanta, Georgia
Erwin A. Rodrigues, MB
Cedars Sinai Medical Center, Los Angeles, California
Kenneth Van Train, BS
Cedars-Sinai Medical Center, Los Angeles, California
Daniel S. Berman, MD
Cedars-Sinai Medical Center, Los Angeles, California

Society of Nuclear Medicine
1850 Samuel Morse Drive, Reston, Virginia 20190-5316

Made in the United States of America.

Library of Congress Cataloging-in-Publication Data

Myocardial perfusion scintigraphy : technical aspects / contributors, Elias H. Botvinick ... [et al.].
p. ; cm. -- (Nuclear medicine self-study program III. Nuclear medicine cardiology ; unit 5)
Includes bibliographical references.
ISBN 0-932004-57-1
1. Myocardial infarction--Radionuclide imaging I. Botvinick, Elias H. II. Society of Nuclear Medicine (1953-) III. Series.
[DNLM: 1. Heart--radionuclide imaging--Examination Questions. 2. Coronary Circulation--Examination Questions. 3. Gated Blood-Pool Imaging--methods--Examination Questions. 4. Radiopharmaceuticals--diagnostic use--Examination Questions. 5. Tomography, Emission-Computed, Single-Photon--methods--Examination Questions. WG 18.2 N964 1997 Unit 5]
RC683.5.R33 N855 unit 5
[RC685.I6]
616.1'207575 s--dc21
[616.1'2407575]

2001020996

Contents

TOPIC 5: **Myocardial Perfusion Scintigraphy—Technical Aspects**

OVERVIEW **5**

CORONARY BLOOD FLOW **5**

Definitions, Units of Measure **5**

Basic Physiology **6**

Specific Lesions and Abnormal States **11**

RADIONUCLIDES **13**

The Perfusion Radiotracers **15**

Linearity with Flow **35**

Evaluation of Ventricular Function **36**

TECHNICAL ASPECTS OF GATED SPECT MYOCARDIAL PERFUSION SCINTIGRAPHY **43**

Overview **43**

Potential Problems with the Method **46**

Variability in the Measurement of Function and Perfusion **47**

STRESS TESTING PROTOCOLS **49**

Dynamic (Treadmill/Bicycle) Exercise: An Indirect Test of Coronary Flow Reserve **49**

Pharmacologic Stress Testing Using Coronary Vasodilators **51**

IMAGING PROTOCOLS **53**

Overview **53**

Thallium-201 Protocols **53**

Technetium-99m Sestamibi and Tetrofosmin Protocols **55**

Dual-Isotope Protocol **58**

Gating **61**

IMAGE ACQUISITION **62**

Planar Imaging **62**

SPECT Imaging **62**

IMAGE PROCESSING AND QUANTITATION **63**

Planar Studies **63**

SPECT Studies **69**

Principles of Display **78**

Standard Software Displays **82**

Current Software **85**

Sources of Error and Quality Control **88**

THE MOST COMMON PLANAR AND SPECT IMAGE ARTIFACTS . . . **95**
General Considerations . . . **95**
Variants of Normal SPECT Analysis . . . **97**
Nonperfusion and Other Indications of Extensive Coronary Disease and Ischemia . . . **99**
Attenuation . . . **100**
Scattered Photons . . . **107**
SPECT Artifacts . . . **108**
Image Interpretation . . . **128**
FLUORODEOXYGLUCOSE IMAGING WITH CONVENTIONAL CAMERAS . . . **128**
Overview . . . **128**
THE CURRENT STATE OF THE TECHNOLOGY . . . **131**
ANNOTATED REFERENCES . . . **132**
QUESTIONS AND CASE EXAMPLES . . . **187**
ANSWERS AND CRITIQUES FOR MULTIPLE-CHOICE QUESTIONS . . . **209**

Editor's Acknowledgment

To me, working to develop this series has been a "labor of love." At the beginning, I doubted that I had the ability to formulate and the energy to complete this work. Toward the middle, while deeply committed to the work but faced with the onslaught of competing modalities, I worried whether there would be practitioners who would read it! Now, as I near the end, I am pleased that the task was undertaken, that it was well supported and that it may serve as a benchmark of effort, if not accomplishment, in the field of clinical teaching.

I asked for, and the Society permitted, the inclusion of many of my teaching tools and a number of contributions related to pathophysiology, metabolism, and technical aspects of the field of cardiovascular nuclear medicine (nuclear cardiology) that are unique to such a clinical set and adds depth. The annotated references and case presentations were demanded by the preset form of the series, but I approached and implemented them with enthusiasm.

There are many to thank: the contributors; my physician, nurse practitioner, nurse, and technologist colleagues; my inspirational students and patients; and the now vibrant field of cardiovascular nuclear medicine. But there is only one person to whom these volumes can appropriately be dedicated and she falls in none of these categories.

Editor's Dedication

My love and gratitude to my best friend and wife, Carroll, who encouraged and supported me and who sacrificed as much as I, simply because of me, to see this effort through.

Myocardial Perfusion Scintigraphy—Technical Aspects

OVERVIEW

In 1973, Zaret et al. (*1*) introduced radionuclide imaging of myocardial perfusion using potassium-43 (^{43}K). For a short period, rubidium-81 (^{81}Rb) appeared to be the agent of choice (*2*). However, both radionuclides had high energies of emission, which was disadvantageous. In the same year, Lebowitz et al. (*3*) introduced thallium-201 (^{201}Tl) for myocardial perfusion imaging. Since these reports, exercise ^{201}Tl myocardial perfusion scintigraphy (MPS) has become an important and widely applied method in the clinical assessment of coronary artery disease (CAD)(*4*). Investigation of the myocardial kinetics of the radionuclide has led to a better understanding of the significance of various patterns of agent redistribution and has shaped ^{201}Tl imaging protocols (*5–7*). Technetium-99m (^{99m}Tc)–labeled radionuclides have been introduced with superior imaging characteristics (*8,9*), making practical the simultaneous evaluation of perfusion and function (*10,11*). SPECT and other technical developments have advanced the field (see Self-Study Program III, *Nuclear Medicine: Cardiology, Topic 1: Physical and Technical Aspects of Nuclear Cardiology*) (*12,13*). Quantitative analysis has objectified image analysis and has provided useful indices for evaluation of CAD (*14*). Tomographic imaging has improved detection and localization of perfusion abnormalities (*14,15*). Pharmacologic stress testing has been developed as an alternative to exercise testing in patients who are unable to exercise adequately (see Self-Study Program III, *Nuclear Medicine: Cardiology, Topic 2: Pharmacologic Stress*) (*16*). Extensive research has established an important clinical role for MPS as a cost-effective method for diagnosis, risk stratification and viability evaluation in CAD (see Self-Study Program III, *Nuclear Medicine: Cardiology, Topic 6: Myocardial Perfusion Scintigraphy—Clinical Aspects*).

CORONARY BLOOD FLOW

Definitions, Units of Measurement

Coronary blood flow is the flow passing through the coronary arteries, and myocardial flow is the flow entering the myocardium. The 2 quantities are usually similar, except for a small amount of myocardial flow that comes from pericardial and mediastinal vessels and in the case of coronary–cameral or coronary–pulmonary arterial fistulas, in which not all flow entering the coronary arteries goes into the myocardium.

Myocardial oxygen consumption or uptake is the amount of oxygen used by the heart. It may be measured per beat or per minute for the whole heart, the left ventricle or per unit mass of tissue (per gram or per 100 g), in milliliters or micromoles. Myocardial oxygen demand is the amount of oxygen that the heart needs. Myocardial oxygen consumption and demand normally are the same, as long as the myocardial oxygen supply is unrestricted. When supply falls below demand, myocardial ischemia occurs.

Myocardial ischemia represents an imbalance between oxygen supply and demand that leads to impaired myocardial oxidative metabolism and myocardial dysfunction. The impairment may be transient ("stunning," "hibernation") or permanent (*17*).

Basic Physiology

Myocardial Oxygen Demand. The heart has one of the highest oxygen consumptions per unit mass of any organ in the body. With exercise or other forms of stress, myocardial oxygen consumption and demand may rise several times above the resting level.

The basic determinants of myocardial oxygen consumption have been worked out in isolated papillary muscle strips and sampling the intact heart (*18*). These determinants include preload and afterload, parameters indirectly related to blood pressure, heart rate, contraction duration and contractility. Most of the energy and oxygen consumption during muscle contraction are used to generate force (internal work), and only about 10% is used for shortening (external work). Another 15% is used for basal metabolism, and about 10% is used in activation, associated with sodium (Na)+K+ adenosine triphosphatase (ATPase) and calcium++ ATPase (*19*). These findings suggest that, in the whole heart, the major consumption of oxygen is used to generate pressure, with lesser amounts being used in ejection (shortening), basal metabolism and cellular activation. Circumferential wall stress is a stronger predictor of myocardial oxygen consumption than pressure and may be calculated by a simplification of the LaPlace relationship for spheres, expressed as:

$$\text{wall stress} = Pr/2h,$$

where P is pressure, r is the radius of curvature and h is wall thickness (*20*). Because changes in pressure and wall stress differ, indices that use pressure are rough predictors of myocardial oxygen consumption, and the 2 measures tend to change in the same direction. These include the double product (peak systolic pressure × heart rate) and the triple product (double product × duration of ejection), which are relatively gross measures and cannot be relied upon to indicate small differences in oxygen demand.

An increase in heart rate affects oxygen consumption, both by increasing the number of contractions per minute and by increasing contractility. Increased contractility in turn increases oxygen consumption per beat, but, at the same time, it decreases ventricular volume and thus wall stress (*21*). Because the right ventricle does not have a single draining vein, less is known about right ventricular myocardial oxygen consumption.

Little is known about the regional distribution of myocardial oxygen consumption across the left ventricular wall. Weiss et al. (*22*) observed slightly greater oxygen extraction and consumption in the left ventricular subendocardial muscle than in other layers.

Myocardial Blood Flow. High left ventricular myocardial oxygen consumption is associated with a high oxygen extraction even at rest, and additional oxygen extraction is restricted by the limitations of the hemoglobin–oxygen dissociation curve. Therefore, when myocardial oxygen demands increase, they are normally met by an increase in myocardial blood flow. In the left ventricle, flows in resting individuals are about 80–100 ml/min/100g and, with increased demands, normally can increase 3–5-fold. Flow in ventricular walls may be inhomogeneous, especially with certain stresses. Flow tends to be less in the outermost third (subepicardial muscle) than the innermost third (subendocardial muscle), with an inner-to-outer (or subendocardial-to-subepicardial) flow ratio calculated in flows per gram that normally ranges from 1.2–1.4 (*23*).

For a given coronary arterial pressure, flow will depend upon the resistance that it meets. The lower the resistance, the higher the flow. Three types of resistance can be found in any region of the ventricle (*24*). The first is the minimal resistance (R_{min}) offered by the vascular bed when it is maximally dilated and the heart is not contracting. The second is the added resistance($R_{beating}$) imposed when the heart beats and compresses the vessels. This effect is inhomogeneous. Finally, when the vessels have tone, this superimposes another resistance, R_{tone}.

R_{min} is lower in left ventricular subendocardium than subepicardium, so that in the arrested heart with maximally dilated vessels, subendocardial flow is much greater than subepicardial flow (*24*), and the inner-to-outer flow ratio may be ≥ 2. Within any layer, however, flow varies greatly, presumably reflecting differences in the resistances of the vascular pathways to small regions of the ventricular wall (*25*).

When the heart is allowed to beat with maximal coronary dilation, systolic intramyocardial pressures modulate the passive flow distributions to reduce subendocardial flows and increase subepicardial flows (*26*). When tone is added to the vessels, the flows are substantially lower than when the vessels are maximally dilated. Great heterogeneity of flows are still found even within a layer, but there is no correlation between flows in the beating heart with or without vascular tone. The inner-to-outer flow ratio is ~1, but, in small regions, flows are determined primarily by local metabolic demands rather than by intramyocardial pressures or vascular resistances, and vary temporally as well as regionally (*27*).

Autoregulation. When the heart is beating and the vessels have tone, each region regulates the flow so that it gets what it needs. This can be studied by cannulating the left coronary artery so that the perfusing pressure can be raised or lowered without altering left ventricular pressure or heart rate, with little alteration in myocardial oxygen consumption or coronary flow demands. When this is done, a plot of pressure versus flow shows the typical pattern that is termed "autoregulation" (*28*) (Fig. 1). Over a wide range within the normal operating pressures, flow changes little as perfusing pressure is raised or lowered. When pressure is raised, flow immediately rises but, because the vessels contract, returns almost to its control value after 20–30 sec. When pressure is lowered, flow immediately decreases but, because the vessels dilate, gradually returns to near normal. At high pressures (>~120 mm mercury [Hg] mean perfusing pressure in acute studies), the flows increase persistently, presumably because the vasoconstriction has been overcome by the high pressure. More interesting and more relevant is what happens at very low perfusing pressures. At a pressure <60–70 mm Hg in anesthetized dogs (*29*) and about 40 mm Hg in conscious

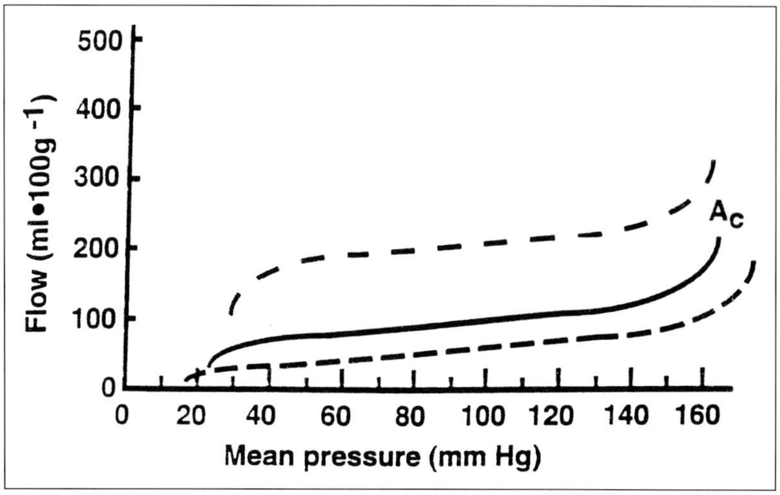

Figure 1 Autoregulation. Typical autoregulation relationships at normal (Ac) higher (above) and lower (below) myocardial oxygen demands. The curved departures from the straight line at high and low pressures are inexact, especially at the higher pressures, because they have not been studied in detail.

dogs, autoregulation fails and flow falls (*28*) (Fig. 2). The flow begins to decrease, because some vessels cannot dilate further and so can no longer compensate for a reduced perfusion pressure. Autoregulation has reached its limits.

Metabolic Regulation. Myocardial oxygen demands are increased by tachycardia, increased pressure and, to a lesser extent, volume work and an increase in contractility. Normal hearts can tolerate very high heart rates, 200–250 beats/min, for short periods (*30*). Tachycardia decreases the total diastolic time per minute and the proportion of diastole per cycle and increases contractility and overall myocardial oxygen consumption. Even when myocardial oxygen demands are increased, however, autoregulation still occurs at the higher flow rate (*31*) (Fig. 1).

Coronary Flow Reserve. At any given pressure, the flow when the vessels have tone is determined by the myocardial oxygen needs at that moment. On the other hand, when the vessels are maximally dilated, flow depends only on vascular resistance and myocardial contraction and is independent of metabolism. If flow is measured at different perfusing pressures when the vessels have tone and again when they are maximally dilated, a typical diagram of coronary conductance, the reciprocal of resistance, results (*29*) (Figs. 3A–D). The higher the conductance, the greater the flow at any perfusion pressure. The normal conductogram (Fig. 3A) shows a relatively horizontal line of autoregulated flow between perfusing pressures of 40 and 120 mm Hg. Autoregulation fails outside those limits. When the vessels are maximally dilated, there is a very steep pressure–flow line. The vertical difference between the 2 lines indicates the extra flow that can be attained at any given pressure by dilating the vessels and is termed the coronary flow reserve (CFR). Like the other flows, it is measured in ml/min/unit mass. It is also possible to derive a dimensionless CFR ratio by dividing maximal flow by autoregulated flow, when flows or velocities cannot be related to a specific tissue mass. Either form of flow reserve gets smaller as the perfusing pressure decreases. When aortic pressure rises, the increased pressure work increases the autoregulated flow, but the increased coronary perfusing pressure increases maximal flow, so that the CFR ratio is unaltered.

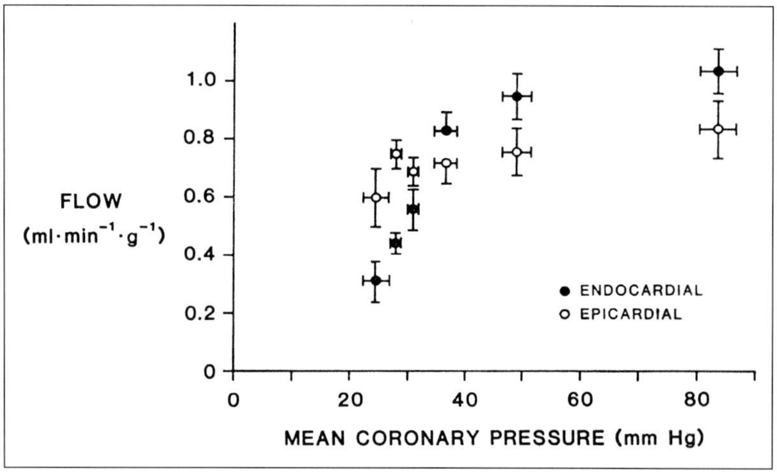

Figure 2 Regional flow relationships. The relation between subendocardial (closed circle) and subepicardial (open circle) flows per gram and mean coronary perfusing pressure is shown. Autoregulation fails at higher pressures in the subendocardium than in the subepicardium. (Reprinted with permission from Canty JM, Jr. Coronary pressure-function and steady-state pressure-flow relations during autoregulation in the unanesthetized dog. *Circ Res* 1988;63:821–836.)

CFR can be reduced when either maximal flow remains unchanged but autoregulated flow increases (Fig. 3B) or when autoregulated flow remains the same but maximal flows are reduced (Fig. 3C). An increase in autoregulated flow will occur in many circumstances, including an increase in heart rate, increased metabolism (as in thyrotoxicosis), increased systolic pressure work, increased contractility or increased preload (dilating the ventricle and increasing wall stress), decreased blood oxygen content (as in anemia), hypoxemia or abnormal hemoglobins (*32*) or with increased wall mass. Some of these conditions may produce changes in maximal flows. Thus, anemia increases maximal flows by reducing blood viscosity but not enough to compensate for the increase in baseline regulated flows. On the other hand, increased heart rate, by reducing the duration of diastole, decreases maximal flows (Fig. 4).

A decreased maximal flow indicates either increased blood viscosity, reduced diastolic perfusion time, increased ventricular diastolic pressure, reduced diastolic perfusion pressure or decreased cross-sectional area (stenosis) of the myocardial vascular bed as a result of large- or small-vessel CAD. Several of these conditions also will be accompanied by an increased autoregulated flow, for example, with rapid pacing or with polycythemia and hypoxemia. Under these circumstances, CFR will be greatly reduced or even absent. This must be considered when evaluating the flow response dynamic or pharmacologic stress in CAD. When CFR is reduced, either because of an increase in autoregulated flow or a decrease in maximal flow, the pressure at which autoregulation fails and pressure dependency starts shifts to the right, that is, toward higher pressures. This is a consequence of the slope of the line of maximal pressure–flow relations. As a result, autoregulation can fail at normal perfusing pressures (Fig. 3D).

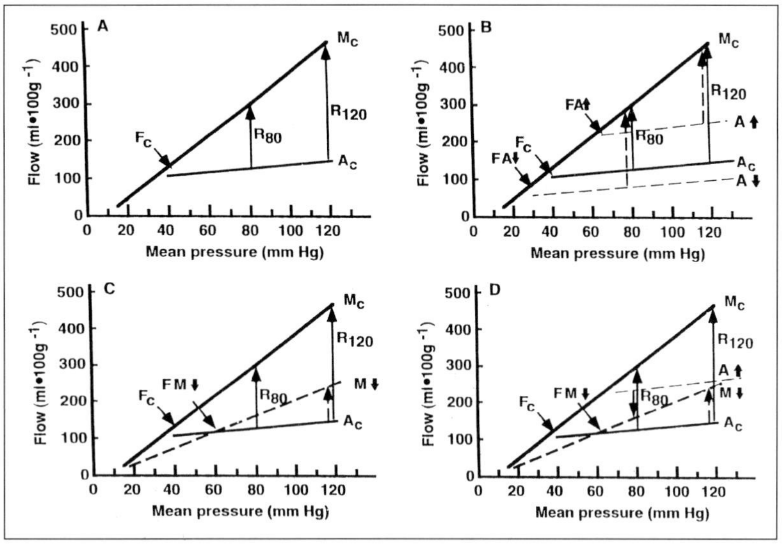

Figure 3 Coronary conductance diagrams. Plots of left ventricular flow (ml/min/100g) against mean coronary perfusing pressure are shown. The higher the conductance, the greater the flow at any perfusion pressure. (A) The normal conductogram. Ac is the control autoregulation line. When autoregulation fails, the curve turns downward at low pressures (not shown) and turns upward at high pressures (not shown). M_c is the control maximal pressure–flow line. Its zero-flow intercept is not shown. The 2 vertical arrows (R_{80} and R_{120}) show the coronary flow reserve (CFR) at 2 different perfusing pressures. The oblique arrow (F_c) shows the approximate pressure at which autoregulation fails at low pressures in the conscious dog. (B) Altered autoregulation. Superimposed on the normal coronary conductogram are dashed lines that indicate autoregulation at increased (A↑) and decreased (A↓) myocardial oxygen consumption. Note that the lower pressure at which autoregulation fails (F_c) is higher when myocardial oxygen consumption is increased (FA↑) and lower when it is decreased (FA↓). Furthermore, the CFR is reduced when myocardial oxygen consumption is increased (shown by the slightly offset vertical dashed arrow next to R_{120}) and is increased when myocardial oxygen consumption is decreased (the slightly offset vertical dashed arrow next to R_{80}). (C) Decreased maximal pressure–flow line. The lower slope of the line of reduced maximal pressure–flow relations (M↓) shows reduced CFR at 120-mm-Hg perfusing pressure (slightly offset vertical dashed arrow next to R_{120}), so that it is now less than the normal reserve at a perfusing pressure of 80 mm Hg. Note, too, that the lower pressure at which autoregulation fails (FM↓) is higher than normal (F_c) when the maximal pressure–flow line has a lower slope. (D) Combined increased myocardial oxygen consumption and decreased maximal pressure–flow line. The symbols are the same as those in A–C. Note that CFR is now absent (downward pointing arrow next to R_{80}), even at a perfusing pressure of 120 mm Hg. In this setting, autoregulation fails at about 125-mm-Hg perfusing pressure. This dire combination is what can be expected in a cyanotic patient with ventricular hypertrophy, arterial hypoxemia and polycythemia.

Regardless of the mechanism, if an altered regional CFR is large enough, it will be evident on MPS. If these conditions apply generally throughout the myocardium, they may not produce any regional heterogeneity and so may not be

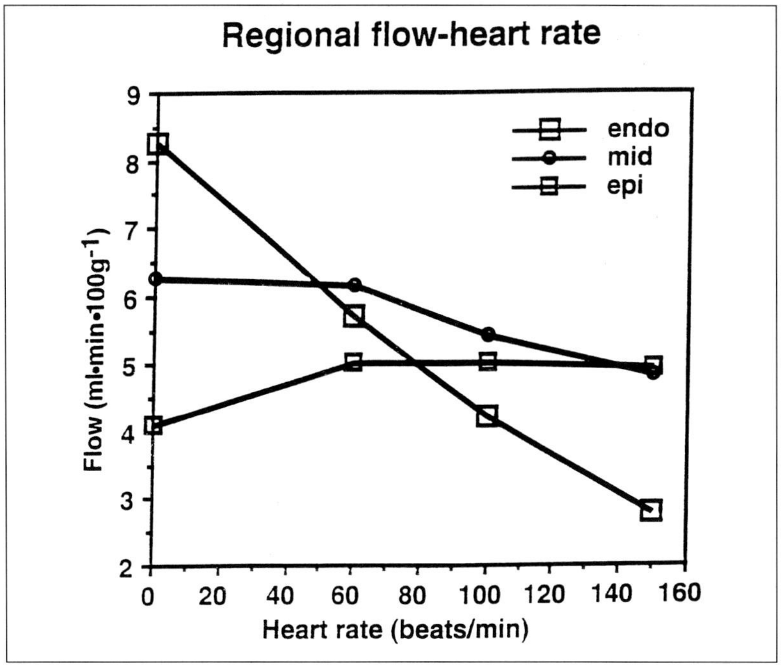

Figure 4 The effect of heart rate on coronary flow. Shown is the decremental effect of heart rate on regional coronary flow when all other factors are controlled. The greatest effect is on endocardial (endo) flow, whereas epicardial (epi) and midmyocardial layers (mid) are less affected. (Adapted from Buckberg GD, Fixler DE, Archie JP, et al. Variable effects of heart rate on phasic and regional left ventricular muscle blood flow in anaesthetised dogs. *Cardiovasc Res* 1975;9:1–11.)

seen with the relative assessment of regional perfusion on current single-photon emission computed tomography (SPECT) but will be evident on quantitative positron emission tomography (PET) perfusion measurements. The development of such quantitation for clinical PET and SPECT is important in maximizing the identification of regional ischemia but less so for the specific case of diffuse homogeneous underperfusion. Diffuse underprofusion, although important to consider, is uncommon and far less common than the simple underestimation of myocardium at ischemic risk. In fact, extensive disease is related to the highest diagnostic image sensitivity and prognostic risk. A normal stress perfusion scan indicates an excellent prognosis and is not commonly related to severe, extensive coronary disease or to events, even in patients who have coronary disease. Further, such extensive ischemia often also presents in association with cavitary dilation, ^{201}Tl lung uptake and the "nonperfusion indicators" of severe, extensive coronary involvement (See Self-Study Program III, *Nuclear Medicine: Cardiology, Topic 6: Myocardial Perfusion Scintigraphy—Clinical Aspects*).

Even when recognized, separating what must be the rare condition of balanced ischemia as a result of extensive multivessel disease from the myriad of other potential factors influencing image findings may be difficult. In addition, the presence of a diffusely reduced CFR that has resulted from a condition other than CAD will make it difficult to appreciate any further regional reduction in CFR from CAD. Again, this seems to be a rare occurence. Shown diagrammatically in Figure 1 of Self-Study Program III, *Nuclear Medicine: Cardiology, Topic 2: Pharmacologic Stress* is the relationship between the percentage of coronary stenosis and the flow through that vessel at rest and with hyperemic stress. In the absence of complicating factors, flow is maintained at rest, even with severe stenosis, because of the dilation of the coronary resistance vessels, the precapillaries and arterioles. With hyperemia, flow in vessels with "significant" coronary lesions fails to augment, as does the normal vessel. It is such induced flow heterogeneity among vessels with varying degrees of pathology that brings image abnormalities.

Pressure–Flow Relations. Bellamy et al. (*33*) observed that when coronary perfusing pressure was reduced progressively, flow ceased at a pressure of ~45 mm Hg during autoregulation and at ~18 mm Hg when the vessels were maximally dilated. Under some circumstances, such as with pericardial tamponade and with very high right or left ventricular end-diastolic pressures, the coronary driving pressure (the difference between inflow perfusion pressure and outflow or backpressure) may be reduced. This has the same effect in reducing CFR as does a decrease in perfusing pressure.

Regulation of Myocardial Vascular Tone. The heart cannot sustain anaerobic metabolism without becoming injured, so myocardial oxygen supply must be tightly regulated. When myocardial oxygen demand increases, flow increases rapidly (within 10–20 sec) to supply the extra oxygen. When myocardial oxygen demand decreases, flow decreases rapidly until oxygen supply and demand are once again in balance. The mechanisms involved in this adjustment are not well understood. The first proposed mechanism concerned intrinsic adenosine, which is produced in proportion to the degree of muscle contraction. The latter causes the breakdown of ATP, and the adenosine monophosphate thereby produced is degraded by the enzyme 5′-nucleotidase to adenosine, a powerful coronary vasodilator. However, elimination of the interstitial adenosine by infusing low-molecular-weight adenosine deaminase, the enzyme that decomposes adenosine, does not alter autoregulation (*34*). Moreover, even in the presence of definite ischemia and reactive hyperemia, infusing adenosine deaminase reduces but does not abolish the hyperemic response. More recently, a number of other potential regulators have been studied, including potent vasodilators such as nitric oxide, substance P, prostacyclin, bradykinin and atrial natriuretic peptides, as well as vasoconstrictors such as neuropeptide Y, endothelin and the adrenergic nerves with their transmitters. Although the specific roles of these various agents in coronary regulation have not yet been documented, nitric oxide does appear to play an important role in the coronary circulation (*35*).

Specific Lesions and Abnormal States

Tachycardia. Heart rates >250 bpm for an extended period may produce a decreased inner-to-outer flow ratio, as a result of a shorter diastolic perfusion time, lowered aortic diastolic perfusing pressure and perhaps a rise in left ventricular diastolic pressure (*36*). Although the absolute flows rise in all layers, CFR becomes reduced in the inner half and, at very high rates, may be absent. It is at this stage that the subendocardial vessels become pressure dependent, and ischemia may result. The inner-to-outer flow ratio decreases. If the ventricle is hypertrophied, then tachycardia causes subendocardial ischemia much more readily. Modest tachycardia, at a rate of 200 bpm, will cause subendocardial ischemia in dogs with coronary stenosis. The tighter the coronary stenosis, the less the increase in heart rate required to cause subendocardial ischemia

Ventricular Hypertrophy. Hypertrophy in adult animals is accompanied by an increase in muscle mass but no corresponding increase in conducting vessels (*37*). In general, the increased wall thickening tends to keep wall tension normal, so that myocardial oxygen consumption per unit mass remains at control values. However, overall ventricular myocardial oxygen consumption is increased in proportion to the increase in muscle mass. Flow increases to supply this increased amount of oxygen and does so by dilating the coronary vascular bed. On the other hand, maximal flow per ventricle is not increased and may even be decreased in the presence of associated small vessel medial hypertrophy or intimal disease, in which CFR tends to be reduced. Similar results have been found in humans (*38*). When the hypertrophy is the result of hypertension, then an uncontrolled blood pressure would bring an increased perfusion pressure, which may result in a normal CFR, with both resting and maximal flows increased proportionally. However, if blood pressure is well controlled or hypotension ensues, CFR again would fall.

Anemia. Anemia increases cardiac output and thus myocardial oxygen consumption and, at the same time, decreases the oxygen-carrying capacity of the blood. This is compensated for by an increased coronary blood flow, which, however, is at the expense of CFR. Studies in dogs have shown that myocardial oxygen supply will be normal at rest at virtually any degree of anemia and at arterial saturations down to 55% (*32*). With exercise, oxygen supply will be inadequate at a hematocrit of 20% when mean arterial pressure is 100 mm Hg and arterial oxygen saturation is 100% and at a hematocrit of 30% when mean arterial pressure is 75 mm Hg.

Hypoxemia. As expected, hypoxemia increases coronary blood flow (*39*). At rest, a saturation of 55% can supply myocardial oxygen needs at all perfusing pressures and in a normal heart at all hematocrits. With maximal exercise, a saturation of 85% is needed to supply the myocardial oxygen needs at a perfusing pressure of 100 mm Hg and hematocrits of 30%–70%. Lower perfusing pressures or saturations cannot supply myocardial oxygen needs at any hematocrit

Coronary Arterial Stenoses. With a localized atheromatous lesion of a major branch of a coronary artery at rest, pressure will drop across the obstruction as a result of the increased resistance it offers to flow. This pressure drop will be greater in diastole, when flow is highest, than in systole. Nevertheless, in both parts of the cycle the coronary perfusing pressure will be decreased. Autoregulation causes the small intramural vessels to dilate and lower their resistance, so that myocardial oxygen demands can be met. CFR, however, will be decreased in this distal bed once the obstruction becomes significant (*40*). If the modest stenosis becomes severe, whether acutely by spasm or by hemorrhage into the plaque or chronically by growth in volume of the plaque, then distal pressures may fall below the level at which autoregulation can occur, and CFR will be absent. Consequently, flow will decrease below the amount needed to supply even the most minimal myocardial oxygen needs, and ischemia will occur, particularly in the subendocardium. The patient may have rest pain and ischemic electrocardiographic (ECG) changes. Such a patient may present with the clinical syndrome of unstable angina. Rest pain indicates severely impaired coronary flow to a region that does not have an increased oxygen demand; if allowed to persist, it is a precursor of necrosis.

If the less severe obstruction gradually increases, resting flow will remain at its previous value but CFR will become progressively reduced (*40*). If the patient with this moderate stenosis exercises, the increased resting coronary vasodilatation will decrease the regional CFR. Pharmacologic stress that increases myocardial oxygen demands or exercise sufficient to raise only modestly the myocardial oxygen needs may then exhaust CFR, producing subendocardial ischemia. These features are the basis for various types of exercise tests and exercise imaging methods to delineate ischemic regions (Table 1). Alternatively, administration of an agent that dilates the coronary resistance vessels without increasing demands will induce heterogeneous flow in the presence of regional variations in the CFR. This is the basis for pharmacologic stress testing with dipyridamole and adenosine.

Gould et al. (*40,41*) have described some important variations in the measurement of CFR. They distinguish between stenosis flow reserve, which is entirely a consequence of the stenosis and the adjacent artery, and metabolic perfusion reserve, which is a function of aortic pressure, heart rate and collateral flow. Stenosis flow reserve can be assessed by quantitative arteriography and the application of

Table 1
BASIS OF EXERCISE AND PHARMACOLOGIC STRESS TESTING

Exercise and dobutamine
- Seek to maximize myocardial oxygen demand
- Demand measured by the double product: heart rate × systolic blood pressure
- Because increased myocardial oxygen demands must be supplied by increased coronary blood flow. Failure to fulfill demands results in ischemia.

Direct coronary dilators
- Seek to maximize this supply in the absence of augmented demand. Perfusion imaging demonstrates heterogeneity in the hyperemic response.

well-validated hydraulic principles. Metabolic perfusion reserve can be assessed by quantitative PET. Subsequently, the authors also distinguished between absolute and relative CFR (*42*). Absolute CFR was defined as maximal flow divided by resting flow. For any given degree of coronary obstruction, this was not constant but varied with aortic pressure and heart rate. By contrast, relative flow reserve (the flow in one myocardial bed compared with that in the bed with the highest CFR) was unaffected by these variations and depended only on the degree of stenosis (Fig. 5). It is only a correlate of relative CFR that is evaluated by conventional scintigraphic methods and MPS. Absolute flow can only be measured with special effort using PET-related tracers (*43*).

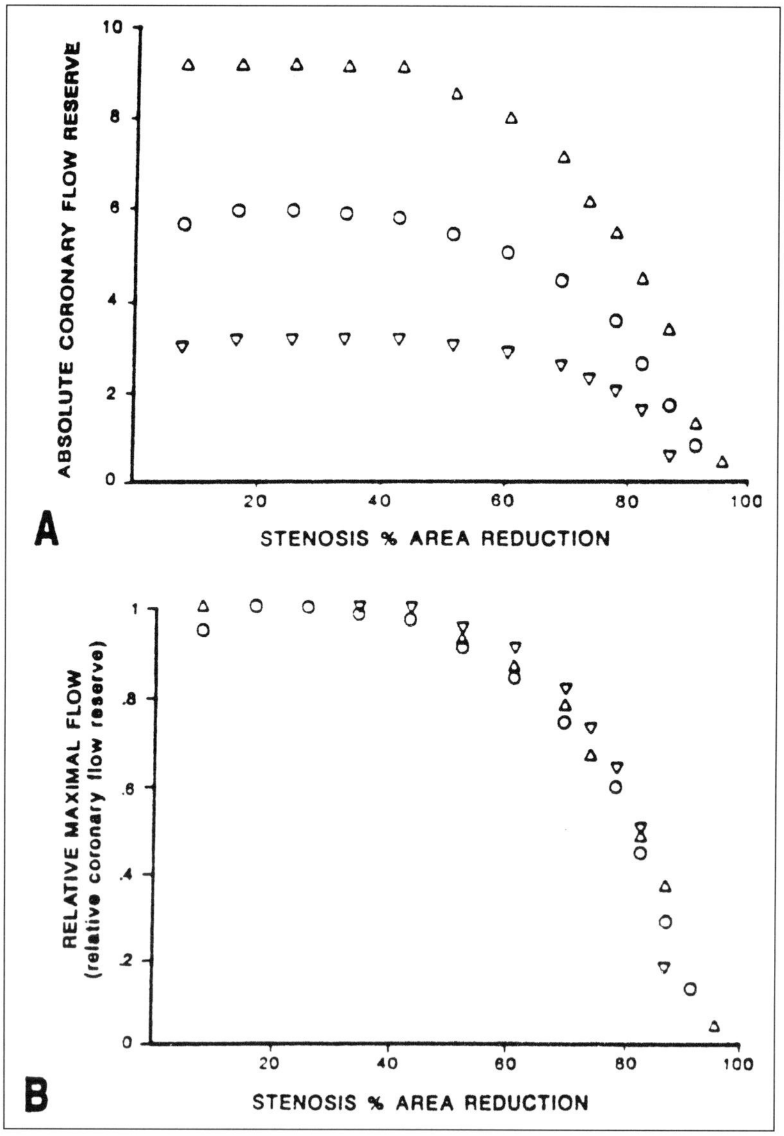

Figure 5 Changes in flow reserve. Changes in absolute coronary flow reserve (A) and relative coronary flow reserve (B) in dogs with progressive experimental coronary stenosis during control (o) state and phenylephrine (∇) and nitroprusside(Δ) infusion. (Reprinted with permission from Gould KL, Kirkeeide RL, Buchi M. Coronary flow reserve as a physiologic measure of stenosis. *J Am Coll Cardiol* 1990;15:459–474.)

RADIONUCLIDES

Overview

Inadequate myocardial blood flow to meet the oxygen demands of the myocardium is the primary abnormality that leads to myocardial ischemia. Because the myocardium has limited energy stores, it requires constant delivery of oxygen and substrates and removal of metabolic wastes to function properly. The high resting resistance of the coronary bed permits compensatory vasodilation for significant stenoses and maintains normal flow at rest (see Self-Study Program III, *Nuclear Medicine: Cardiology, Topic 2: Pharmacologic Stress*) (Fig. 5). However, with stress testing, seeking to augment coronary flow by increasing myocardial demands or with direct coronary dilation, the augmentation in blood flow in a stenotic coronary artery often is blunted. With relatively increased flow demands, ischemia will result, and indicators of ischemia, reduced perfusion, diastolic dysfunction, systolic dysfunction, ECG changes and pain will appear (Fig. 6), a sequence known as the "ischemic cascade." The perfusion indicator on stress testing is the earliest and has proven the most diagnostic and prognostic sign. It is critically important for clinical decision making.

If demands are quickly reduced to baseline or if a complete coronary occlusion is quickly released in the studied animal or in humans at angioplasty,

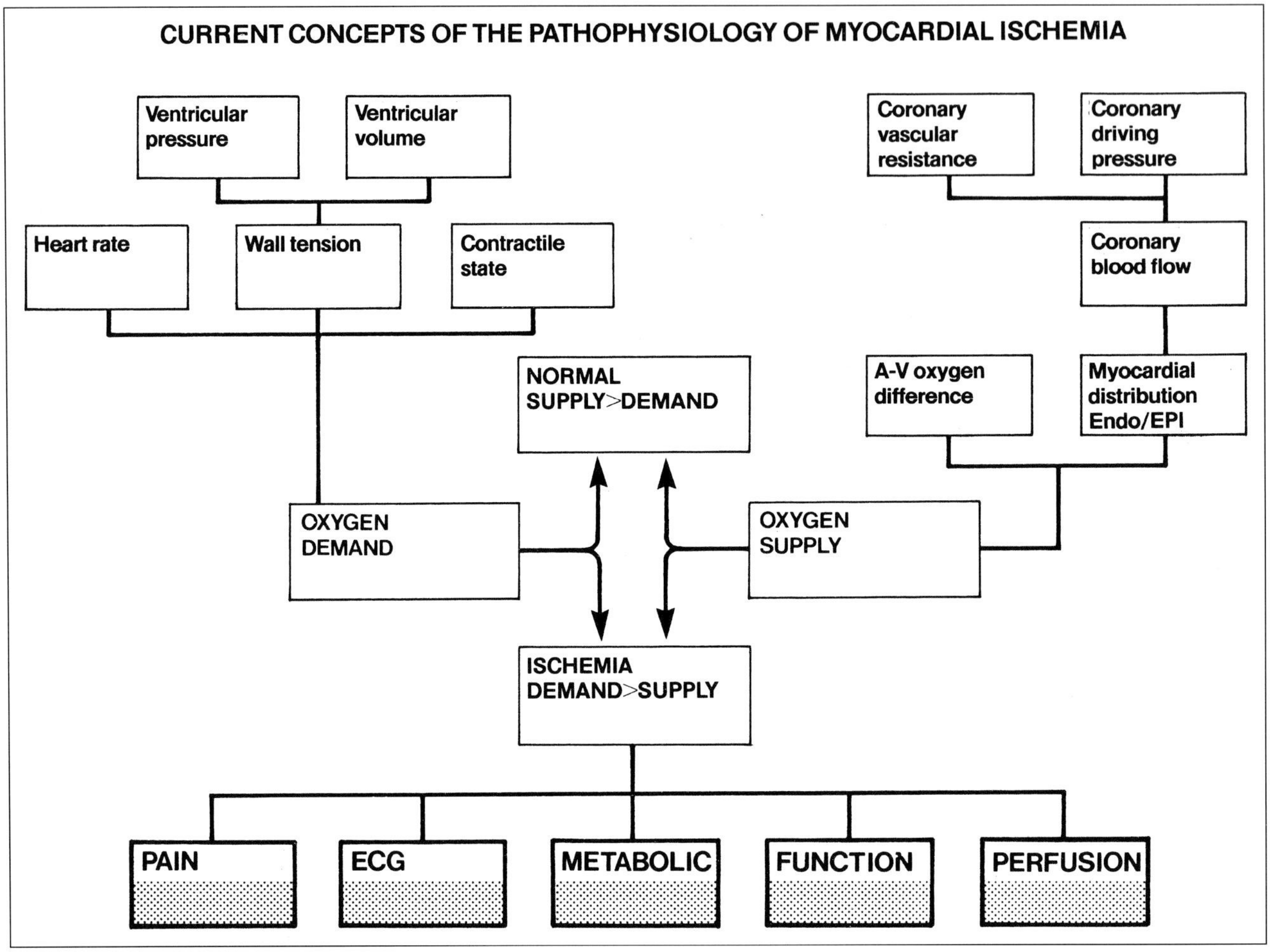

Figure 6 Ischemic indicators. Shown is a schematic diagram of the factors that control myocardial oxygen demand and support myocardial oxygen supply. The bottom line presents 5 ischemic endpoints that may occur when demand exceeds supply. Metabolism requires intracoronary sinus sampling and is insensitive with localizing difficulties. Pain and electrocardiographic (ECG) changes are often nonspecific, ambiguous or insensitive. Stress-induced wall-motion abnormalities once challenged perfusion defects as the scintigraphic endpoint of choice. Today, stress echocardiography is based on induced wall-motion abnormalities read subjectively. The perfusion ischemic endpoint is available only with scintigraphy, is reproducible and quantitative and may be used with ischemic and nonischemic stress methods. (Courtesy of W.W. Parmley, University of California at San Francisco, San Francisco, CA)

ischemia and its indicators are quickly reversed and contractile function will return, ECG changes will return to baseline and chest pain will resolve. If perfusion is restored with some delay, contractile function may remain depressed, even for weeks ("stunned myocardium"). With persistent but modest flow reduction or repeated episodes of stunning, contractile function may remain chronically depressed in the presence of viable myocardium ("hibernating myocardium"). If reduced blood flow is not restored or with prolonged supply/demand imbalances, irreversible damage will occur, leading to myocardial necrosis and the eventual replacement of myocytes with dysfunctional scar. With sufficient myocardial loss, left ventricular dilation (remodeling) and heart failure will ensue, with an adverse long-term prognosis.

Because of the clinical value and potential for pathophysiological changes, it is important to detect and accurately evaluate the primary ischemic indicator.

This will be evident as a relative blunting of the hyperemic response and a diminution in the CFR. This will be seen either in relation to a supply/demand imbalance and true induced ischemia or, as generally seen with direct coronary dilators, as an induced relative reduction of perfusion without ischemia. Regardless of the mechanism, the perfusion endpoint can identify the flow abnormality, making MPS an extremely useful clinical tool.

The Perfusion Radiotracers

Early Agents. Previously, ^{43}K or ^{81}Rb were used as radiotracers (*1,2*). Both are nonallergenic, with magnitude and distribution of localization in the myocardium that permit the evaluation of regional perfusion and related parameters. However, problems related to high emission energy and relative unavailability, as a result of brief half-lives and cyclotron production, made them impractical for clinical use.

Thallium-201

Physical Characteristics and Kinetics. Thallium was introduced in 1973 (*3*). Although the overall use of technetium-based perfusion agents has overtaken ^{201}Tl, at this time ^{201}Tl is the single most commonly used radionuclide for the evaluation of myocardial perfusion, closely followed by ^{99m}Tc methoxyisobutyl isonitrile (sestamibi) and ^{99m}Tc tetrofosmin. Delivered as the chloride, ^{201}Tl is a paradox of pharmaceutical chemistry. In large doses, it is an ingredient of rat poison and the murder weapon in an Agatha Christie novel (*44*). Yet it is a true radiotracer and entirely innocuous in the imaging dose administered.

Thallium-201 is a cyclotron-produced radionuclide and must be transported to the site of application. Shipping is facilitated by the long, 73-hr physical half-life, which also makes possible delayed imaging after 4 and 24 hr, important aspects of the ^{201}Tl perfusion imaging protocol (see Self-Study Program III, *Nuclear Medicine: Cardiology, Topic 1: Physical and Technical Aspects of Nuclear Cardiology*). This long physical half-life and the biologic half-life give ^{201}Tl a significant effective half-life, placing practical limitations on the size of the administered dose and making first-pass and gated SPECT functional analysis problematic. Thallium-201 has emission energies of 69–80 keV (93% abundance), 135 keV (2% abundance) and 168 keV (8% abundance). The radionuclide decays by electron capture to ^{201}Hg, which emits x-rays in the range of 70 keV that are used for imaging. Thallium-201 has a radiation exposure of 0.24 rad/mCi, similar to that of a flat and upright film of the abdomen.

Mechanism of Thallium-201 Localization. The distribution of the thallous ion, a cation, is predominantly intracellular (*3,5–7*), and its transport across the cell membrane is an energy-requiring process dependent on the Na+/K+ ATPase pump (*6,7,45*) (Fig. 7). When injected intravenously, the initial regional myocardial concentration of ^{201}Tl is determined by the product of regional myocardial blood flow and myocardial extraction fraction. Because the myocardium receives ~5% of the cardiac output and because the myocardial extraction fraction for ^{201}Tl is 87% (*45,46*), ~4% of the ^{201}Tl administered goes to the heart and the remainder distributes to the other body organs, again in proportion to their flow and extraction (*47*). Myocardial extraction fraction is linearly related to regional myocardial blood flow (*46,47*), except at very low or very high flow rates. At very low flow rates, extraction fraction increases, whereas at very high flow rates, such as might be induced by exercise, cardiac pacing or coronary vasodilators, myocardial extraction fraction decreases and results in a "roll off," or a reduction in myocardial uptake of ^{201}Tl relative to increasing regional coronary flow (*48–51*) (Fig. 8). In experimental animals, myocardial

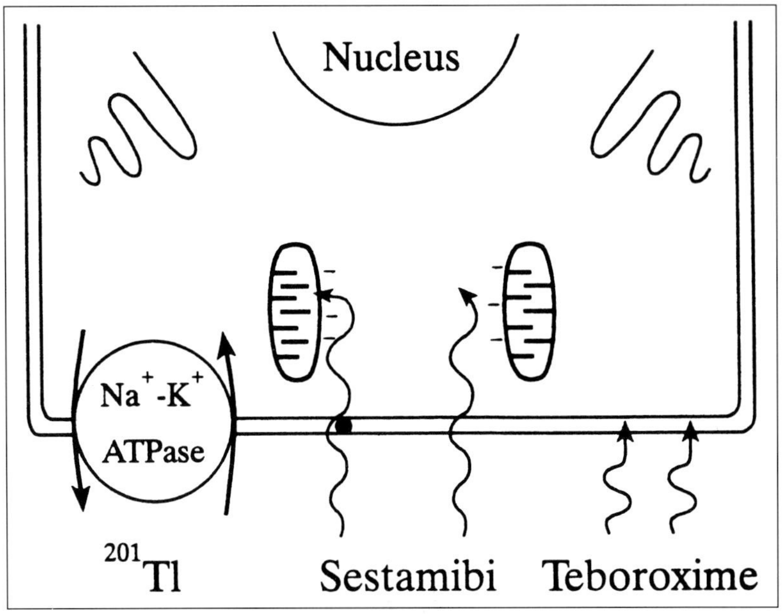

Figure 7 Cellular entry. Shown diagrammatically is the method of cellular entry of thallium-201, technetium-99m (^{99m}Tc) sestamibi and teboroxime. Thallium-201 passes the cell membrane via an energy-dependent mechanism utilizing a Na+/K+ adenosine triphosphatase (ATPase) transmembrane pump. This differs from the mechanism of diffusion that serves as the basis for passage of the ^{99m}Tc-based agents. Sestamibi appears to bind to mitochondria, redistributes little and behaves much like a microsphere. Teboroxime appears to be membrane bound, which explains its persistence in the area of even disrupted myocytes, its excellent relationship to vessel patency but its poor relationship to regional viability. Technetium-99m tetrofosmin appears to pass the cell membrane and localize intracellularly, as shown here for sestamibi. (Reprinted with permission from Liu P. New technetium-99m imaging agents. Promising windows for myocardial perfusion and viability. *Am J Cardiol Imaging* 1992;6:28–41.)

extraction of ^{201}Tl has been shown to be potentially affected by other factors, such as hypoxia, cardiac glycosides and certain other drugs (*45,47, 51,52*). However, once localized within the cell, ^{201}Tl will not be released by hypoxia or ischemia (*45*). Overall, perfusion is normally homogeneous after ^{201}Tl injection (Fig. 9), and defects on the initial myocardial images are produced predominantly by regional disparity in myocardial flow distribution, whether injection is made at rest, during exercise or after administration of a coronary vasodilator (*53*) (Fig. 10). Although this evident disparity in regional perfusion may or may not relate to pathologic ischemia, in practice the additional role played by myocardial ischemia, hypoxia or drugs in producing image defects appears to be minor.

Myocardial Distribution. After this initial distribution phase, redistribution of ^{201}Tl takes place, so that ^{201}Tl defects, corresponding to hypoperfused but viable regions, normalize over several hours, whether ^{201}Tl injection is made during exercise (*48*) or at rest (*54–56*) (Figs. 11,12). The redistribution phenomenon is a consequence of both the accumulation of ^{201}Tl in hypoperfused zones and the loss of thallium from the normal myocardium (*6,13, 20,54–58*) (Fig. 13). During this redistribution phase, ^{201}Tl enters the myocardium from the systemic pool (input), and it also leaves the myocardium (output or intrinsic washout). The difference between input and output is reflected in the net myocardial washout rate (Fig. 14). The local concentration of ^{201}Tl changes until equilibrium is reached and the ratio between output and input becomes constant (*59*). The intrinsic washout rate has been determined experimentally to be monoexponential, with a half-life of 75 min (*60*), whereas the net washout rate of ^{201}Tl after exercise injection has been shown to have a half-life of ~4 hr (*61*). Several factors other than ischemia may influence the intrinsic and net ^{201}Tl washout rates. The initial concentration of ^{201}Tl in the myocardium and the "gradient" between the myocardium and blood are important determinants of washout rate. Similarly, image target-to-background ratio probably plays a significant role in the practical calculation of washout. Washout of ^{201}Tl appears faster when the radionuclide is injected at high levels of exercise than when injected at lower exercise heart rates (*62–65*), with pharmacologic vasodilator stress or at rest (*66*). In contrast, alterations in myocardial blood flow after ^{201}Tl has been administered do not alter its distribution but do affect myocardial clearance of the agent and the calculated washout rate (*67,68*). Slow myocardial clearance is an image correlate of induced ischemia (*69*). The rate of clearance of ^{201}Tl from the blood also affects myocardial washout rate, which in turn influences the time course of ^{201}Tl defect reversibility (*70,71*). Glucose loading and eating soon after ^{201}Tl injection shifts flow to the stomach, lowers blood ^{201}Tl concentration and is thought to lead to a high frequency of nonreversible defects in viable regions (*72*).

Assuming that adequate time has been allowed for the ultimate redistribution pattern to be established, ^{201}Tl defects may be categorized as reversible, partially reversible, nonreversible or as exhibiting reverse redistribution, based on the change in image radionuclide distribution on the exercise or pharmacologic stress and delayed images, generally acquired 4 hr after administration. In reversible defects, the net myocardial washout rate of ^{201}Tl is slower in the region of the defect than in normal areas. This ultimately leads to equalization of the concentration of ^{201}Tl in initially normal and abnormal regions. This reversibility, whether after resting or exercise injection, is associated with the presence of viable myocardium. The time period for redistribution may vary, and complete redistribution may require up to 24 hr (*72,73*) (Figs. 15, 16). This phenomenon of late reversibility has important implications for the differentiation of viable from nonviable myocardium and has influenced the design of imaging protocols (*74*) (Fig. 17).

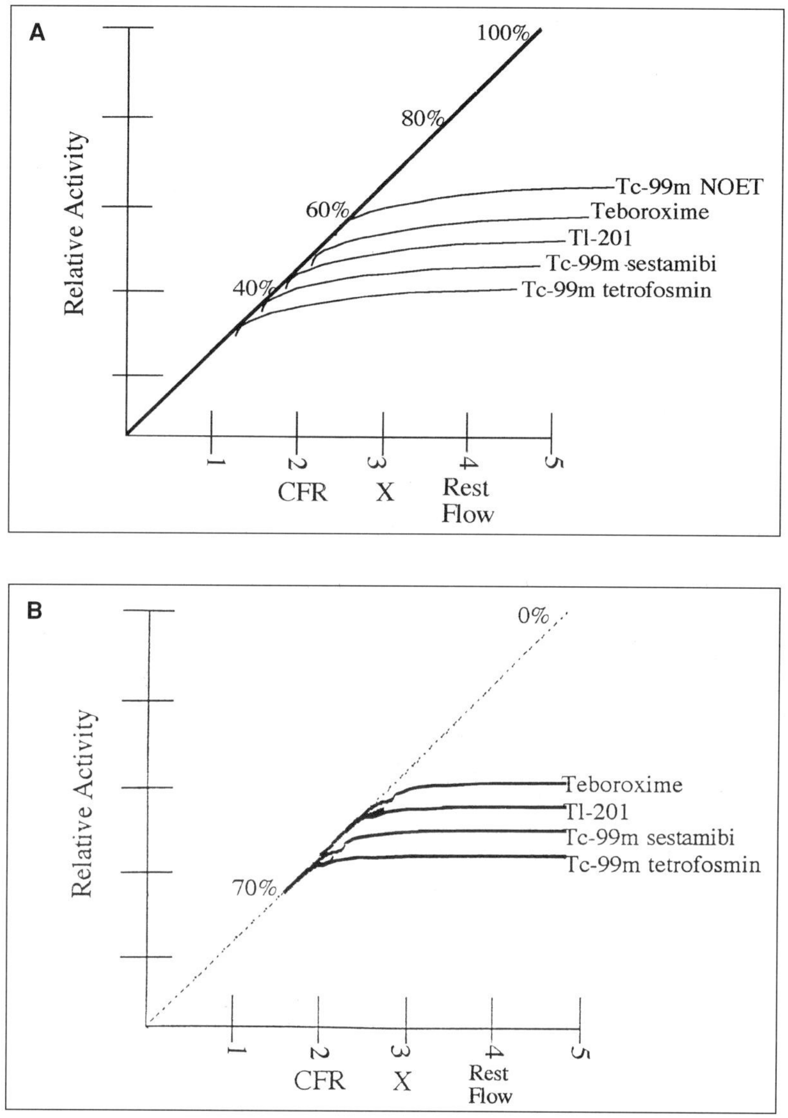

Figure 8 Linearity with flow. Shown diagramatically for a variety of the available and proposed perfusion agents is the relationship between their myocardial uptake and regional myocardial blood flow or coronary flow reserve (CFR), measured in multiples of resting flow (CFR × rest flow). Each agent departs from the diagonal line of complete flow linearity at the approximate limit of their specific linearity with flow. (A) The line of linearity is labeled with the percentage of the CFR reflected by a linear flow relationship at any given level. (B) The approved perfusion agents are similarly plotted, but now the range of percent stenosis related to the CFR is approximated. All agents have a high sensitivity for tight lesions. However, less severe, less flow-limiting agents will be best identified by agents with greater flow linearity. As is evident here, agents with better linearity with flow are needed. The preservation of radionuclide distribution in a linear relationship to flow is an important indicator of success of a marker of regional myocardial perfusion. When the blunted hyperemic flow response exceeds the level of tracer linearity with flow, the tracer concentration and image intensity match those of the normal flow response and so cannot be identified as abnormal. The greater the tracer flow linearity, the higher it can track the blunted hyperemic response. Greater obstruction brings greater abnormalities of the hyperemic response. Differences in flow linearity relate to the ability of the tracer to identify abnormal responses in less stenotic vessels in the higher range of the abnormal flow response. Thus, all other factors being equal, the greater the linearity with flow, the greater the ability of the agent to identify less severe but significant lesions and the higher its expected sensitivity.

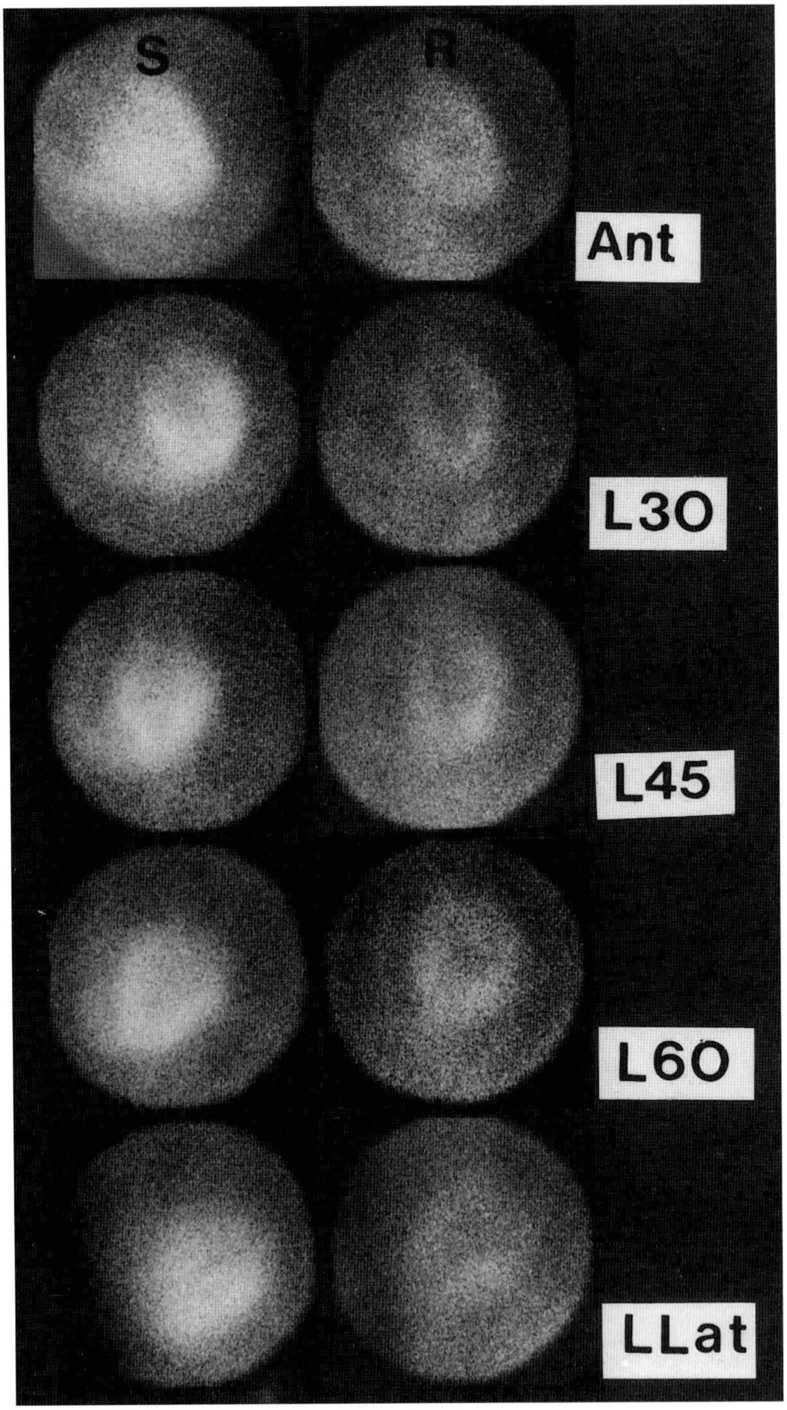

Figure 9 Normal planar perfusion scintigram. Shown are normal planar thallium-201 perfusion images acquired at stress (S, left column) and 4 hr later with redistribution (R, right column). Images are shown in 5 projections: anterior, 30° left anterior oblique (L), 45° L, 60° L and left lateral (LLat) from above downward. Redistribution images acquired for the same duration and displayed at the same intensity scale are nonetheless much less intense than the poststress images, as a result of the high washout rate. The low background level indicates a high level of related exercise, with perfusion shifting from the soft tissues of the chest to the exercising muscles. The radionuclide is distributed homogeneously through the left ventricle but reduced in the less massive right ventricle and left ventricular base (Reprinted with permission from Botvinick E, Dae M, O'Connell JW, Ortendahl D, Hattner RS. The scintigraphic evaluation of the cardiovascular system. In: Parmley WW, Chatterjee K, eds. *Cardiology.* Philadelphia, PA: JB Lippincott; 1991:1–121.)

In partially reversible defects, the concentrations of ^{201}Tl in the normal and defect regions approximate one another during the redistribution phase but do not equalize. This pattern is believed to occur in myocardial regions that contain a mixture of nonviable and viable but ischemic myocardium.

In nonreversible or fixed defects, the initial ratio of ^{201}Tl concentration between the abnormal and normal regions is maintained over time, because net washout rates for ^{201}Tl are similar in the normal and abnormal zones. Nonreversible defects are usually associated with the presence of an element of myocardial scar. However, the level of regional perfusion and regional ^{201}Tl uptake in fixed defects has been shown to be directly related to the level of regional viability and the likelihood of functional reversibility (*75*).

In regions demonstrating apparent reverse redistribution, the relative intensity of the defect compared with that in the normal region decreases over time, and the defect appears more prominent at rest. This may relate to an accelerated washout rate of ^{201}Tl from the defect zone (*76*). This pattern may be observed in the setting of nontransmural myocardial infarction associated with a patent infarct related coronary artery, more commonly after revascularization (*76*), and may result from higher-than-normal blood flow to the residual viable myocardium in the partially infarcted zone (Figs. 18–21). This finding has been related to regional viability (*77,78*) or admixed viable and nonviable tissue (*79*). Most recently, Pace et al. (*80*) presented evidence suggesting that the phenomenon of reverse redistribution is itself "reversible" or variable. They found that reverse redistribution was found preoperatively in 27 of 47 (57%) patients before coronary bypass graft surgery (CABG) and in 60 of 564 (11%) myocardial segments. Among these, 40% showed normal systolic function, 32% were hypokinetic and 28% were dyskinetic. After surgery, 18 of 26 (69%) revascularized dyskinetic segments that had shown previous reverse redistribution demonstrated improved systolic function. Is the finding a reliable indicator of regional viability or simply a variable finding without a strong relationship to any physiologic process? A study by Soufer et al. (*81*) demonstrated that reverse redistribution was not generally related to the presence of CAD or coronary-related risk. It is probable that it most commonly represents a variant of normal and may relate to varying technical factors, such as background activity and camera angulation, as well as regionally increased and varying washout rates in some normal areas (*4,76,82,83*). An entirely normal stress perfusion image suggests that associated reverse redistribution is probably technical in origin and not an indicator of pathology.

Image Defects and Anatomy. Early on, sophisticated animal experiments demonstrated the important influence of left ventricular wall motion and volume on the apparent distribution of the perfusion radiotracer (*46,84*). After the intravenous administration of ^{201}Tl and microspheres to normal canines, aortic obstruction brought acute ventricular dilation and an

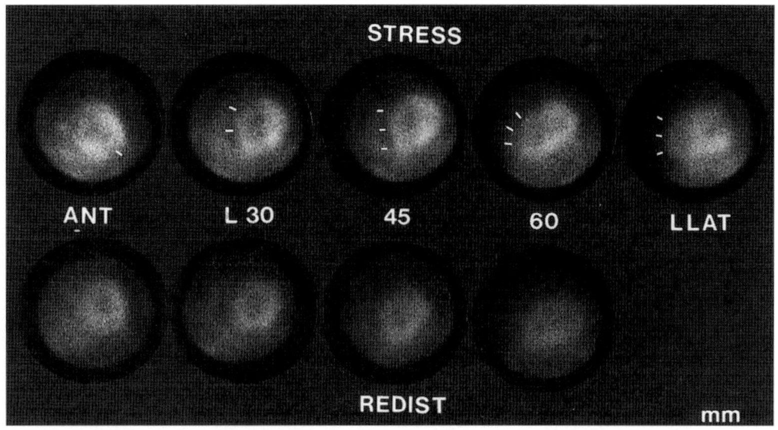

Figure 10 Stress-induced ischemia. Shown are analog planar images after stress (STRESS) and at redistribution (REDIST) in anterior (ANT), 30°, 45°, and 60° left anterior oblique (L) and left lateral (LLAT) projections in a patient with extensive apical, anterior and septal ischemia (arrows). The fainter but more homogeneous distribution of radiotracer after redistribution (REDIST) is shown in the bottom row, indicating normal perfusion at baseline viability. (Reprinted with permission from Botvinick E, Dae M, O'Connell JW, Ortendahl D, Hattner RS. The scintigraphic evaluation of the cardiovascular system. In: Parmley WW, Chatterjee K, eds. *Cardiology.* Philadelphia, PA: JB Lippincott; 1991:1–121.)

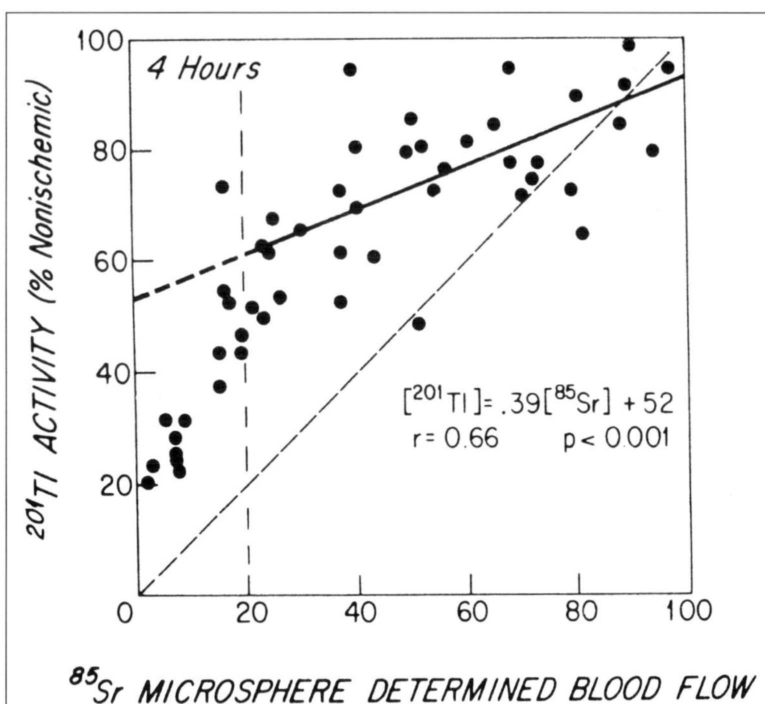

Figure 11 Correlation of thallium-201 (^{201}Tl) uptake with regional flow in rest-redistribution. Relationship between ^{201}Tl activity (% nonischemic) and initial strontium-85 microsphere-determined blood flow (% nonischemic) in the zone of chronic low flow from dogs killed 4 hr after administration of ^{201}Tl. The light dashed line represents the line of identity. The regression line (solid line) is depicted for ischemic flows of 20%–100% of nonischemic flow and has been extrapolated to 0 flow (dashed portion). The increase above the line of identity reflects the degree of rest-redistribution. (Reprinted with permission from Pohost GM, Okada RD, O'Keefe DD, et al. Thallium redistribution in dogs with severe coronary artery stenosis of fixed caliber. *Circ Res* 1981;48:439–446.)

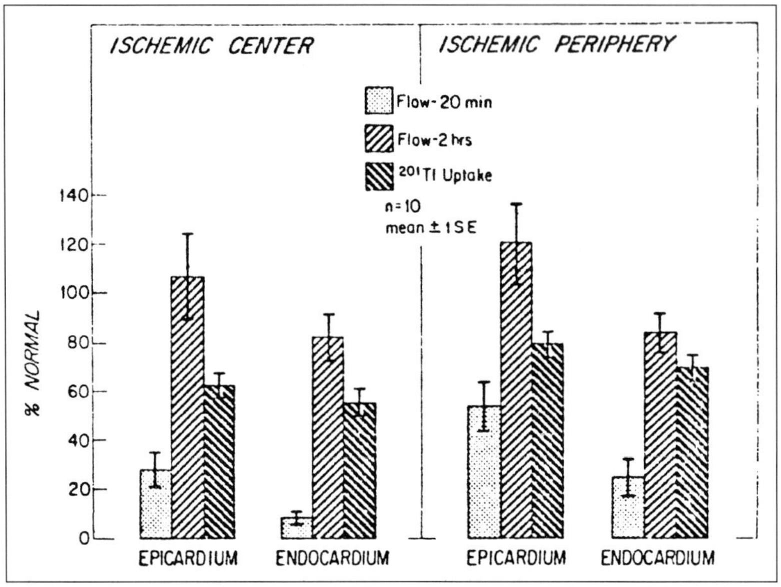

Figure 12 Thallium-201 (^{201}Tl) redistribution, serial tissue samples. Regional myocardial blood flow is expressed as the percentage of normal in epicardial and endocardial samples taken from central and peripheral ischemic zones in 10 dogs after 20 min of coronary occlusion and 100 min of reperfusion. Thallium-201 was administered after 10 min occlusion and was counted 2 hr later and similarly expressed. Thallium-201 uptake in ischemic zones is significantly higher than flow (stippled bars) at the time of ^{201}Tl administration, indicating redistribution of the tracer during the 100-min reperfusion. However, ^{201}Tl activity after 2 hr of redistribution is still less than reperfusion flow, also counted after 2 hr. Note the greater effect on the subendocardium. (Reprinted with permission from Pohost GM, Zir LM, Moor RH, et al. Differentiation of transiently ischemic from infarcted myocardium by serial imaging after a single dose of Tl-201. *Circulation* 1977;55:294–302.)

apparent perfusion defect on planar imaging. However, the post mortem analysis of radionuclide and microsphere data revealed continued homogeneous tracer distribution. This phenomenon, the production of apparent perfusion defects with variations in ventricular size and motion, is associated with partial volume effects and other technical factors but not with true perfusion defects. This effect is seen with SPECT as well, where it is enhanced by the imperfect nature of the tomographic method. More recent studies have confirmed this phenomenon, which is applicable to all such tracers (*46,84,85*).

Reliance on perfusion defect analysis alone as an index of myocardial hypoperfusion frequently leads to underestimation of the extent of disease in patients with multivessel coronary involvement (*86–96*) (Fig. 22). This difference between image and anatomy primarily relates to the stress applied, which may not be sufficient to cause ischemia or heterogeneous perfusion in all areas, and to the pathophysiologic nature of scintigraphy, which differs from the anatomic nature of coronary angiography. This limitation may also result, in part, from the contribution of collaterals and to the fact that the initial ^{201}Tl distribution reflects relative rather than absolute reduction in myocardial blood flow. MPS presents its data in terms of regional heterogeneity. Thus, in a patient with multiple regions of ischemia, areas with less hypoperfusion may appear relatively normal compared with the most severely hypoperfused segments. Furthermore, those rare patients with extensive CAD and rather uniform reduction in myocardial perfusion during optimal stress fail to exhibit any perfusion defect on the initial ^{201}Tl images. This has been reported to occur with a frequency of ~1% of all patients with CAD who undergo planar imaging (*96,97*) and is even less frequent with SPECT (Fig. 23).

Detection of ischemic regions, not associated with a relative perfusion defect, is often possible through the use of a spatially distributed regional indicator of absolute myocardial hypoperfusion, such as the regional myocardial washout rate of ^{201}Tl (*96,97*). This washout rate can be analyzed independently for each myocardial region by comparing the percentage of regional loss of ^{201}Tl occurring between the immediate postinjection study and the delayed redistribution study with the calculated quantitative value previously established in a normal reference population (*13,14,76,90,91*). A slower-than-normal regional washout rate may then identify regions with less-than-normal perfusion (*91,92,96*). Washout analysis has not been applied to SPECT studies, because it has been

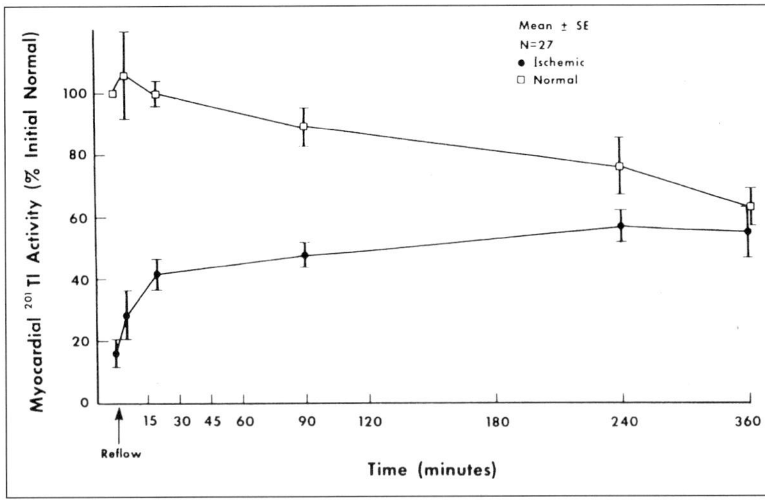

Figure 13 Another example of redistribution with simultaneous sampling of normal and ischemic regions. The serial determination of myocardial thallium-201 (^{201}Tl) activity is shown, expressed as a percentage of initial ^{201}Tl activity in normal (above) and ischemic (below) regions in 5 groups of dogs (n = 27), with coronary occlusion for 20 min and reperfused for 5, 20, 90, 240 and 360 min. For each sample, the initial value of ^{201}Tl activity in the region was obtained before reperfusion, and all values represent the mean plus or minus its standard error for all dogs. Near-equalization of ^{201}Tl concentration in normal and underperfused regions is observed after 4 hr. (Reprinted with permission from Beller GA, Watson DD, Ackell P, et al. Time course of thallium-201 redistribution after transient myocardial ischemia. *Circulation* 1980;61:791–797.)

shown that relatively normal SPECT images are quite rare in the setting of widespread CAD and more rare with apparent ischemia. Also, tomography helps to maximize the visibility of ischemia and associated flow-related defects. However, with both planar and SPECT studies, normal images are associated with low coronary risk, even in the presence of CAD.

Nonperfusion image indicators of widespread ischemia, such as lung uptake, cavitary dilation and basal uptake, indicating generalized distal myocardial underperfusion, may be present in cases of extensive CAD and associated ischemia (*98*) (Fig. 24). When associated with a normal image, they may indicate widespread ischemia. Such phenomena are rare in practice, and most normal scans acquired with adequate stress, even with nonperfusion indicators or in the presence of CAD, have been found to be associated with a good prognosis and a low incidence of coronary events (*99*). The explanation for this high predictive value of a negative test probably lies in the fact that the image portrays the areas of significant ischemia or ischemic potential, and this measure appears to correspond better with prognosis than do stress ECG changes or "significant lesions." In fact, image findings have been reported to identify a spectrum of CAD-related prognoses, even in the presence of a markedly positive exercise ECG (*100–104*). Here, the differences between pathophysiologic image data and anatomy must be considered.

In spite of the established relationship between anatomically severe and extensive disease and prognosis, some work has shown that coronary events, often based in coronary occlusion, do not correspond to the severity of coronary narrowing but occur frequently with less severe stenoses (*105–107*). Image, ECG and other data that document the relationship between the pathophysiologic significance of lesion severity and the clinical outcome belie such studies. Although the explanation is not clear, the facts suggest that the image identification of severe disease represents the "tip of the iceberg" and is associated with the frequent presence of extensive, nonobstructive atheroma. Image identification, then serves as a marker for the full extent of atheromatous involvement and the likelihood of unstable disease: the "total ischemic burden" (*108*). That is, the more severe and extensive the scintigraphic abnormality, the more extensive the related coronary disease and the more likely the existence of a lesion that could progress to occlusion.

Ischemia and Other Causes of Slow Washout. Low achieved exercise heart rate is associated with submaximal myocardial hyperemia and submaximal myocardial ^{201}Tl uptake and washout (Table 2). For this reason, slower-than-normal

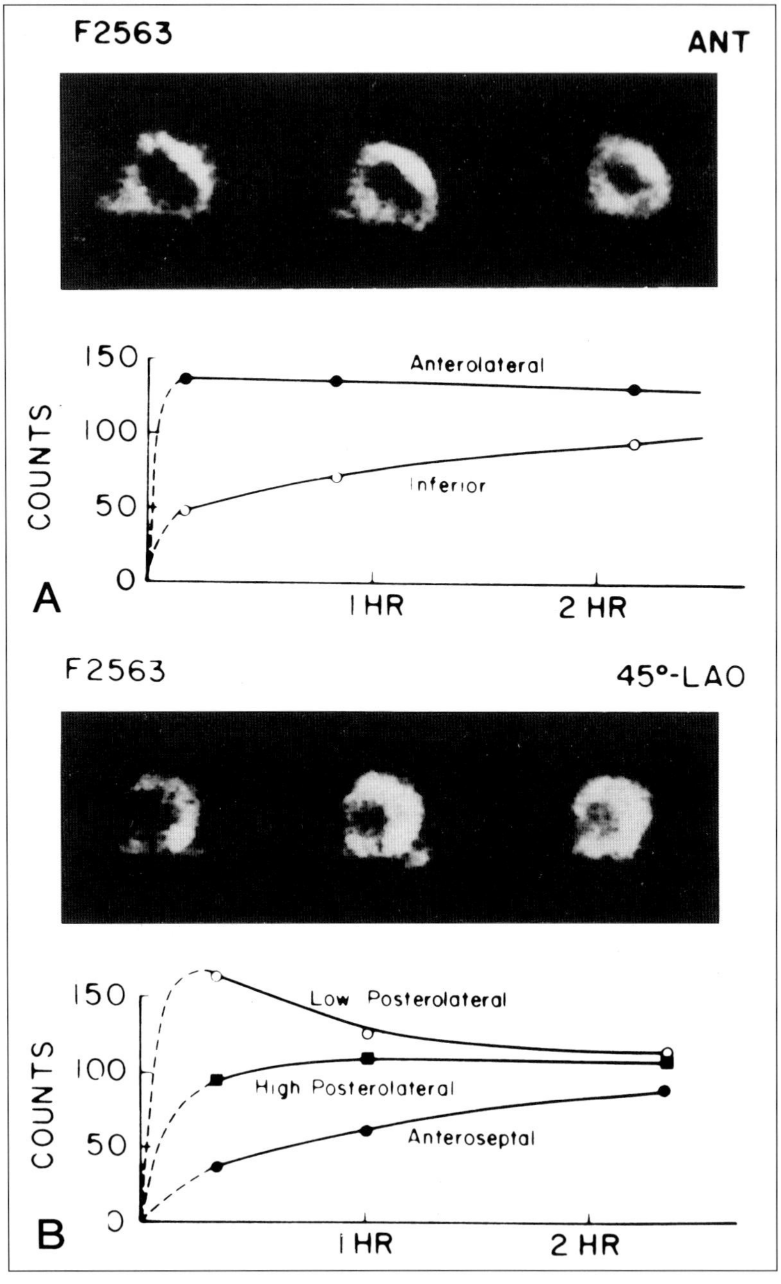

Figure 14 Myocardial washout of thallium-201 (^{201}Tl). Planar perfusion images acquired serially over the course of 2 hr after the stress administration of ^{201}Tl in anterior (A) and left anterior oblique (LAO) (B) projections are shown. Normal regions lose activity rapidly, whereas visually abnormal regions show flat or upsloping curves of serial regional radioactivity. Other regions, such as the high posterolateral wall in the LAO projection, may appear visually normal, yet their true relation to abnormal perfusion is exposed by the generation of an abnormal (flat) washout curve. (Reprinted with permission from Watson DD, Campbell NP, Read EK, et al. Spatial and temporal quantitation of planar thallium myocardial images. *J Nucl Med* 1981;22:577–584.)

regional myocardial ^{201}Tl washout rates may occur in the absence of CAD, when the patient is injected at a suboptimal heart rate (estimated at 85% of maximal predicted for age) (*62–71*). Subcutaneous infiltration of the ^{201}Tl dose delays initial myocardial uptake, with resultant lower peak tissue levels and a slower washout rate compared with those seen with the rapid intravenous delivery of the ^{201}Tl dose. Infiltration adds a reservoir for myocardial uptake and can hasten redistribution, making rapid poststress imaging even more critical (*109*). Arm vein uptake in the absence of a subcutaneous infiltration has been seen in up to 53% of patients in whom ^{201}Tl was injected into veins other than the medial antecubital vein. The slow myocardial ^{201}Tl washout rate that results from this condition is most likely the result of the same phenomenon that causes slow myocardial ^{201}Tl washout rate after subcutaneous infiltration of the dose. Calculation of the washout rate of ^{201}Tl in low-count-rate studies may be erroneous because of the high statistical noise. This condition is encountered when the ^{201}Tl dose is less than the recommended amount (0.44 mCi/kg; total not to exceed 4 mCi), when the myocardial image is acquired for too brief a period or when significant soft tissue attenuation is present as a result of obesity, overlying diaphragm, pectoral muscles or breasts. In the case of breast attenuation, the actual recorded counts in 1 or multiple myocardial segments may be reduced and may cause false-positive slow washout or evident defects in these segments, sometimes mimicking the distribution of segmental CAD (Fig. 25).

Attention to the details of the exercise and imaging protocols is crucial for a reliable determination of myocardial washout of ^{201}Tl. For reliable washout rate analysis, each view should be acquired for an identical time during both the initial and 4-hr redistribution studies. It is important that ^{201}Tl be injected 1 min before peak exercise.

If ^{201}Tl is injected after exercise or if exercise is terminated too quickly after injection, an erroneously slow washout rate of ^{201}Tl may be observed before thallium extraction. In these circumstances, ^{201}Tl is delivered to the myocardium during the phase of recovery from maximum hyperemia rather than during maximum hyperemia. If the start of imaging is delayed too long after ^{201}Tl injection or the sequence of imaging is other than that used in the established normal database, or, of course, if another radionuclide is employed, false-positive slow regional myocardial washout rates may again occur (*62–66,69–71,91–93,95,96*). Each of these errors also results in underestimation of induced perfusion defects. Because washout may not be linear with time, increasing the redistribution imaging time falsely lowers the calculated ^{201}Tl washout, and failing to recognize a prolonged time delay for the onset of redistribution imaging may lead to an erroneously increased washout value. The recommended specific imaging protocol for each variation of ^{201}Tl imaging or those for other radiotracers should be followed closely to obtain reliable results from related quantitation software. Provided technical factors are optimal, regional ^{201}Tl myocardial washout rate is relatively homogeneous compared with regional uptake values and varies little, regardless of projection or the mass of myocardium involved.

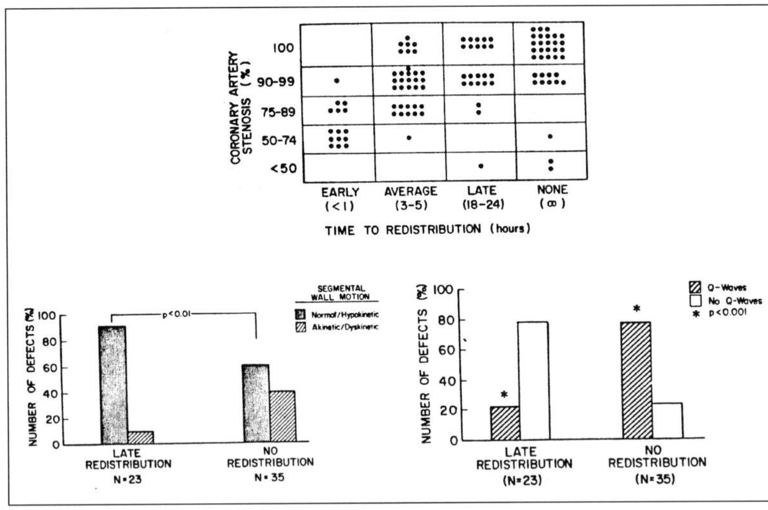

Figure 15 Delayed redistribution. The relationship between the time to full perfusion image redistribution and the degree of coronary stenosis is shown. The time to redistribution is directly related to the degree of narrowing. Late redistributing segments, unlike those not redistributing, are more likely viable and usually demonstrate preserved regional wall motion and no specific electrocardiographic evidence of infarction (Reprinted with permission from Gutman J, Berman D, Freeman M, et al. Time to completed redistribution of Tl-201 in exercise myocardial scintigraphy: relationship to the degree of coronary artery stenosis. *Am Heart J* 1983; 106:989–996.)

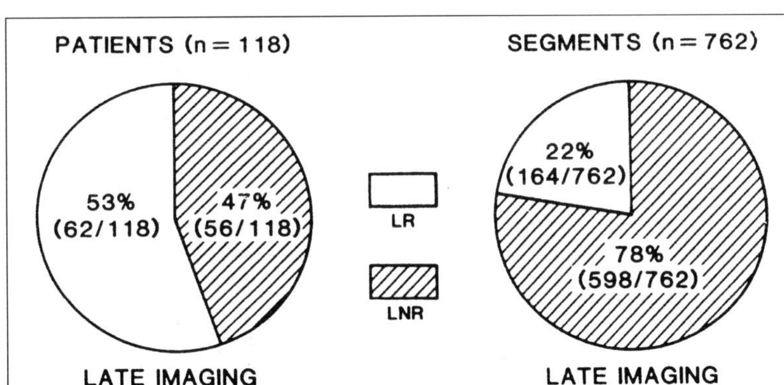

Figure 16 The importance of late reversibility. In this study of 118 patients with fixed thallium-201 (^{201}Tl) defects after 4 hr, a high frequency of late reversibility (LR) was noted in studies and in segments among patients who underwent 18–72-hr ^{201}Tl redistribution imaging. Delayed ^{201}Tl redistribution may be of great value for assessment of fixed defects in selected cases after reinjection and is easily adapted to the dual-isotope rest ^{201}Tl/stress technetium-99m protocol. LNR = late nonreversibility. (Reprinted with permission from Yang LD, Berman DS, Maddahi J, et al. The frequency of late reversibility in SPECT thallium-201 stress redistribution studies. *J Am Coll Cardiol* 1990;15:334–340.)

Technetium-99m–Labeled Agents. Thallium-201 is suboptimal for MPS. The low photon energy of the primary emission of ^{201}Tl (68–80 keV) is strongly scattered and attenuated and is not well suited to standard gamma cameras, which perform best at the 140-keV photopeak of ^{99m}Tc. Furthermore, the longer 73-hr half-life of ^{201}Tl limits the injected dose to 3–4 mCi, resulting in relatively low-count-density images. Many of the limitations of ^{201}Tl have been overcome by the development of ^{99m}Tc-labeled perfusion agents, with their permitted 20- to 30-mCi dose and 6-hr physical half-life (*110,111*).

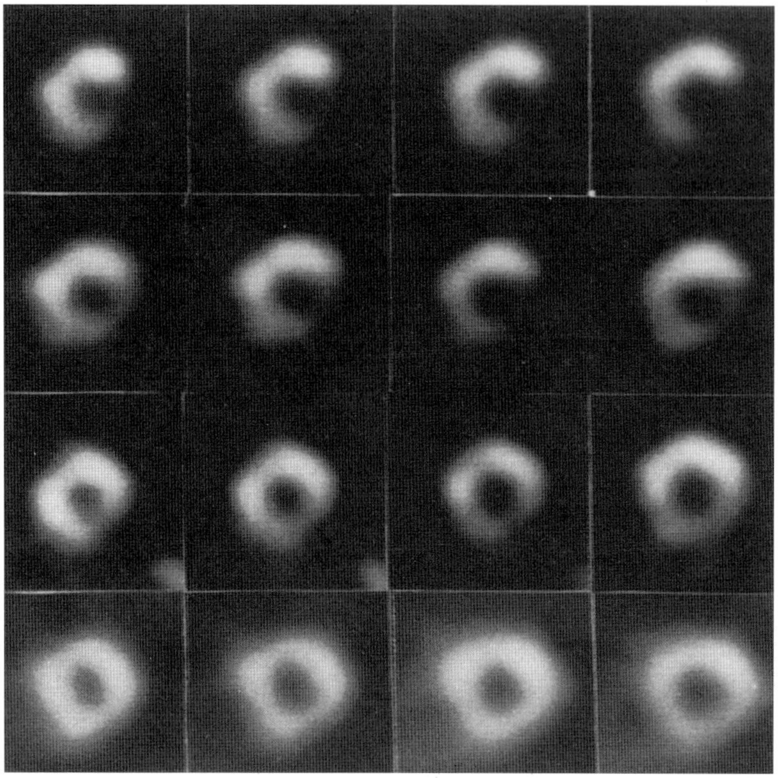

Figure 17 Late 24-hr redistribution. Shown from above downward are midventricular short-axis thallium-201 (^{201}Tl) SPECT slices acquired immediately, 4 and 24 hr after stress. Redistribution, barely appreciated at 4 hr, is seen well after 24. The lower panel is acquired in the same patient with stress performed after revascularization. Only the 24-hr ^{201}Tl image gave evidence of viability and potential improvement after revascularization. Today, the reinjection method makes 24-hr imaging unnecessary in many cases. (Reprinted with permission from Kiat H, Berman DS, Maddahi J, et al. Late reversibility of tomographic myocardial thallium-201 defects: an accurate marker of myocardial viability. *J Am Coll Cardiol* 1988;12:1456–1463.)

Technetium-99m Isonitriles. Localization and Kinetics. Among several compounds that have been evaluated in this group and which all distribute intracellularly according to perfusion (*112–116*), ^{99m}Tc sestamibi exhibits the best biological properties for clinical application (*51,106–123*) (Figs. 8,26,27). Technetium-99m sestamibi, with primarily biliary excretion, has transient hepatic labeling (*109–112,115,124*) with more prompt, yet suboptimal, hepatic excretion and less pulmonary uptake than its predecessors ^{99m}Tc-t-butyl isonitrile (^{99m}Tc TBI) (*125–127*) and ^{99m}Tc carboxyisopropyl isonitrile (CPI) (*114,128–130*). CPI had excellent myocardial uptake, but its utility was blunted by significant hepatic uptake that served as a tracer reservoir for late myocardial delivery (*114,130*). In addition, unlike ^{201}Tl, ^{99m}Tc sestamibi demonstrates minimal lung uptake (*112–115,124–129*). These features result in a high myocardial target-to-background ratio (*131,132*). The generator production of ^{99m}Tc and the ready availability of the agent from regional dispensaries or with local reconstitution of the powdered agent make it available at all hours. Needing heating for preparation, a more user-friendly microwave protocol has been approved. Technetium-99m sestamibi has been shown to be safe in humans (*124,126,127*), is approved for perfusion scintigraphy and is widely used. Table 3 compares the kinetics and other physical characteristics of ^{201}Tl with the ^{99m}Tc-labeled agents.

Technetium-99m sestamibi is a positively charged particle with transport independent of ATP-related active transport. Because of its great lipophilicity, it gains cellular access by passive diffusion across the cell membrane and binds to mitochondria (*110,111,119,120,133,134*). Like ^{201}Tl, its initial myocardial uptake is directly related to myocardial blood flow over a wide range of flow rates (Figs. 7,8), with a similar but somewhat earlier "roll-off" (or loss of linearity) in uptake occurring at high flow rates (*47–52,109,116,118,121,128,134–136*) (Figs. 28,29). Although the peak extraction fraction of ^{99m}Tc sestamibi is lower than that of ^{201}Tl (*128*), net extraction and overall myocardial retention are similar in the 2 agents (Fig. 30).

Because of the short, 6-hr half-life of ^{99m}Tc and the relatively prompt hepatobiliary and renal excretion of ^{99m}Tc sestamibi, 10 times as much ^{99m}Tc-sestamibi as ^{201}Tl can be injected to yield a similar radiation dose (0.05 Gy) to the target organ, the small intestine. The recommended maximum single-day dose of ^{99m}Tc

sestamibi is ~30 mCi. Whenever a technetium-based agent is employed at high dose, the added related data rate can be used to shorten acquisition or add to image data density. Because of the higher dose administered, ^{99m}Tc sestamibi studies often result in a far higher image count density per unit time than does ^{201}Tl, with greater contrast resolution and high photon flux. The physical and biological behavior of sestamibi requires a different approach to its application. The user must be aware of its physiologic extracardiac localization, which requires alterations of the acquisition protocol to permit optimal myocardial visualization and avoid apparent abnormalities of intracardiac distribution. Until recently, ^{99m}Tc sestamibi usually was imaged after the passage of time and the ingestion of milk or a milk substitute to empty the gall bladder. However, too often this brought increased interfering background activity in the adjacent bowel. Imaging is now performed earlier and without milk, to encourage persistence in the more remote gall bladder. Table 4 compares the advantages and disadvantages of ^{201}Tl and the available ^{99m}Tc-based perfusion agents.

Evaluation of Ventricular Function. This high dose and resultant high data density permit the performance of first-pass studies (Figs. 5,31), and the resultant data density and stability of the localized dose provide more optimal ECG gating of planar or tomographic images for functional evaluation (*10,11,137–142*) (Figs. 11,32,33). First-pass (*10,137–139*) and gated ejection-fraction (*11,140–142*) imaging using sestamibi and other technetium-based agents, parallels well the conventional first-pass and gated blood-pool methods. Gated perfusion images, appearing as beating myocardial slices, characterize well regional and global left ventricular function. First-pass acquisition can be performed during stress; gated imaging is a poststress acquisition. If we want function evaluation with perfusion imaging, should we apply the first-pass or the gated method?

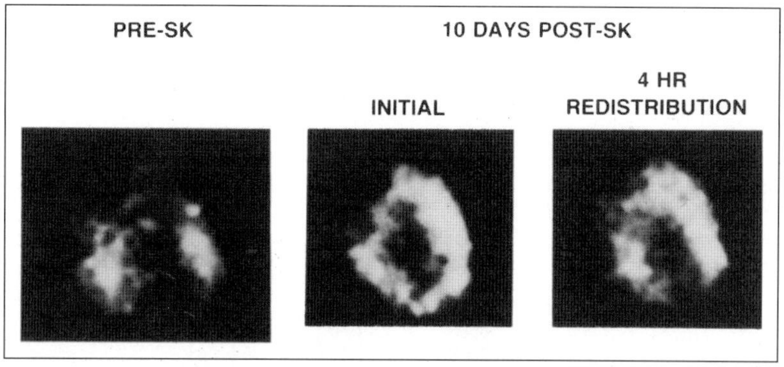

Figure 18 Reverse redistribution after streptokinase infusion. Serial planar thallium-201 (^{201}Tl) images are shown, acquired before streptokinase infusion (PRE-SK) and 10 days after SK (POST-SK) at rest (initial) and at 4-hr redistribution. Extensive anterior and inferior defects are evident on the pre-SK image, whereas the rest image obtained after reperfusion is normal. The delayed ^{201}Tl image, however, demonstrates recurrence of the apical and distal inferior defect. This so-called reverse redistribution has been said, in some cases, to indicate nontransmural infarction with patency of the infarct related vessel. (Reprinted with permission from Weiss AT, Maddahi J, Lew AS, et al. Reverse redistribution of Tl-201: a sign of non-transmural myocardial infarction with patency of the infarct-related coronary artery. *J Am Coll Cardiol* 1986;7:61–67.)

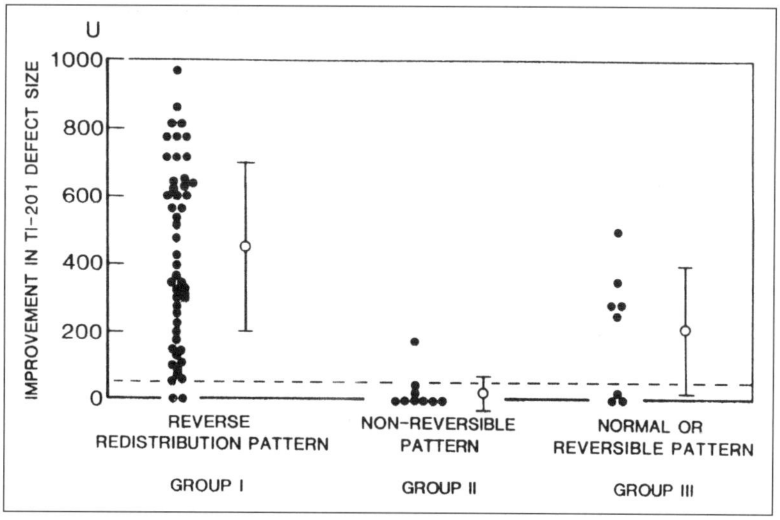

Figure 19 Frequency of reverse redistribution. The relationship between the improvement in quantitative thallium-201 (^{201}Tl) defect size over the 10 days after streptokinase therapy and the pattern of ^{201}Tl redistribution is shown. Improvement clearly was most prominently related to the presence of reverse redistribution. (Reprinted with permission from Weiss AT, Maddahi J, Lew AS, et al. Reverse redistribution of Tl-201: a sign of non-transmural myocardial infarction with patency of the infarct-related coronary artery. *J Am Coll Cardiol* 1986;7:61–67.)

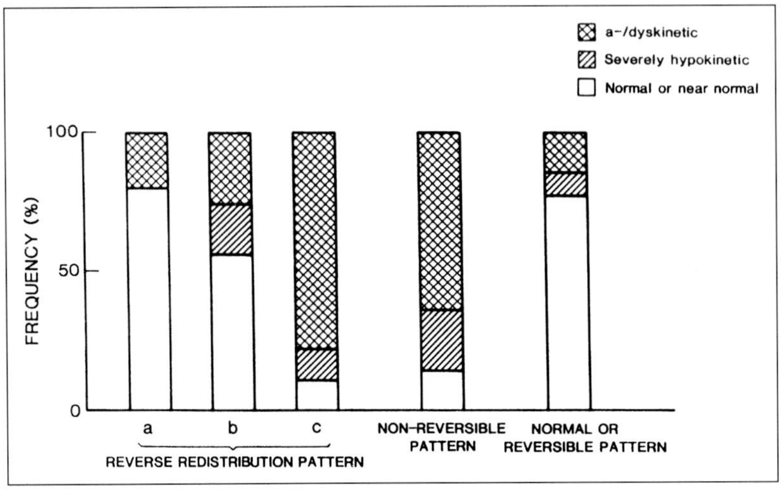

Figure 20 Relationship of reverse redistribution to regional wall motion. The relationship between segmental redistribution patterns and the character of regional wall motion is shown. Reverse redistribution was seen across the spectrum of wall motion, from normal to dyskinetic and in equal frequencies. However, the degree of reverse redistribution was greatest (a) with normal wall motion and minimal (c) with severe wall-motion abnormalities (Reprinted with permission from Weiss AT, Maddahi J, Lew AS, et al. Reverse redistribution of Tl-201: a sign of non-transmural myocardial infarction with patency of the infarct-related coronary artery. *J Am Coll Cardiol* 1986;7:61–67.)

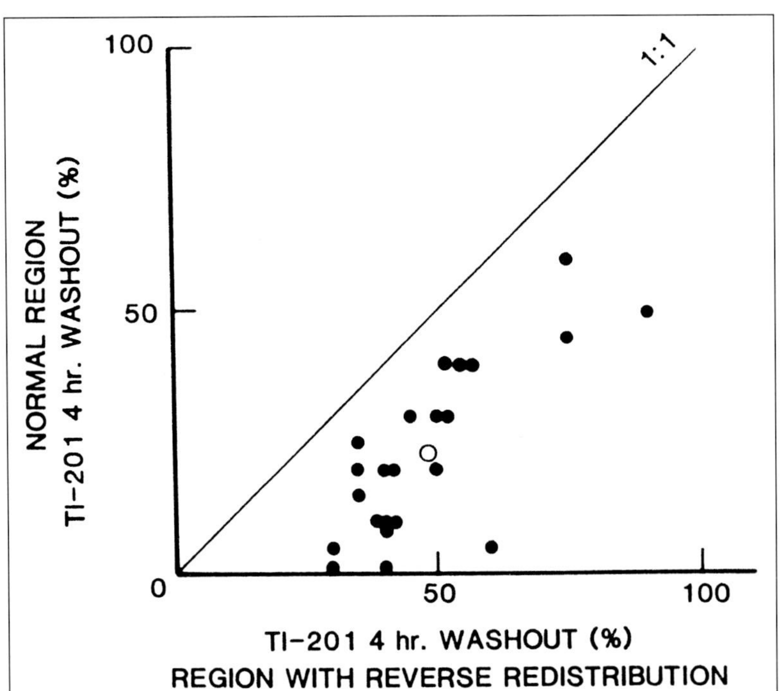

Figure 21 Accelerated washout with reverse redistribution. Accelerated washout in regions with reverse redistribution is shown. Reverse redistribution after thrombolysis was related to patency of the infarct-related vessel, improvement in rest thallium-201 defect size and normal or near-normal wall motion. Although the finding clearly relates to a successful thrombolysis, the conclusion that reverse redistribution is related to a nontransmural infarction appears tenuous. Accelerated washout is the antithesis of the expected finding in infarcted regions. (Reprinted with permission from Weiss AT, Maddahi J, Lew AS, et al. Reverse redistribution of Tl-201: a sign of non-transmural myocardial infarction with patency of the infarct-related coronary artery. *J Am Coll Cardiol* 1986;7:61–67.)

When framed after list-mode acquisition, first-pass analysis can be applied to generate a scintiventriculogram. This is contingent on the presence of a regular rhythm, which is also required for gated studies, now always acquired in frame mode. When gated acquisition is set for a fixed time in the presence of a grossly irregular rhythm, the variable number of accepted beats in each frame yields variable counts per frame and variable regional myocardial intensities, corrupting the SPECT perfusion data. In this case, image defects may relate to irregularities of the gated acquisition and not to perfusion abnormalities. This may be overcome if acquisition time is varied to accommodate equal numbers of cycles or even total counts per projection frame. With expanding computer capabilities, list-mode acquisition of gated studies will permit postacquisition processing like that currently applied to first-pass studies. This could provide a separate gated study for the analysis of functional data and an ungated study with uncorrupted perfusion data. Gated studies are performed with a variety of algorithms on standard equipment, but first-pass data need rapid acquisition on a state-of the-art camera supporting rapid count rates. The first-pass protocol is also more demanding and requires a well-informed, steady and cooperative patient and a well-coordinated team to administer the bolus radionuclide injection at the appropriate time and with the best patient position. Even with these optimal conditions, a significant failure rate may be expected. The method utilized depends on availability of appropriate equipment, as well as operator

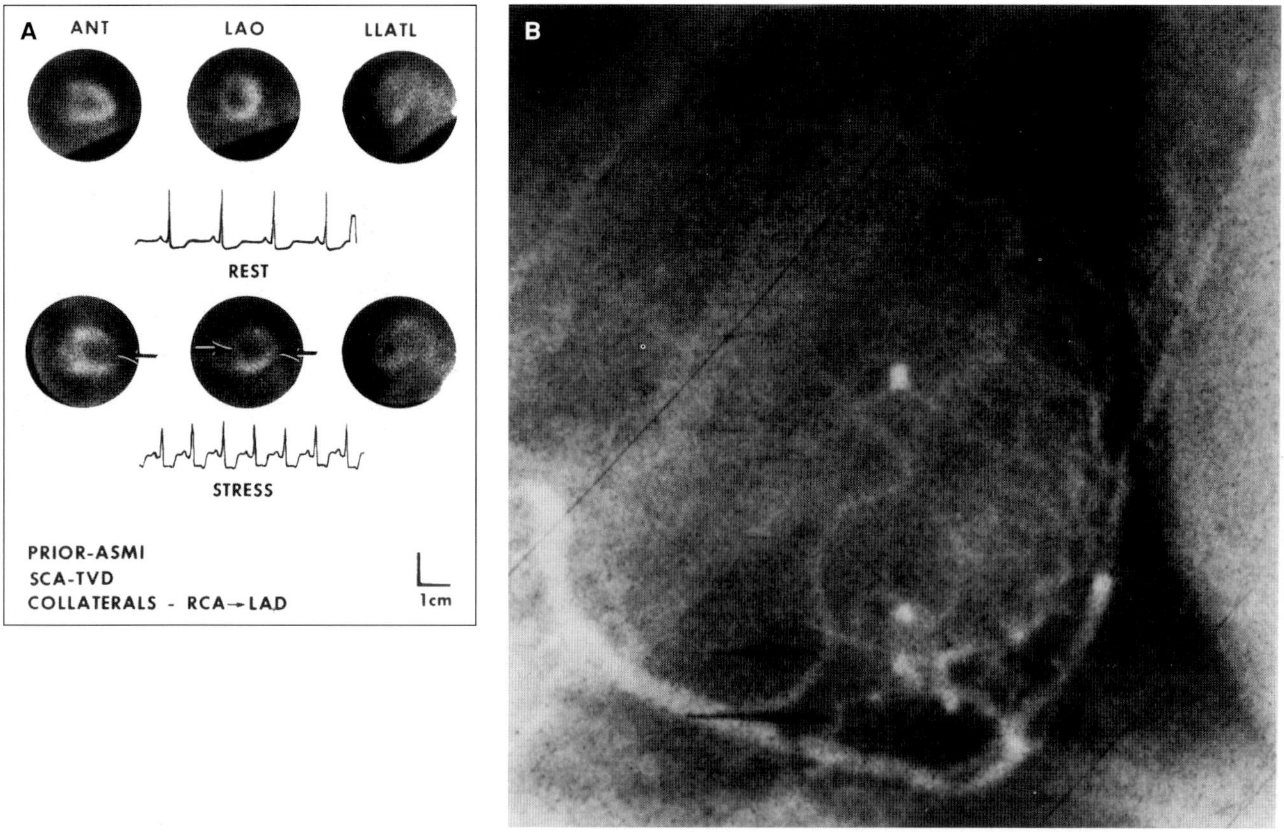

Figure 22 High-risk planar pattern. (A) Stress and rest thallium-201 perfusion images of a patient with triple-vessel disease (TVD) on selective coronary angiography (SCA) are shown. A previous anteroseptal myocardial infarction (ASMI) is evident in the rest images. Extensive defects in the stress image indicate ischemia in the distribution of multiple vessels and extensive myocardium at risk. The inferior wall appears normal, although the right coronary artery (RCA) is also stenotic. This suggests the relative nature of the method or relates to the fact that the RCA ischemic threshold was not reached. The RCA territory was, in fact, probably the best perfused, because the vessel served as a collateral to the left anterior descending (LAD) coronary artery, as shown in (B). (Reprinted with permission from Dash H, Massie B, Botvinick E, et al. The noninvasive identification of left main and three-vessel coronary artery disease by myocardial stress perfusion scintigraphy and treadmill electrocardiography. *Circulation* 1979;60:276–285.)

expertise (technical and medical), software available, the profile of the referred patient population and the clinical question to be addressed. Both methods certainly can be applied in the same patient. Table 5 compares first-pass with post-localization gated perfusion imaging for evaluation of ventricular function.

Characteristics for Clinical Use. Technetium-99m sestamibi and ^{201}Tl appear closely parallel in their localization in infarcted myocardium (*129,132,143,144*). However, some studies in ischemic animal models and in patients suggest a variable sestamibi infarct defect size compared with that of ^{201}Tl, in which ^{201}Tl seems to better assess the true extent of ischemia and viable myocardium. Such localization differences may adversely affect assessment of the true extent of myocardium at ischemic risk (*113–115,145*). However, ^{99m}Tc sestamibi has been tested widely and compares well with the clinical results of ^{201}Tl. The excellent imaging characteristics of the agent have made it popular for imaging of extracardiac pathology.

Reversibility and Viability. Technetium-99m sestamibi, with its obvious advantages over ^{201}Tl in physical characteristics of higher energy and shorter half-life and its ready availability, is especially useful for the evaluation of acute

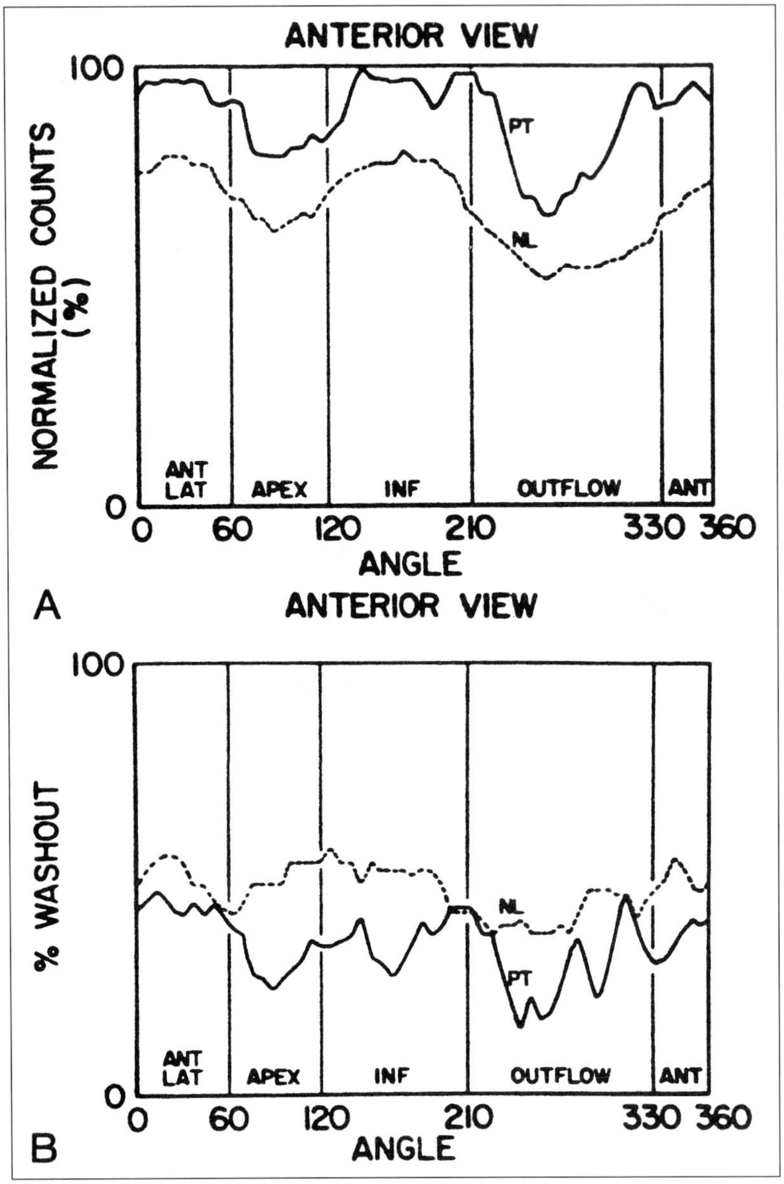

Figure 23 Advantages of washout analysis. The radial distribution of counts (A) in the anterior projection is normal. However, radial washout (B) analysis is abnormal in all segments, indicative of global ischemia in the presence of what might appear to be a normal perfusion image. (Reprinted with permission from Abdulla A, Maddahi J, Garcia E, et al. Slow regional clearance of myocardial Tl-201 in the absence of perfusion defects: contribution to detection of individual coronary stenoses and the mechanism for its occurrence. *Circulation* 1985;71:72–80.)

coronary syndromes (Tables 3,4). In contrast to ^{201}Tl, ^{99m}Tc sestamibi demonstrates minimal myocardial redistribution over time (*116,128,129, 146,147*) (Fig. 34), permitting defect analysis later after tracer injection and making it a potentially better agent for prolonged SPECT imaging (Fig. 35). Lack of significant redistribution also allows more flexibility in the time of image initiation after injection. This is desirable in certain clinical conditions, for example, in patients who present with evolving myocardial infarction and in whom thrombolytic therapy is planned (*148,149*) (Fig. 36). In these patients, the evaluation of the size of jeopardized myocardium is important. Here, ^{99m}Tc sestamibi may be injected before or simultaneously with initiation of thrombolytic therapy, but images may be obtained after completion of thrombolytic therapy, when the patient is stabilized and can more easily undergo imaging (*127–130*). This lack of redistribution necessitates 2 separate injections of ^{99m}Tc sestamibi, during exercise and at rest, for the assessment of reversibility of myocardial perfusion defects, which raises questions regarding its sensitivity as a viability agent. Technetium-99m sestamibi clearly has the ability to determine regional viability of dysfunctional myocardium, but its equality to ^{201}Tl localization in this regard is still questioned. Extracted by passive diffusion instead of active transport, sestamibi shows little evidence of redistribution (*119,120,127,129,146*). Although cellular sestamibi uptake is clearly viability dependent and depolarization of myocyte or mitochondrial membranes (mimicking ischemia) inhibits cellular uptake and retention of the agent (*117,150*), it is not inhibited by other imposed conditions that mimick the metabolic deficiencies of ischemia (*151*).

However, some studies have shown sestamibi uptake similar to that of ^{201}Tl, localizing in viable myocardium late after administration and characterized by models of stunning (*151–152*) (Fig. 37) and hibernation (*153–156*). Several studies performed in animals demonstrate an excellent relationship between ^{99m}Tc sestamibi distribution and regional perfusion (*141,145,154*), as well as with ^{201}Tl uptake (*152*). Three studies correlate ^{99m}Tc sestamibi uptake with histopathologic estimates of tissue viability in heart explants (*155*) and after CABG (*157,158*). The range of positive (45%–91%) and negative (59%–100%) predictive values for viability assessment with sestamibi are similar to those with other methods. Beller et al. (*118*) and Sinusas et al. (*159*) saw regional sestamibi fall dramatically only in the presence of cellular necrosis (Fig. 38). Gimple and Beller (*160*) also demonstrated reduced ^{99m}Tc-sestamibi uptake compared with that of ^{201}Tl in regions with severe, sustained flow reduction and related dysfunction, when imaged after 2 hr of ^{201}Tl redistribution, but found comparable uptake of the 2 radionuclides in the presence of more modest flow reduction. Also, Dae et al. (*145*) found a generally but not completely identical autoradiographic distribution of the 2 radionuclides after their simultaneous administration in a variety of interventions in animals. Nonetheless, taking into account imaging and technical differences, numerous patient studies that have compared ^{201}Tl with ^{99m}Tc sestamibi distribution have found similar image defect size (*161,162*).

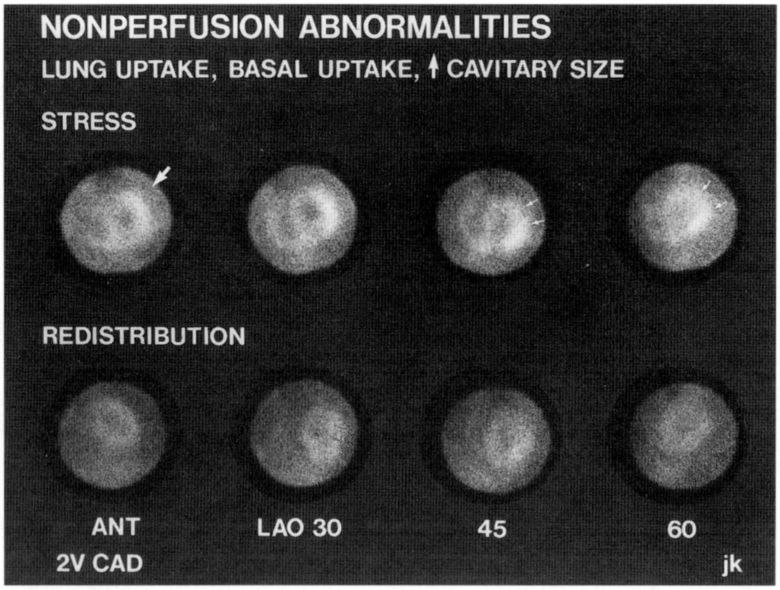

Figure 24 Example of supplementary indicators. Stress and redistribution images are shown, illustrating nonperfusion or supplementary indicators of ischemia. Here, lung uptake (arrow, upper left), basal uptake (arrows, upper right) and cavitary dilation are seen. Especially when viewed in relation to perfusion abnormalities, they suggest extensive myocardium at ischemic risk. (Reprinted with permission from Canhasi B, Dae MW, Botvinick EH, et al. Interaction of supplementary indicators of ischemia and stress electrocardiography in the diagnosis of multivessel coronary disease. *J Am Coll Cardiol* 1985;6:581–589.)

Boronic Acid Adducts of Technetium-99m Oximes. The second group of ^{99m}Tc-labeled myocardial perfusion agents includes boronic acid adducts of technetium oximes (BATO compounds) (*163*). The most promising BATO compound was teboroxime (*164*). Leppo and Meerdink (*165*) studied the myocardial transport of 2 technetium-labeled BATO compounds and ^{201}Tl during varying levels of coronary flow in an isolated blood-perfused rabbit heart model. This study showed that, at a wide range of coronary flow rates (.3–2.4), mean teboroxime extraction was 25% higher than that of ^{201}Tl. The mean capillary flux for teboroxime was also 46% higher than that of ^{201}Tl. Maublant et al. (*166*) showed, in an experimental cell culture model, that ^{99m}Tc teboroxime has faster uptake and greater myocardial cell accumulation than ^{201}Tl and ^{99m}Tc sestamibi. They also showed that, in general,

Table 2
CAUSES OF SLOW THALLIUM-201 WASHOUT

Injection with submaximal hyperemia (at suboptimal heart rate or with pharmacologic stress)
Injection after exercise
Infiltration of the injected dose
Arm vein uptake
Injection in the postprandial state
Low count rate studies: low injected dose, high background or significant attenuation
Stress and delayed images acquired for varying times
Long delay in acquisition of redistribution imaging
Errors in image quantitation

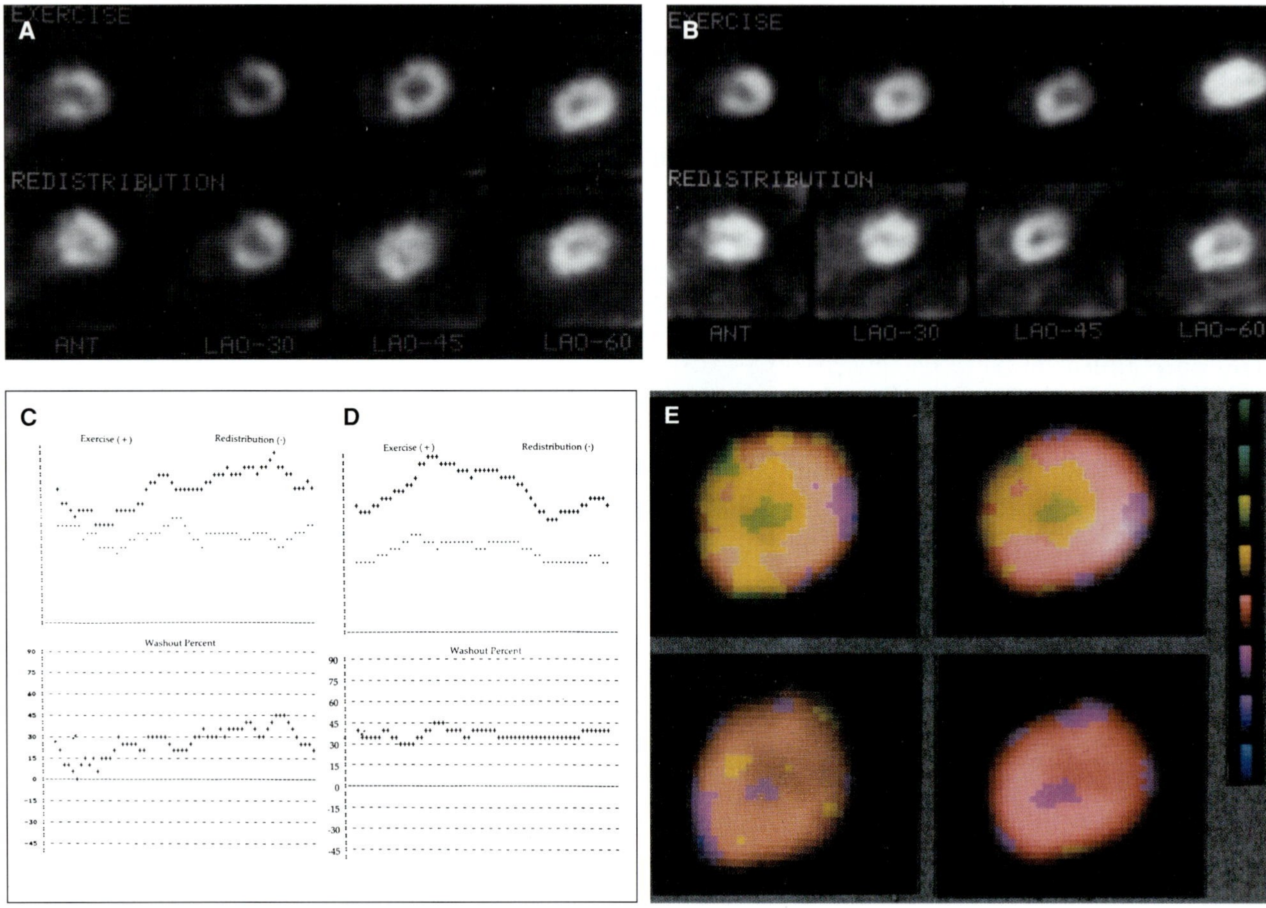

Figure 25 Planar perfusion image washout analysis. (A) Computer-enhanced planar thallium-201 images are presented after stress (above) and at redistribution (below) in (left to right) anterior, 30° left anterior oblique (LAO), 45° LAO and 60° LAO projections in a patient with chest pain, before percutaneous transluminal coronary angioplasty (PTCA). There seems to be a subtle decrease in activity at the left ventricular (LV) apex in the anterior projection and in the septum in 30° and 45° LAO projections. Also, the LV cavity appears larger in the poststress images. These findings resolve in the post-LAD PTCA study shown in (B). (C) Radial counts distribution is shown from the 12 o'clock position, progressing counterclockwise, after stress (crosses) and at redistribution (dots) in the LAO 45° projection for the initial study. Regional radioactivity and the difference between stress and redistribution radioactivity are least in the septal region at left. Below is the radial distribution of percent washout, in which the lower limit of normal varies regionally from about 25%–35%. Again, washout is reduced in the septal region at the left. The normalized post-LAD PTCA exercise, redistribution and washout radial counts distributions are shown in (D). (E) Color washout functional images in the 45° LAO projection from the same patient are shown before (left) and after (right) LAD PTCA. These images are color coded for regional washout, with red-violet-blue as normal and yellow-green as abnormal. The pre-PTCA study reveals gross washout abnormalities in the region of the septum, extending over the lateral wall and the region of the cavity. In fact, washout is being measured not in the cavity but in the overlying myocardium. Apparent cavitary dilation seems often to relate to this relative perfusion distribution. The full distribution of washout abnormalities and their normalization after intervention are best appreciated using washout analysis and the functional image display. (Reprinted with permission from Botvinick E, O'Connell JW, Dae M, Hattner R, Schechtmann N. Analysis of thallium-201 "washout" from parametric color-coded images. *J Nucl Med* 1988;29:302–311.)

teboroxime is the least and ^{201}Tl the most sensitive to metabolic inhibition at the cellular level. Uptake persisted, even in the face of cell lysis. These findings raise questions about the ability of the agent to serve as a viability marker (*166*). In open-chest dogs, Stewart et al. (*167*) showed relatively high extraction of teboroxime after intracoronary injection and demonstrated that myocardial washout of teboroxime appeared to be flow related and quite rapid. Johnson et al. (*168*) and Gewirtz (*169*) demonstrated in animal models the potential clinical value of the rapid clearance of teboroxime in quantitating the degree of flow limitation in individual coronary stenoses of varying severity.

Studies in animals and in humans have shown that myocardial uptake of teboroxime is rapid and high, so that, unlike results with other agents, the myocardium is very well visualized only 2 min after injection (*163,170*). Myocardial clearance of the agent is also rapid, with biexponential halftimes of 2 (68%) and 78 min (32%) (*167,171*) and differential, flow-dependent washout proportional to regional flow (*172*). These properties necessitate the completion of imaging within 10–15 min from the time of injection (*173*). To perform SPECT imaging with teboroxime, imaging must begin 2 min after injection and be completed in about 13 min. Shortening of the time between injection and initiation of imaging may be feasible only if dipyridamole or adenosine pharmacologic stress testing is used instead of exercise (*173*). Heller (*174*) applied planar teboroxime imaging during coronary balloon occlusions and after percutaneous transluminal coronary angioplasty to demonstrate its localizing ability and the rapid documentation of vascular patency. Shortening of SPECT acquisition time would also be necessary, because rapid washout would present varying regional data to the camera over time, in breach of a basic rule of SPECT acquisition. SPECT acquisition could be successfully performed only if a continuous acquisition mode or 3-head camera (*175*) were used.

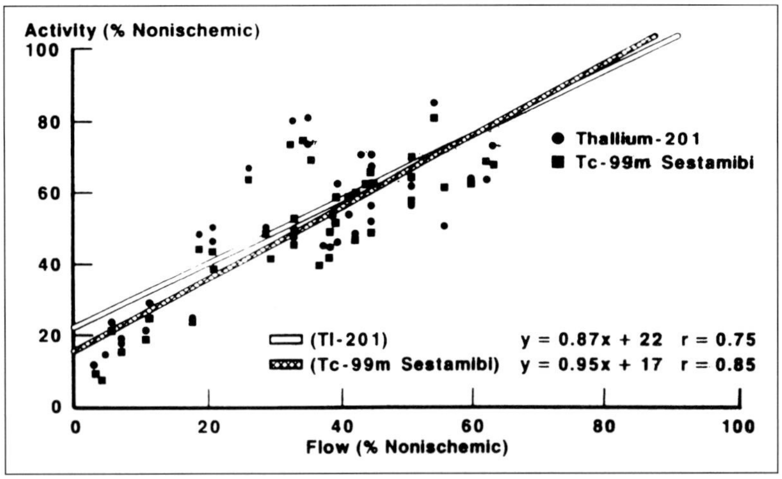

Figure 26 Sestamibi versus microspheres. The correlation of thallium-201 and technetium-99m sestamibi with microsphere myocardial blood flow over a range of 5%–70% of nonischemic flow is shown. The linear correlation of the 2 agents with flow is evident. (Reprinted with permission from Sinusas AJ, Watson DD, Cameron JM Jr, Beller GA. Effect of ischemia and post-ischemic dysfunction on myocardial uptake of technetium-99m labeled methoxyisobutyl isonitrile and thallium-201. *J Am Coll Cardiol* 1989;14:1785–1793.)

Teboroxime has been shown to be safe (*173*), accurate and is approved by the U.S. Food and Drug Administration (FDA). The clearance of this neutral, membrane-bound agent could permit regional flow calculation, employing rapid SPECT acquisition, a 3-head camera and an established method (*176*). Although the agent is tightly membrane bound and has been found to persist even in cells that have been chemically lysed (*165*), it may be help to determine the presence of a patent coronary vessel after thrombolysis, regardless of the viability of the related myocardium (*177,178*). However, the poor relation of teboroxime distribution to myocardial viability and the technical difficulties presented by its accelerated kinetic behavior make SPECT imaging problematic and make teboroxime the least popular among approved myocardial perfusion imaging agents (*177,179,180*). It is not now actively marketed.

Other Technetium-99m–Based Myocardial Perfusion Agents

Tetrofosmin and Furifosmin. Tetrofosmin, a diphosphine compound (*181,182*), furifosmin (Q-12) (*183*) and a similar agent, Q-3 (*181,184*) are new ^{99m}Tc-based, cationic myocardial perfusion agents (*8,182,185*). Although of different chemical classes, each behaves kinetically and localizes in myocardium, similar to ^{99m}Tc sestamibi, with little redistribution.

Like sestamibi, tetrofosmin passes the myocardial membrane by passive diffusion and localizes in mitochondria, remaining essentially unchanged in distribution for 6–8 hr. However, clinical application demonstrates its washout even 2 hr after administration in some patients, a characteristic that could require protocol adjustments. Technetium-99m tetrofosmin is also a marker of

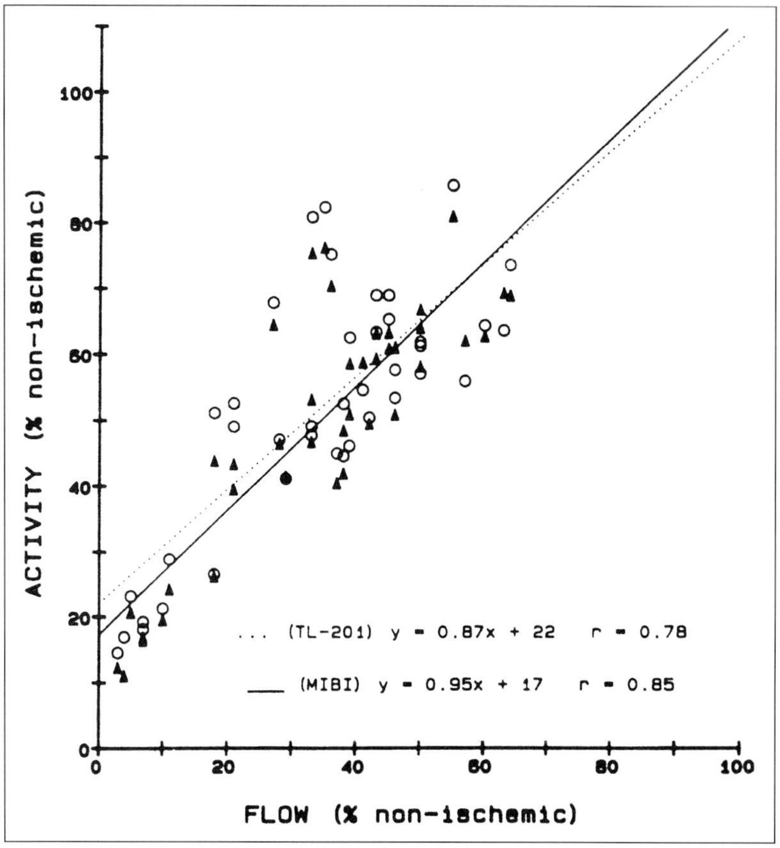

Figure 27 Thallium-201 (^{201}Tl) and technetium-99m (^{99m}Tc) sestamibi in regions with reduced flow. Shown are ^{201}Tl (open circles) and ^{99m}Tc (closed circles) activities versus flow in central ischemic endocardial samples taken from dogs and including coronary regions subtended by a chronic stenosis with endocardial flow reduction ≥40%. Although many methods can identify regions with flow reduction below normal resting levels, as evident in in acute infarction, only perfusion scintigraphy can track linearly, within limits, the level of the hyperemic response. It is an insufficiency of the hyperemic response that forms the basis for the clinical stress-related identification of induced ischemia and related coronary stenoses. This linearity and its limits are presented in figures elsewhere in this text. (Reprinted with permission from Sinusas AJ, Watson DD, Cameron JM Jr, Beller GA. Effect of ischemia and post-ischemic dysfunction on myocardial uptake of technetium-99m labeled methoxyisobutyl isonitrile and thallium-201. *J Am Coll Cardiol* 1989;14:1785–1793.)

cell membrane integrity. Like sestamibi, this is a cationic lipophilic complex that is extracted in proportion to blood flow and taken into viable cells that are required for uptake and retention, with limited redistribution. In general, a 90% concordance between relative tetrofosmin uptake and that of ^{201}Tl compared well with the 93% concordance of ^{201}Tl and sestamibi uptake (*186*). Unlike sestamibi, tetrofosmin requires no heating for its brief preparation, making it more appealing for laboratories, which are all struggling to increase efficiency. This feature, combined with the slightly lower price, contributes to overall reduced costs. In large population centers, the radiopharmaceutical is prepared and distributed in unit doses by distribution centers. Tetrofosmin is stable in the vial for 8 hr and demonstrates excellent myocardial-to-background activity, even minutes after a stress injection. The agent is safe and is administered, as are all radiopharmaceuticals, in tracer doses that do not interfere with biologic processes. Tetrofosmin shares many characteristics with furifosmin, but washes out even less rapidly and, like sestamibi, has been dubbed “an ionic microsphere” because of its perfusion-related localization and long myocardial dwell time. It has been successfully tested, has been FDA approved and is gaining increased clinical application.

Unlike sestamibi, these agents have reduced biliary excretion and rapid hepatic clearance (*181*). Thus, interference from gall bladder or intestinal background should be less of a problem when imaging myocardial perfusion (Tables 3,4). This also promises earlier imaging, at 15–30 min instead of the 30–45 min required for sestamibi after exercise and 60–75 min after dipyridamole and at rest. The related heart–lung count ratios for sestamibi, tetrofosmin and furifosmin are 0.6–0.9, 0.7–1.2 and 1.1–1.4, respectively. In addition, the extraction rate of these agents is reduced, and the myocardial uptake of furifosmin (1.3%–1.5% of the injected dose) is less than that for tetrofosmin (1.5%–1.7%), sestamibi (2.2%) and ^{201}Tl (4%). Therefore, given equal doses, these agents require a relatively increased acquisition time to get similar counting statistics and myocardial image quality. The reduced extraction fraction of ^{99m}Tc-based sestamibi and tetrofosmin and their reduced linearity with flow, have been shown to influence diagnostic sensitivity in limited studies (*187*). Yet most other studies show the promise of these agents for both diagnosis and prognosis when compared with ^{201}Tl. These agents have demonstrated diagnostic sensitivity and specificity equal to that of ^{201}Tl (*188–195*). In infarcts, defect size appears equal to that identified with sestamibi, and a recent study demonstrated quantitative tetrofosmin localization to parallel PET estimates of regional viability (*196*). The varied physical characteristics of tetrofosmin are acceptable if they produce similar diagnostic accuracy. However, even this agent sometimes needs special preparation to avoid high background levels (*197*).

Table 3
ATTRIBUTES AND KINETICS OF THALLIUM-201 AND CURRENT TECHNETIUM-99M BASED AGENTS

		Technetium-99m	
	Thallium-201	**Sestamibi**	**Tetrofosmin**
Chemical nature	Element	Isonitrile	Diphosphine
Charge	Cation	Cation	Cation
Potassium analog	Yes	No	No
Active transport	Yes	No	No
Production method	Cyclotron	Generator/kit	Generator/kit
Myocyte localization	Cytoplasm	Mitochondrial membrane	Mitochondrial membrane
IC state	Free cation	Bound (IC "μsphere")	Bound (IC "μsphere")
Ease of preparation	NA	Moderate	Simple
Myocardial distribution	Proportional to flow*	Proportional to flow	Proportional to flow
Emission energy (keV)	69–83†,135,167	140	140
Half-life (hr)	73	6	6
Dose (maximum, mCi)	4	30	30
Effective dose	2.6 rem/2 mCi	1.1 rem/mCi	0.8 rem/mCi
Peak extraction	High	Lower	Lowest
Net extraction	All		Similar
Excretion	Renal	Biliary	Less biliary
Linearity with Flow	High	Lower	Lowest
Postinjection time to imaging	Immediate	Delayed	Modest delay
Count density	Low	High	High
Contrast resolution	Low	Higher	Higher
Redistribution	Yes	No	No
Lung uptake	Prominent	Minor	Minor
Gated SPECT	No	Yes	Yes
First-pass studies	No	Yes	Yes
Attenuation/scatter	High	Moderate	Moderate
Marker for viability	Excellent	Good	Good

*Early after administration.
†98% abundance.
When imaged later. IC = intracellular; μsphere = microsphere; NA = not applicable.

In an isolated rat heart model, furifosmin demonstrates accelerated early clearance, in 5–10 min (*198*). This feature may be of value to viability assessment, but, like teboroxime, it may again present problems related to imaging time. The kinetics of ^{99m}Tc sestamibi were compared with those of tetrofosmin and furofosmin in isolated perfused rat heart. Overall, furifosmin has a lower extraction fraction and myocardial retention than ^{201}Tl but with little washout, similar to tetrofosmin. However, retention is lower than that for tetrofosmin and E_{max} and E_{net} (the maximal and final tissue levels) are both lower. All protocols should be faster with furifosmin. However, its reduced myocardial uptake and localization may then present the need to increase the imaging time to get good counting statistics, reducing somewhat any temporal advantage. Hendel et al. (*199*) were part of a multicenter trial that evaluated and demonstrated the accuracy of furifosmin compared with that of ^{201}Tl. Other limited studies support this diagnostic accuracy (*183,195*). Furifosmin has not yet received extensive clinical investigation and is not yet FDA approved.

Some are skeptical about the number of new agents in development and the methods of evaluation (*192*). However, rather than a jumble of different

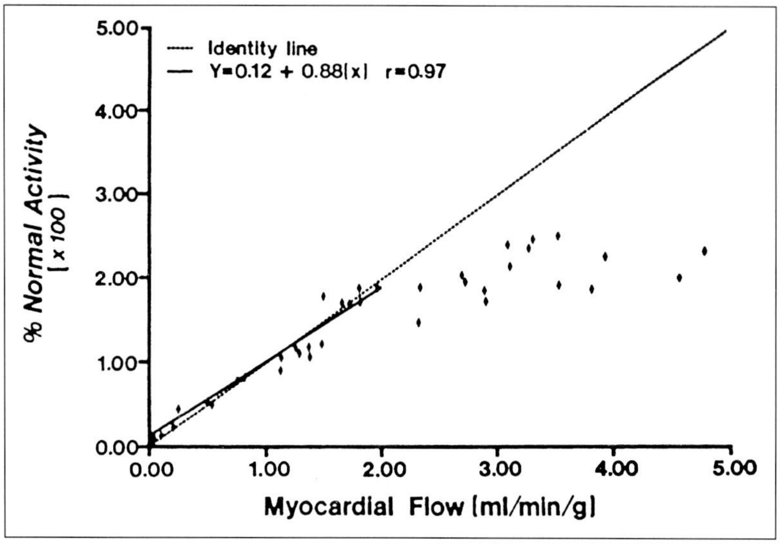

Figure 28 Relation of technetium-99m (^{99m}Tc) sestamibi to the hyperemic flow response. The relationship of microsphere blood flow versus ^{99m}Tc sestamibi activity is plotted as the percentage of normal in the circumflex bed after standard dipyridamole infusion in dogs fitted with mild-to-moderate left circumflex coronary stenoses. The solid regression line sits on the dashed line of identity. Technetium-99m sestamibi distribution linearity is evident only up to flow rates slightly exceeding 2.0 ml/min/g. The plateau reached for flows above this value indicates that regions perfused by less severe lesions that permit flow augmentation beyond this point will display relatively normal intensity levels. The level to which activity linearly tracks flow (linearity with flow) sets the limit of identifiable restriction of the hyperemic response and, with it, the degree of related coronary stenosis. (Reprinted with permission from Glover DK, Okada RD. Myocardial kinetics of Tc-MIBI in canine myocardium after dipyridamole. *Circulation* 1990;81:628–637.)

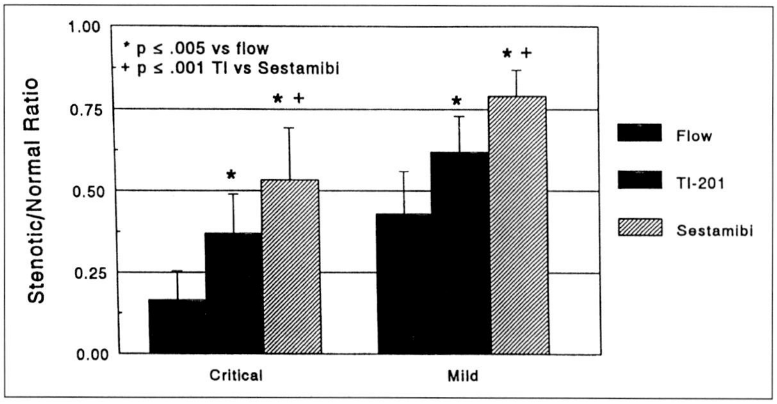

Figure 29 Thallium-201 (^{201}Tl) and technetium-99m (^{99m}Tc) sestamibi uptake in stenotic beds after a dilator. Shown is the stenotic-to-normal uptake ratio of blood flow, ^{201}Tl activity and sestamibi activity in dogs receiving adenosine infused according to the standard protocol, with either a critical or a mild left anterior descending coronary artery stenosis. Thallium-201 and (even more so) sestamibi activity underestimate flow abnormalities. (Reprinted with permission from Glover DK, Ruiz M, Edwards NC, et al. Comparison between Tl-201 or Tc-99m sestamibi uptake during adenosine-induced vasodilation as a function of coronary stenosis severity. *Circulation* 1995;91:813–820.)

compounds, the varying characteristics of these agents present a range of choices to be used alone or in combination for specific advantages resulting from their specific features. Cost, as well as efficacy, will play an important role in their popularity and resultant applications.

Technetium-99m N-NOET and Nitromidazole. In more primitive stages of evaluation are bis(N-ethoxy,N-ethyl dithiocarbamato nitrido ^{99m}Tc V (NOET) (*200,201*) and ^{99m}Tc nitromidazole (*202*). The former is a new cardiac perfusion imaging agent with the highest linear relationship to flow among all agents so far evaluated, whereas the latter promises to be a "hot spot" label for ischemic and viable myocardium. NOET is a member of a new group of cardiac imaging agents with technetium nitrido cores. It is a neutral lipophilic compound with a high myocardial uptake in animals (*203*) and the property of redistribution (*204,205*). NOET has traits similar to ^{201}Tl, including redistribution, and the additional advantages of its ^{99m}Tc label. Initial problems with its formulation have led to a delay in its evaluation and approval. Fagret et al. (*204*) demonstrated a strong relationship between the distribution of NOET and ^{201}Tl and the findings on coronary angiography.

The effect of ischemic injury on the cardiac transport of NOET and that of ^{201}Tl were studied in isolated rabbit hearts (*206*). Although less sensitive than ^{201}Tl to mild ischemic injury, the reduced extraction and retention of NOET with severe ischemic injury make its uptake a potential viability marker.

Linearity with Flow

Tetrofosmin distributes intramyocardially with reduced linearity to flow (see Fig. 8) compared with sestamibi and a lower flow-rate "cutoff" value, above which there is no further extraction (Figs. 39,40). Sestamibi distribution itself has a lower linearity with flow than does ^{201}Tl. Generally, stress MPS identifies abnormal flow reserve and related stenoses by the flow heterogeneity developed in response to a hyperemic stress. The more severe the stenosis, the less its related ability to augment flow and the greater the induced difference from the normal response and related flow heterogeneity. The less severe the stenosis, the greater its related ability to augment flow and the less the induced difference from the normal response and its related flow heterogeneity. The more severe the stenosis, the lower is the potential hyperemic response and the less extensive is the linearity with flow required to identify the related flow abnormality. The less severe the stenosis, the greater is the potential hyperemic response and the more extensive is the linearity with flow required to identify the related flow abnormality. The cutoff value sets the level of hyperemia that can be differentiated from normal and is a limit of method sensitivity associated with the level of lesion stenosis that can be identified by the induced flow heterogeneity. Agents that are less linear with flow have a reduced ability to recognize higher abnormal levels of induced hyperemia, will have more difficulty in identifying mild or moderately severe stenoses and, theoretically, will be able to identify only lesions with more severe stenoses than can an agent with a higher flow cutoff and greater linearity with flow. The agent with the higher cutoff value could differentiate and separate normal from higher but abnormal levels of the hyperemic response and would be more sensitive and able to identify less severe stenoses. NOET shows promise as the perfusion agent with the best linearity to flow.

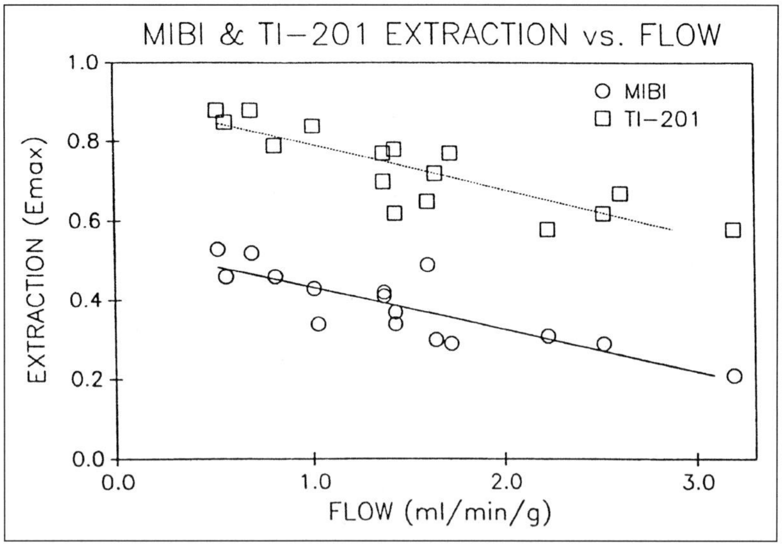

Figure 30 Radionuclide extraction. The relationship between the extraction of thallium-201 (^{201}Tl) and technetium-99m sestamibi at increasing levels of coronary blood flow is shown. Although both tracers demonstrate a reduction in extraction as flow increases, the fractional extraction (E_{max}) is higher for ^{201}Tl. (Reprinted with permission from Leppo J, Meerdink DA. Comparison of the myocardial uptake of technetium-labeled isonitrile analogue and thallium. *Circ Res* 1989;65:632–639.)

Table 4

ADVANTAGES AND DISADVANTAGES OF TECHNETIUM-99M-BASED PERFUSION AGENTS COMPARED WITH THALLIUM-201

Advantages	Disadvantages
Improved availability	Kinetics (no major reversibility)
Reduced radiation exposure	Reduced lung uptake
Increased dosage	Hepatic/splanchnic labeling
Reduced attenuation	Protocol
Improved resolution	Reduced linearity with flow
Stable localization; end diastole/ thrombolysis	Relation to viability?
Combined function and perfusion	
Permits dual-isotope imaging	
Cost?	

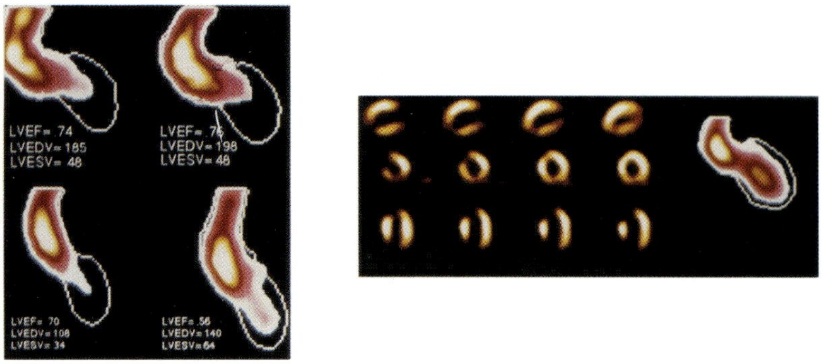

Figure 31 Sestamibi first-pass evaluation. In the left panel are normal (upper) and ischemic (lower) responses to exercise (right), with the rest study on the left. The ischemic response is characterized by an exercise-induced increase in left ventricular end-diastolic and end-systolic volumes (LVEDV and LVESV, respectively), with a fall in LV ejection fraction (EF) and a deterioration in regional wall motion. Here, a prominent left atrium with exercise, lower, suggests induced mitral regurgitation. In the right panel are vertical long-axis (top), short-axis (middle) and horizontal long-axis (bottom) images from a rest sestamibi study with inferior, apical and distal septal infarction. The associated stress first-pass study at right reveals wall-motion abnormalities in these regions and also in the anterior wall. This identifies ischemia in another major vascular territory, not evident on the perfusion image. (Reprinted with permission from Port SC. Recent advances in first pass radionuclide angiography. *Cardiol Clin* 1994;12:359–372.)

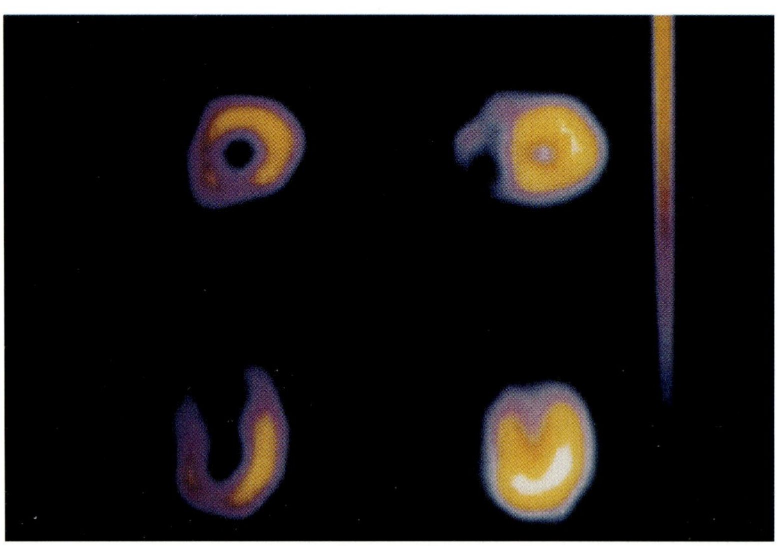

Figure 32 Gated sestamibi imaging. End-diastolic (left) and end-systolic gated technetium-99m sestamibi perfusion images in a normal heart in selected short-axis (top) and horizontal long-axis (bottom) SPECT slices. Inward systolic motion is evident, as well as brightening, or increased intensity during systole. The latter, a result of partial volume effect, is well correlated with myocardial thickening. (Reprinted with permission from Botvinick E, Dae M, O'Connell JW, Ortendahl D, Hattner RS. The scintigraphic evaluation of the cardiovascular system. In: Parmley WW, Chatterjee K, eds. *Cardiology.* Philadelphia, PA: JB Lippincott; 1991:1–121.)

Evaluation of Ventricular Function

The simultaneous evaluation of myocardial perfusion and function offers great potential advantages, including: (1) functional data may be useful in identifying and discounting attenuation artifacts, especially with unexplained or equivocal perfusion defects, and adds an element of redundancy with the security of parallel results; (2) 2 pieces of important pathophysiologic data are provided in a single study, with the application of a single radionuclide and reduced acquisition time for increased yield—a cost-effective strategy; (3) function evaluation provides another measure of regional pathophysiology, and some early evidence demonstrates an improvement in diagnostic sensitivity and specificity; (4) it provides information regarding the functional consequences of a perfusion defect and thus may add to risk stratification; (5) it provides directly comparable, registered data sets, applied with the same technology and the same physiology, for the best determination of size and severity of perfusion defect and related regional and global left ventricular function after infarction, and this promises improved risk stratification and evaluation of myocardial viability; and (6) functional maps summarizing perfusion and function data may be compared directly, and combined function–perfusion polar maps are possible and could be advantageous for the comparison of function and perfusion in a myocardial region as part of viability evaluation.

When function abnormalities exceed those of perfusion, a noncoronary cause is suggested. Some possibilities include noncoronary cardiomyopathy or related small-vessel, hypertensive or valvular heart disease. Function evaluation presents an important quantitative measure of the effects of treatment (see Self-Study Program III, *Nuclear Medicine: Cardiology, Topic 6: Myocardial Perfusion*

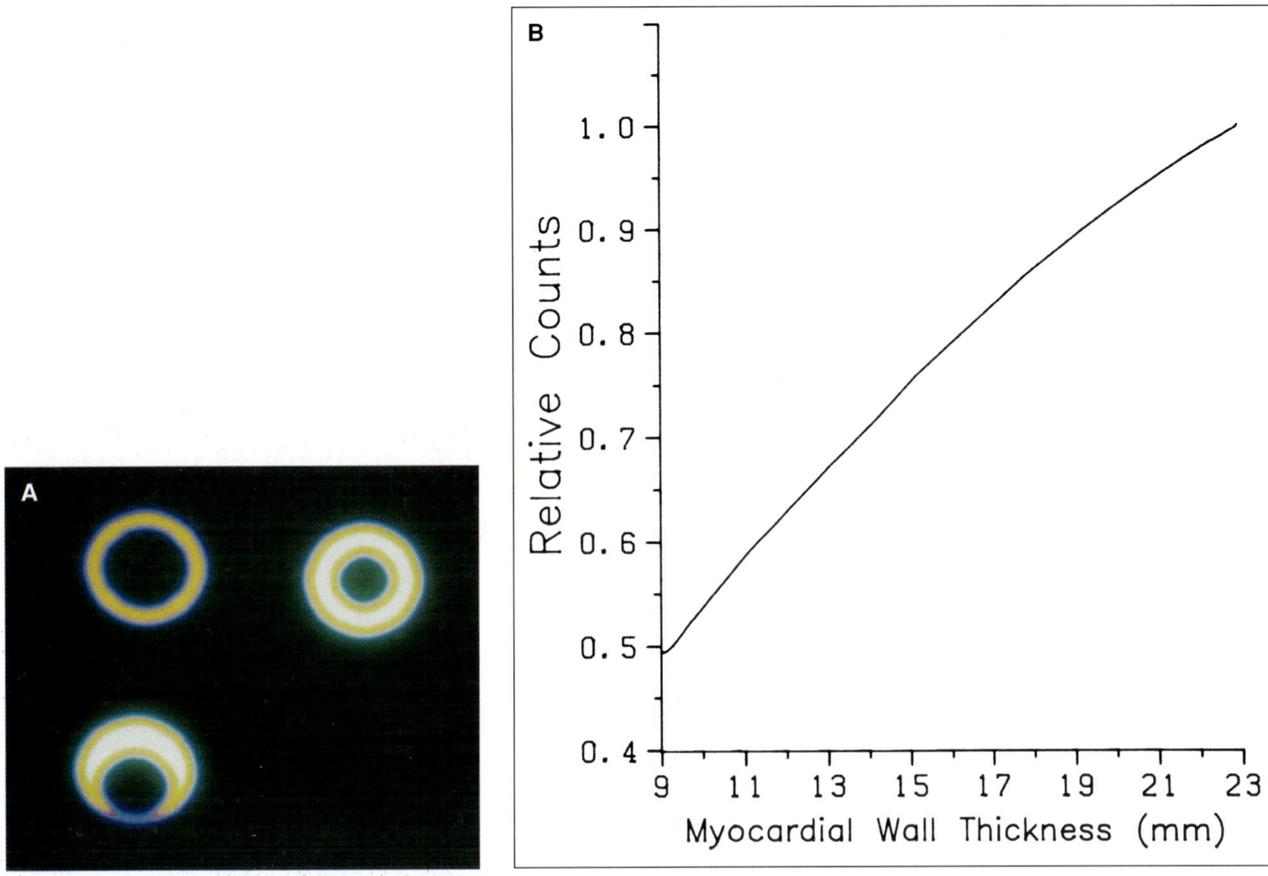

Figure 33 Intensity versus thickness. (A) A cylindrical phantom of varying thickness but with uniform tracer concentration is shown. The upper panels image thin-walled (left) and thick-walled (right) phantoms with homogeneous wall thickness, and below is the image of a phantom with varying wall thickness, thinner at the bottom and progressively increasing toward the top. Of note is the variable intensity across the phantom, which parallels regional wall thickness. This image simulates a short-axis SPECT slice and demonstrates the reason for increasing intensity and relative counts with systolic thickening. The (near) linearity of this relationship is demonstrated in (B). (Reprinted with permission from Galt JR, Garcia EV, Robbins W. Effects of myocardial wall thickness on SPECT quantification. *IEEE Trans Med Imaging* 1990;9:144–150.)

Scintigraphy—Clinical Aspects). Function evaluation with MPS can be performed by first-pass or gated methods (Table 5).

First-Pass Studies. First-pass studies must be acquired at a rapid frame rate during the bolus intravenous administration of the radiotracer (Figs. 13,41). This is the oldest and best established nuclear cardiology method, providing an assessment at rest and with exercise in an inexpensive manner. However, accurate calculation of the left ventricular ejection fraction (LVEF) from a first-pass injection made during vigorous treadmill exercise is technically demanding and, because of patient motion, cannot be achieved in all patients. Treadmill activity gives increased vertical motion with 5%–10% or more studies that cannot be interpreted. Although bicycle exercise limits translation motion of the chest, patients and physicians are less accustomed to this form of stress. The method is potentially capable of determining wall motion and LVEF with exercise, among the most important and well-established prognostic measures in CAD.

With this method, it is best to use a digital multicrystal camera for highest counting statistics (1×10^6 cps) in order to achieve adequate data rates

Table 5
PRACTICAL COMPARISON OF FIRST-PASS AND GATED PERFUSION METHODS FOR EVALUATION OF VENTRICULAR FUNCTION

First-pass
Needs technetium-99m (^{99m}Tc)-based agents
Needs state-of-the-art, high-sensitivity cameras (detectors)
Technically demanding camera requirements/protocol
Performed with radionuclide administration
Can be performed with stress but not always possible
May be performed with rest and stress
Left ventricular wall motion, volumes and ejection fraction
Can provide right ventricular ejection fraction and wall motion
Evaluates features of background-free blood pool
Gated
May be performed with thallium-201- or ^{99m}Tc-based agents
Uses conventional cameras
Always delayed after radionuclide injection and after stress
May be performed with rest and stress
Left ventricular wall motion, volumes and ejection fraction
Provides left ventricular wall thickening
Accuracy dependent on endothelial border definition

(200,000–300,000 cps). However, such a device, with its extra-thick crystals, is not optimal for conventional imaging, and excellent first-pass studies can be acquired with the counting statistics of current digital cameras. From such first-pass studies, right ventricular ejection fraction (RVEF), LVEF, end-diastolic, end-systolic and stroke volumes can be calculated, as well as cardiac output, pulmonary blood volume and peak emptying and filling rates, although regional wall motion, LVEF and ventricular size are the critical and most reproducible measures.

A high-quality, compact bolus is needed for the study. The method may be applied with the same-day rest–stress ^{99m}Tc sestamibi (tetrofosmin) protocol using 10 and 30 mCi for rest and stress studies, respectively, or the 2-day protocols with 25-mCi doses. A bolus of 10 mCi may be applied for the first-pass bolus with the multicrystal camera and lower doses with conventional cameras. A large antecubital or external jugular vein provides access for the bolus injection, with a short plastic catheter attached to a 20-ml syringe fitted with a 20-g needle. A 30-sec acquisition time is applied, bracketing the injection time. Sampling is conducted at a frequency of at least 40 frames/sec at 25-msec intervals with high temporal resolution. This gives good definition of end diastole and end systole. This short data acquisition period is well suited for exercise evaluation. Some individuals continue to use ^{201}Tl for this purpose, but images often cannot be interpreted, and ^{201}Tl is not recommended. Standard data processing algorithms have been developed with motion correction software focused on an americium-241 (^{241}Am) or iodine-125 (^{125}I) marker placed on the chest. Correction must be made for field nonuniformity, background and counts lost in dead time. A temporal filter is applied to reduce statistical noise.

Perfusion imaging is a relative method, and its regional evaluation is at least theoretically affected by the relative intensity of associated segments. In addition, it may be abnormal in the absence of ischemia. Abnormal wall motion is a more absolute indicator of regional ischemia, is not so affected by adjacent segments and theoretically may more resemble an assessment of total coronary blood flow. LVEF is a parameter that has been strongly associated with mortality after infarction and in CAD in general. LVEF as a predictor of cardiac death and perfusion as an indicator of both death and infarction present a strong combination of prognostic parameters. Added function evaluation could have diagnostic and prognostic value where rare symmetrically reduced perfusion is clarified by widespread function abnormalities, as in small vessel or diffuse severe coronary disease, and so may improve the sensitivity of the method. However, it is known that normal perfusion studies in the presence of widespread severe CAD are rare and that a normal MPS is

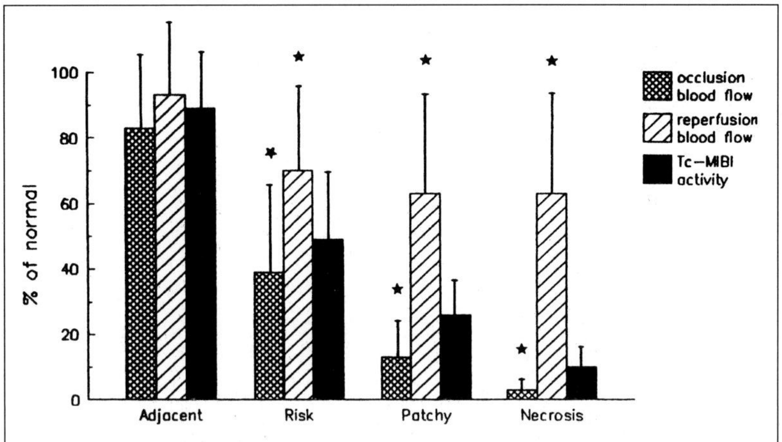

Figure 34 Sestamibi redistribution. Occlusion and reperfusion microsphere blood flows are measured in an area of necrosis, distal to a complete occlusion, and are shown with adjacent regions of patchy necrosis and ischemic risk, as well as the area outside the risk region in an animal model. After occlusion and reperfusion, flow is much improved, although not normal. Yet sestamibi activity has changed little, indicating little redistribution. (Reprinted with permission from De Coster PM, Wijns W, Cauwe F, et al. Area at risk determination by technetium-99m hexakis-2-methoxyisobutyl isonitrile in experimental reperfused myocardial infarction. *Circulation* 1990;82:2152–2162.)

associated with an excellent prognosis. In fact, studies have shown that rest, stress or poststress wall-motion abnormalities in CAD generally correlate well with regional perfusion defects.

Gated Evaluation of Left Ventricular Function. Gated SPECT studies became feasible when increased computer power made it possible to acquire 8–16 separate images through the cardiac cycle in each of 32–64 SPECT projections. In this process, 8–16 SPECT MPS images are made, each at a different phase of the cardiac cycle. Gating was performed in only 3% of MPS studies in 1993 but that figure rose to >40% in 1997 and >60% in 2000 (Figs. 32,42). Gating ^{201}Tl MPS was shown to be feasible, especially if using multidetector systems to reduce acquisition time and reduce the effects of redistribution and shifting radionuclide patterns on SPECT acquisition (*207*). LVEF is calculated by the direct measurement of end-diastolic and end-systolic volumes from anatomic regions defined by an endocardial edge-detection algorithm. LVEF has been calculated by a number of workers using different methods (*208–211*) and seems best applied to the high-count stable distribution of the ^{99m}Tc based perfusion tracers sestamibi and tetrofosmin.

Two major algorithms are available as part of the Emory University (Atlanta, GA) Toolbox and the Autoquant software developed by workers at Cedars-Sinai Hospital (Los Angeles, CA) (*207,210–215*). The approach of Germano et al. (*210*) used the threshold of a Gaussian function precalibrated to a myocardial phantom to locate the endocardium. Although this results in only a good approximation of the endocardial border, which is actually beyond system resolution, the relative tolerance of the LVEF calculation to modest edge variation makes the method clinically useful. It was the first to permit fully automated "end-to-end" functional processing of both sestamibi and ^{201}Tl studies (*216*). In another method, validated independently by Cooke et al. (*212*) and Vansant et al. (*217*), a geometric model is applied. Here, the left ventricular center is localized from maximal-count circumferential profiles, and the end-diastolic myocardial thickness is assumed to be 1 cm throughout. Systolic myocardial thickening is then taken from a Fourier analysis of counts variation in which wall thickness is taken as proportional to intensity, for reasons that will be noted. This results in localization of endocardial and epicardial borders and permits the calculation of an accurate automated LVEF as well as volume, thickness and mass measures and the generation of a 3-dimensional model of the left ventricle (*218*). Faber et al. (*214*) have validated this method in 80 patient studies, using the first-pass technique. In addition, Cooke et al. (*212*) have demonstrated the relative reproducibility of the LVEF by this method

A STRESS Tl-201 MYOCARDIAL PERFUSION IMAGING PROTOCOLS

DYNAMIC OR
PHARMACOLOGIC
STRESS
Tl-201
(3-4mCi)
/__(20min)__SPECT_____4hours_____SPECT__reinject__SPECT
1mCi Tl-201
(if needed)

or

DYNAMIC OR
PHARMACOLOGIC
STRESS
Tl-201
(3-4mCi)
/__(20min)__SPECT___4hours___reinject__SPECT__24hrs__SPECT
1mCi Tl-201 (if needed)
(if needed)

B REST - REDISTRIBUTION Tl-201 PROTOCOL

REST Tl-201
(3-4mCi)
/___(10min)___SPECT____(4-24hrs)____SPECT

This rest-redistribution protocol is an excellent method for the determination of myocardial viability.

C Tc-99m Sestamibi/Tetrofosmin Same Day Protocols

DYNAMIC OR PHARMACOLOGIC STRESS Tc-99m (6-7mCi) — REST Tc-99m (25-30mCi)
/____(15-30min)____SPECT____2-4hours___/___30-60min___SPECT

OR

REST Tc-99m (6-7mCi) — DYNAMIC OR PHARMACOLOGIC STRESS Tc-99m (25-30mCi)
/____(30-60min)____SPECT____2-4hours___/___15-30min___SPECT

D Tc-99m Sestamibi or Tetrofosmin Seperate Day Protocols

DAY 1: DYNAMIC OR PHARMACOLOGIC STRESS Tc-99m (25-30mCi)
/____(15-30min)____SPECT

DAY 2: REST Tc-99m (25-30mCi)
/____(30-60min)___SPECT

OR

DAY 1: REST Tc-99m (25-30mCi)
/____(30-60min)____SPECT

DAY 2: DYNAMIC OR PHARMACOLOGIC STRESS Tc-99m (25-30mCi)
/____(15-30min)___SPECT

E Tl-201 REST/Tc-99m STRESS PROTOCOL

REST Tl-201 (3-4mCi) — DYNAMIC OR PHARMACOLOGIC STRESS Tc-99m (25-30mCi)
/___(10min)___SPECT_/_(15-30min)__SPECT

F ACUTE INFARCTION Tc-99m SESTAMIBI PERFUSION IMAGING PROTOCOL

ON PRESENTATION
PRIOR TO THROMBOLYSIS(PTCA)

REST
Tc-99m
(25-30mCi)
/_____Thrombolysis____(<4hrs)____SPECT

ONE DAY TO ONE WEEK LATER

REST
Tc-99m
(25-30mCi)
/____(30-60min)____SPECT

Figure 35 Perfusion imaging protocols. (A) Stress thallium-201 (^{201}Tl) myocardial perfusion imaging protocols. These protocols take 4–6 hr to complete. The initial protocol presented requires 3 SPECT studies in a single day, a major task for patient and laboratory. This is necessitated by the fact that images that normalize at 4 hr may again become abnormal with reinjection. For this reason, it is best to reinject only those with persistent abnormalities after 4 hr. To determine this, a prereinjection SPECT image must be acquired. Alternatively, in the second protocol, the need for reinjection is determined from limited planar images taken after 4 hr. Even the suggestion of persistent defects after 4 hr will bring reinjection and the second SPECT set. If defects persist, 24-hr SPECT imaging is performed and has been found to demonstrate and the stability of the calculation with varying assumed wall thickness, in which the assumption of a 1.5-cm end-diastolic wall thickness brought only a 6% (relative) error in calculated LVEF. They further explored the tolerance of the method, demonstrating its continued accuracy even when counts were reduced to 5% of their normal level! The method has also has been well correlated with left ventricular volumes and mass calculated from gated magnetic resonance (MR) imaging studies (*216–219*). A recent study demonstrated the heterogeneity of myocardial wall motion and thickening and suggested the need for segmental normal values (*223*). Studies in animals and humans demonstrated the potential inaccuracies of the gated SPECT perfusion method for LVEF and size evaluation (*220,224*).

Such software and others for gated SPECT imaging are widely available, and >50% of labs perform gating as a standard part of stress MPS studies. Each image in the projection set is acquired in synchrony with the 12-lead ECG. High spatial and contrast resolution is achieved as a result of the high count density available with a 30-mCi dose of ^{99m}Tc-labeled radiotracer. By this method, a rest or poststress measure of left ventricular function may be acquired very dependably. It allows an assessment of the state of perfusion at the time of injection and the state of function at the time of imaging. Although several recent studies support the value of gated ^{201}Tl studies, a significant percentage of gated ^{201}Tl studies (measured by some to be as high as 30%) are suboptimal, and quality control in this area, although important, is insufficient (*225*).

In acquisition parameters, a trade-off must be made between high temporal or high spatial resolution, based on the time taken to acquire each frame and its resultant count density. Although planar studies can be performed with 24 frames/cycle, little data can be gleaned from gated planar images, because the endocardium is not seen or approximated. With SPECT, the frame number may require reduction in order to handle all the additional data related to the multiple projection angulations needed to compile the tomographic slices. Even more problematic is the need to gain adequate data density in each frame during each projection, where a higher frame number reduces acquisition time and data density. For these reasons, most systems permit only 8 frames/cycle and some allow 16. However, a low frame rate may blunt LVEF calculation, especially at low heart rates, because of insufficient sampling. Acquisition at 16 frames/cycle also may be helpful if seeking highly resolved end-diastolic frames. The choice of 8 or 16 frames/gated cycle need not affect acquisition time, unless data per frame are unduly reduced or irregular rhythms increase bad beat rejection. The study may be acquired and then processed electively, if and when the gated data are needed for review.

reversibility in those occasional defects that might remain (or become) abnormal after the second SPECT set. (B) Rest-restredistribution ^{201}Tl protocol. This protocol is an excellent method for the determination of myocardial viability. (C) Technetium-99m (^{99m}Tc) sestamibi/tetrofosmin same-day protocols. The rest–stress sequence is preferred, because the stress-first sequence may result in the overdiagnosis of fixed abnormalities. These protocols usually take 4–6 hr, unless the time between radionuclide administrations is reduced. (D) Technetium-99m sestamibi or tetrofosmin separate-day protocols. These protocols require prolonged evaluation, which may not be acceptable in many clinical situations. When stress is performed first and is found to be normal, the subsequent rest study need not be performed, and the protocol thus will be abbreviated. (E) Thallium-201 rest/^{99m}Tc stress protocol. This protocol takes 90–120 min and can be completed in half a day. Subsequent images may be acquired at 24 hr in the ^{201}Tl window to assess ^{201}Tl redistribution in order to assess viability. (F) Acute infarction ^{99m}Tc sestamibi perfusion imaging protocol. This protocol takes advantage of the kinetic features of sestamibi to permit imaging of the effects of thrombolysis.

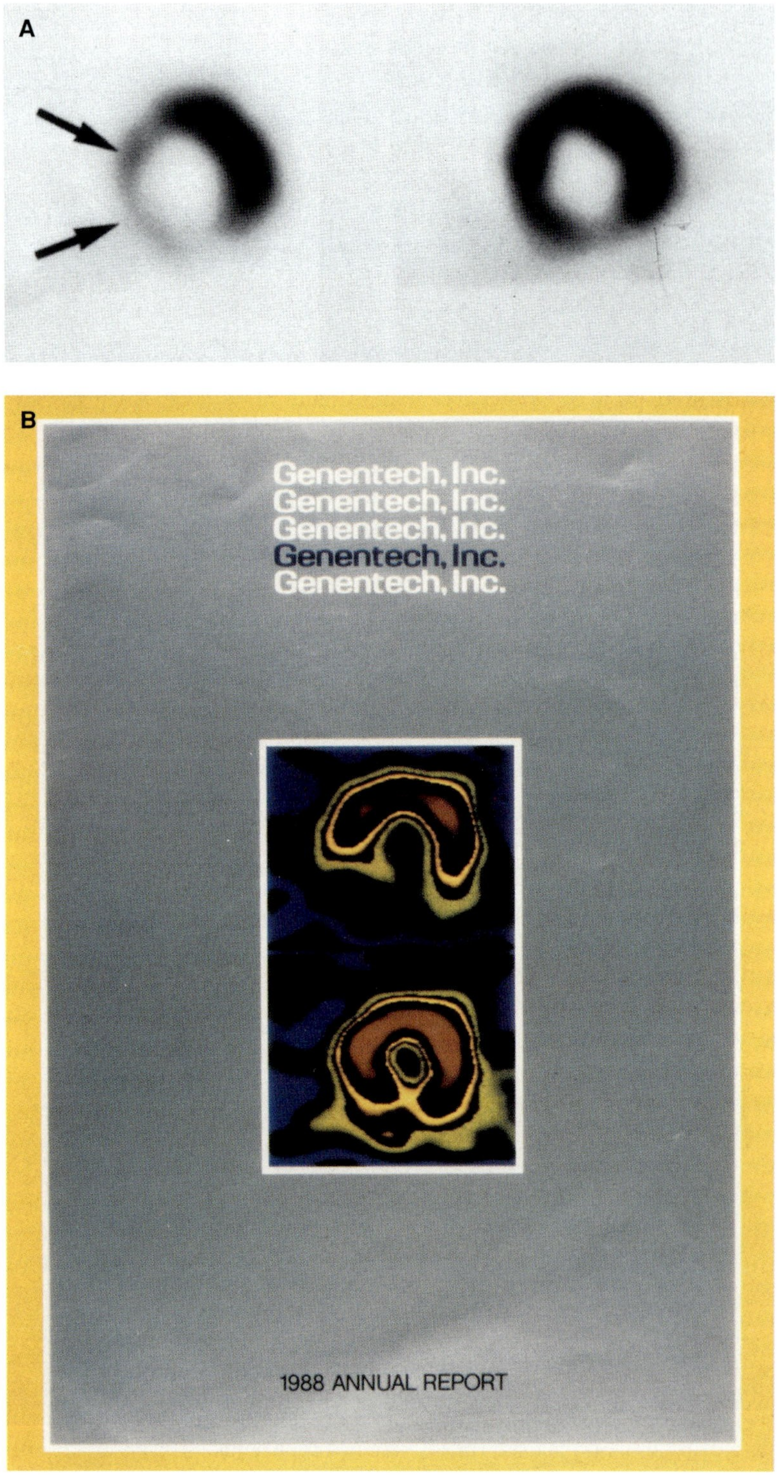

Figure 36 Perfusion after thrombolysis. (A) SPECT technetium-99m sestamibi mid-ventricular short-axis slices pre- (left) and post-(right) thrombolytic therapy are shown. The initial image was acquired after thrombolysis, with administration on presentation, and shows the state of perfusion at the time of injection. The postinfusion image was acquired the day after the procedure. Because sestamibi is little redistributed, it can be administered on admission and before thrombolysis or percutaneous transluminal coronary angioplasty (PTCA). Subsequent images may be acquired within a 4–5-hr window and will reflect the state of perfusion at the time of injection, before reflow. A subsequent image, made later to allow for perfusion normalization, will reveal the state of reperfusion. Both after thrombolysis and after PTCA, defects have been evident in the early hours to days after instrumentation, in spite of apparent anatomic success. It is best to wait as long as possible or for recurrent symptoms before evaluating the state of perfusion. However, recent studies with intracoronary ultrasound and Doppler methods suggest that early image defects indeed are associated with persistent abnormalities in vascular reactivity and the coronary flow reserve. These may improve over time, with consequent resolution of image defects. Thus, early image defects may not always indicate a lesion but may relate to physiologic abnormalities and are also predictive of subsequent occlusion after PTCA. This appears less common with stents. Technetium-99m sestamibi has become a major tool in the evaluation of the benefits of thrombolytic and PTCA trials after infarction. In such trials, application of the perfusion endpoint permits the attainment of definite results with far fewer patient numbers than the evaluation of the survival endpoint. (Reprinted with permission from Gibbons RS. Technetium-99m sestamibi in the assessment of acute myocardial infarction. *Semin Nucl Med* 1991;21:213–222.) (B) A single slice from a perfusion scintigram performed in a patient with an acute coronary occlusion (top). The bottom image is acquired after infusion of tPA (thromboplastin activator). The figure was chosen by Genentech, Inc., to demonstrate the effectiveness of their new product, tPA. (Reprinted from Genentech, Inc. *1988 Annual Report.* South San Francisco, CA: Genentech; 1988.)

Alternatively, the gated data may be summed and rapidly processed as a single study, as is done with current state-of-the-art devices. Gated SPECT studies yield wall motion analysis, wall thickening (increased intensity in systole), LVEF, end-diastolic, end-systolic and intermediate images and left ventricular volumes.

LVEF and volumes calculated by gated ^{99m}Tc sestamibi and tetrofosmin MPS compare well with similar evaluations made by other established methods (*219–231*). The gated SPECT method is widely available, well validated and has been shown to add significantly to perfusion-related findings. Rozanski et al. (*232*) have presented normal values for LVEF and volumes for different clinical subgroups. Gated evaluation of left ventricular function should be a routine part of clinical perfusion scintigraphy.

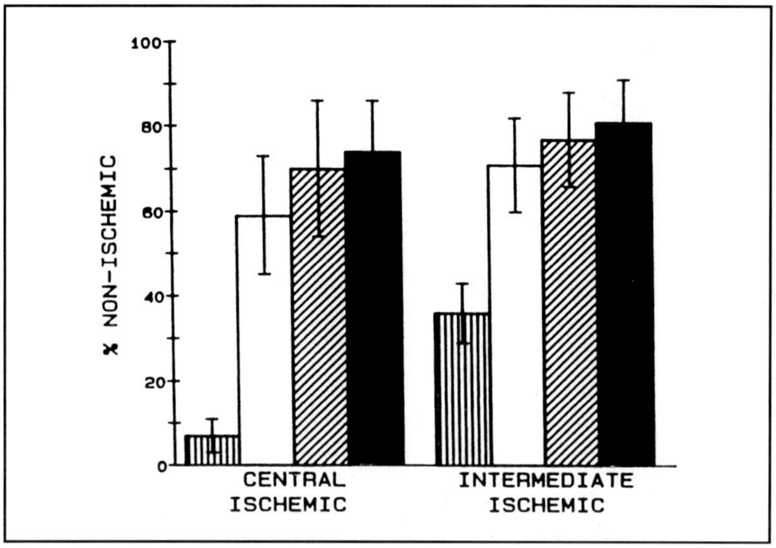

Figure 37 Thallium-201 (^{201}Tl) and technetium-99m (^{99m}Tc) sestamibi in "stunned" myocardium. The relationships between regional blood flow and myocardial ^{201}Tl and sestamibi activity in dog myocardium stunned with reperfusion after 15 min of coronary occlusion are shown. Illustrated is the level of regional flow with occlusion (vertically hatched bars) and after reperfusion (open bars), as well as ^{201}Tl (diagonally hatched bars) and ^{99m}Tc sestamibi (solid bars) activity in 29 endocardial samples from the central ischemic region and 21 endocardial samples from an intermediate ischemic region. Each value is expressed as the percentage of nonischemic values. Reperfusion ^{201}Tl activity levels, as well as those of ^{99m}Tc sestamibi, were comparable, with reperfusion flow in all ischemic segments. (Reprinted with permission from Sinusas AJ, Watson DD, Cannon JMJ, et al. Effect of ischemia and postischemic dysfunction on myocardial uptake of technetium-99m-labeled methoxyisobutyl isonitrile and thallium-201. *J Am Coll Cardiol* 1989;14:1785–1793.)

TECHNICAL ASPECTS OF GATED SPECT MYOCARDIAL PERFUSION SCINTIGRAPY

Overview

We seek to apply all factors to maximize image quality. Gated SPECT studies present functional information such as wall motion, myocardial thickening and LVEF, in addition to perfusion information (*212,233*). Gated SPECT imaging represents a combination of planar, multigated blood-pool techniques imposed on a standard myocardial SPECT acquisition. This results in a separate gated myocardial perfusion study for each projection. The high photon flux of ^{99m}Tc sestamibi or tetrofosmin makes it possible to acquire perfusion studies in gated mode. These agents are available with any full ^{99m}Tc-based protocol or with the rest ^{201}Tl/stress ^{99m}Tc protocol. Gated ^{201}Tl SPECT is also possible, but the low count rate usually requires an unacceptably long acquisition time. Rarely, stunning at the time of poststress acquisition presents evidence of reduced left ventricular function compared with function evaluation at true baseline. Poststress function data may be compared with baseline values available from other studies but are best compared with values acquired at gated rest perfusion imaging. For this reason, a gated rest study could be of value. An abnormal stress perfusion image in the presence of normal wall motion suggests the presence of a reversible defect, without the need to perform the rest image acquisition (*234*).

Although gating of planar images is certainly possible and yields an impression of regional and global function, the true cavity is never delineated and myocardium is never assessed in its transmural distribution. Apparent cavity size is affected by the thickness and radiointensity of overlying myocardium. Wall thickness is even more affected by these factors. Although SPECT images are derived from similar planar data, reconstruction techniques permit a more accurate representation of structure, although not completely unencumbered by the artifacts of superimposed anatomy. The actual cavity is reconstructed from the approximation presented at multiple angulations, and a variety of functional parameters may be evaluated.

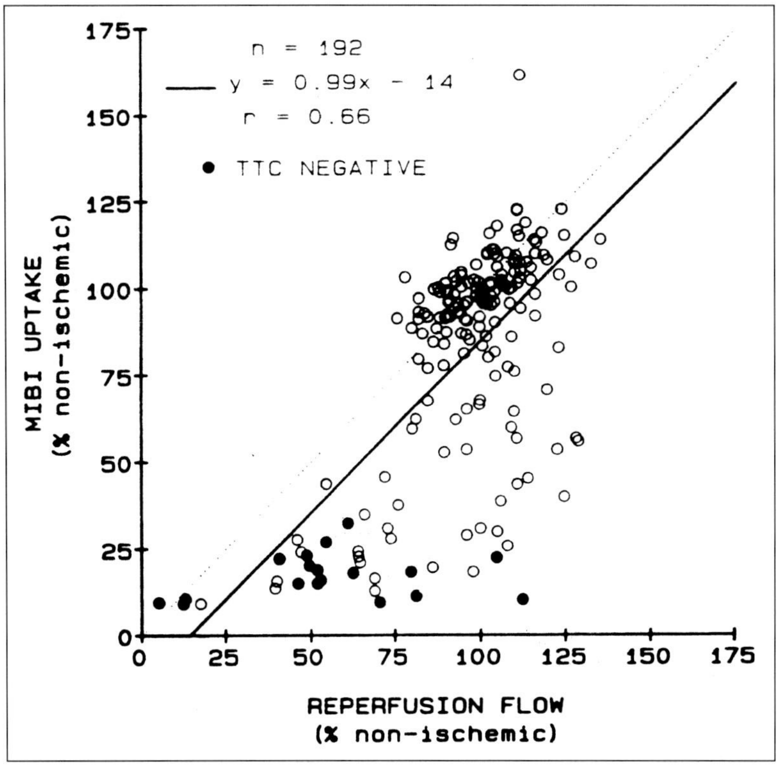

Figure 38 Technetium-99m (^{99m}Tc) sestamibi does not behave as a microsphere. Myocardial ^{99m}Tc sestamibi (MIBI) activity is expressed as the percentage of nonischemic activity versus reperfusion flow in dogs that received ^{99m}Tc sestabimi during reperfusion. The frequent finding of solid circles (2′3′5-triphenyltetrazolium chloride [TTC]-stained negative nonviable samples) associated with a spectrum of reperfusion flows indicates that localization is not solely flow related. The substantial impairment of ^{99m}Tc sestamibi uptake despite significant increases in reperfusion flow in necrotic regions indicates that the agent is not distributed as a microsphere. However, there is also a considerable lack of linearity between reperfusion flow and sestamibi activity in relation to viable segments. (Reprinted with permission from Sinusas AJ, Trautman KA, Bergin JD, et al. Quantification of area at risk during coronary occlusion and degree of myocardial salvage after reperfusion with technetium-99m methoxyisobutyl isonitrile and thallium-201. *Circulation* 1990;82:1424–1437.)

Gated acquisition employs the frame mode to divide the cardiac cycle into many short time intervals of equal duration. Intervals usually range from 20–60 msec, depending on heart rate and the number of frames per cardiac cycle. At a heart rate of 60 bpm (1000 ms/beat), 25 frames/cycle will result in images that are each 40 msec in duration, and 8 frames/cycle yield 125-msec frames. An ECG sensor box sends a signal to the computer when it detects the R wave, indicating the beginning of the cardiac cycle. The computer then initiates acquisition of the first frame and contributes image data to each successive frame for identical amounts of time. Frame duration is set before study acquisition, based on the R–R interval and the number of frames desired. At the end of the last frame, the heart should be once again at end diastole, the beginning of the next contraction cycle, and the computer will be ready to contribute data to the first frame at the onset of the new cycle when it detects the next R wave. Each frame is pooled with its corresponding frames in successive cycles in each projection to accumulate sufficient counts to represent the myocardium as a separate image at each interval during the cardiac cycle. Each frame requires sufficient data density to permit the reconstruction of adequate SPECT images in that time interval. This is possible using conventional ^{99m}Tc agent dosages without altering the duration of acquisition, provided that the number of frames per cardiac cycle (the frame rate) is kept relatively low. Acquiring more frames per cardiac cycle requires more cycles and an increased acquisition time to accumulate the same count density in each image.

Blood-pool or other gated planar functional studies generally require at least 16 frames/cycle to gain sufficient temporal resolution to present a valid representation of ventricular volume changes and wall motion. Because such data must be repeated, stored and processed for each SPECT projection stop, practical limits have set a peak of 8–16 frames for MPS SPECT. The acquisition of more frames would require more time per frame to accumulate similar data, a compromise that would increase acquisition time and the possibility of motion artifacts. Alternatively, the data accumulated in half the time must provide adequate statistics for function evaluation. Although 16 frames provide greater regional accuracy, 8 frames have been shown to be sufficient to provide acceptably accurate regional and global functional data (*212*) and require less computer memory, acquisition and processing time. Because computer memory is limited, longer acquisition times are not desirable and 8 frames/cycle provide adequate functional evaluation, gated SPECT images usually are produced with the acquisition of 8 frames through the cardiac cycle and with each planar projection image acquisition (*235*). A full SPECT series is constructed for each frame in the projection image set, initially in transaxial slices and then, as for the nongated set, in vertical, horizontal and short-axis slices. These are then played sequentially in a closed-loop cine format for the visual appreciation of motion, and end-diastolic and end-systolic image sets are analyzed for quantitative LVEF, regional wall motion and thickening. During processing, it is possible to collapse the gated images in each projection and degate into 1 static image that is identical to the image produced by standard ungated SPECT. This is called degating, removing the effects of gated acquisition. Degating provides access to both gated and ungated data from the same study.

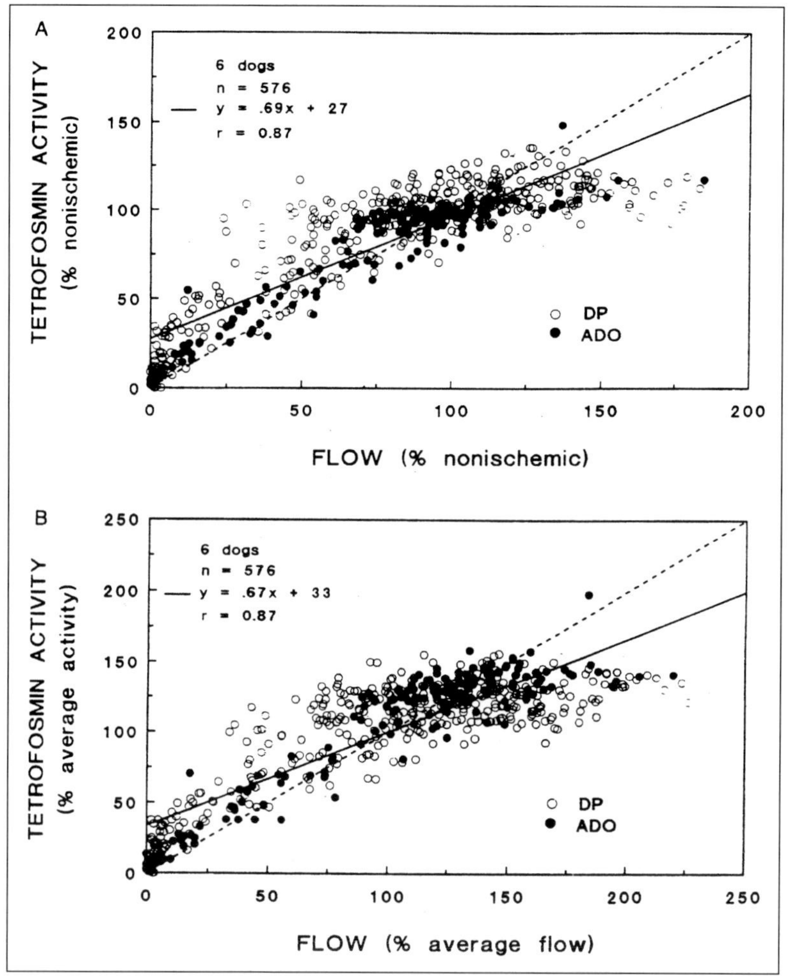

Figure 39 Tetrofosmin linearity with flow. Shown are normalized technetium-99m tetrofosmin activity and microsphere flow after dipyridamole (DP) or adenosine (ADO) stress in 6 dogs with coronary occlusion. (A) Values are normalized to nonischemic myocardial activity and flow. (B) Mean values for each dog. (Reprinted with permission from Sinusas AJ, Shi QX, Saltzberg, et al. Technetium-99m tetrofosmin to assess myocardial blood flow: experimental validation in an intact canine model of ischemia. *J Nucl Med* 1994;35:664–671.)

Because objects smaller than 2× the spatial resolution (~26 mm) demonstrate maximal counts proportional to object thickness and because the projected myocardial cross-section is generally less than 2× the system spatial resolution, regional intensity is proportional to myocardial thickness. This "partial volume effect" may also be thought of in terms of the extent that the myocardium fills a pixel. With systolic thickening from 8–12 mm, pixel filling is greater. Greater pixel filling translates into increased pixel intensity (Figs. 32,33,43). Visually, the contracting, thickening wall appears to brighten or move up the color scale in systole. Thickening or brightening, then, is gross evidence of regional myocardial viability but cannot exclude partial thickness or nontransmural infarction. The relationship between regional pixel intensity and thickening has been documented in phantoms and in correlations with echocardiographic findings (*212*). Evidence of wall motion and thickening may be important for CAD diagnosis and appears to add to diagnostic specificity (*236,237*). Here, normal motion and thickening in the presence of a fixed defect suggest an artifact of motion or attenuation rather than a true infarction (Fig. 44).

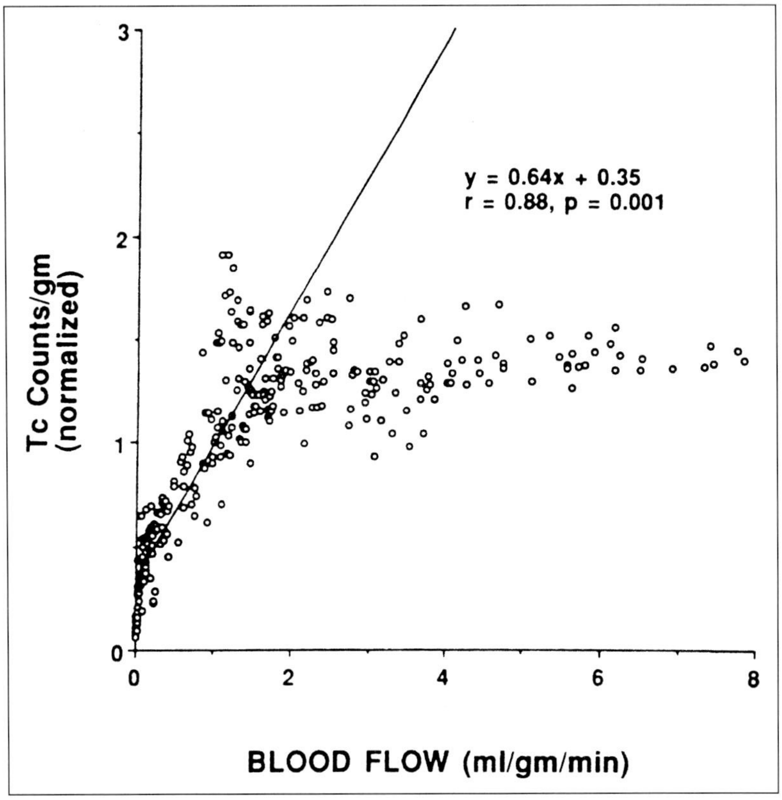

Figure 40 Furosifosmin linearity with hyperemic flow. Presented is a plot of the hyperemic response of microsphere myocardial blood flow compared with sample technetium-99m Q12 activity in dogs with left circumflex coronary artery occlusions. Q12 was administered at the peak of intravenous dipyridamole administration. There is a clear plateau in uptake at flows >2.0 ml/min/g. (Reprinted with permission from Gerson MC, Millard RW, Roszell NJ, et al. Kinetic properties of ^{99m}Tc-Q12 in canine myocardium. *Circulation* 1994;89:1291–1300.)

The evaluation of perfusion in isolated end-diastolic frames of the gated study might provide some advantages (*237–239*). To gain the maximum benefit in the assessment of stress end-diastolic images, these should be compared with rest end-diastolic images and both rest and stress images must be gated, or specificity will be lost (*240*).

Potential Problems with the Method

Parameters of Gated Acquisition. As with gated blood-pool studies, irregular rhythms add ambiguity to image interpretation, so beats outside the imaging window are rejected. A trigger acceptance window is a time interval that includes the median R–R interval and sets the temporal R–R boundaries for acceptance of image data. This window is set to permit analysis of beats with similar related ventricular volumes, wall motion and ejection fraction, because these vary with R–R interval. With bad beat rejection, a narrow acceptance window causes computer rejection of cycles outside that window and prolongs the study. Gated studies may require unacceptably long acquisition times in patients who have irregular heart rates, because a large percentage of beats will be rejected. Wider acceptance windows are less selective and will decrease the acquisition time. Although it is desirable to acquire data from a singular R–R population, it is counterproductive to set a small acceptance window in the presence of a sinus arrhythmia or other rhythm, when all beats are of similar origin and functional effect. A broad window will still preserve data integrity without unduly prolonging the study.

Quality control methods to assess the adequacy of gating and the cycles and counts accepted in each frame are not yet available, with current reliance entirely on ECG monitoring and the observations of the technologist. Standards of "normal" have not yet been established. Guidelines for the optimal gating protocol, acquisition and processing options are not yet available (*13*). Unlike tools currently available for monitoring the adequacy of blood-pool acquisition as beat-length histograms with a record of the proportion of beats accepted, no such methods apply to gated MPS. Moreover, list-mode acquisition that would enable the selection of uniform beat length for postacquisition analysis cannot be performed. Eight-frame acquisition is the standard, but more frequent sampling may be required in some cases in which LVEF may be underestimated. Normal values for regional wall motion and thickening have not yet been established, and a standard static image display of regional wall motion and thickening in comparison with perfusion has not been agreed upon (*13*).

Variability in the Measurement of Function and Perfusion

General Considerations. The radionuclide and imaging protocol employed, the manner of image processing and other factors that influence the ability to resolve the myocardial wall all affect the accuracy of LVEF determination. Of course, the failure of the edge-detection algorithm to discern the endocardial border will cause significant errors in the calculation of LVEF and volumes. Heart rate also is important. Variability in angular data acquisition rate caused by irregularities in heart rate and counts registered in different projection images can cause apparent perfusion image defects.

The Influence of Ventricular Volume. Limited image resolution with underestimation of end-systolic volume is the likely reason for the overestimation of LVEF in small ventricles (*13,241*). Because of the lower count rate, lower emission energy and increased scatter in ^{201}Tl compared with ^{99m}Tc-based images, this should be a greater problem with gated ^{201}Tl studies. Varying myocardial resolution as a result of intrinsic physical tracer differences and varying levels of processing may be the reason for the reported varying LVEF with ^{201}Tl and ^{99m}Tc perfusion images (*242*).

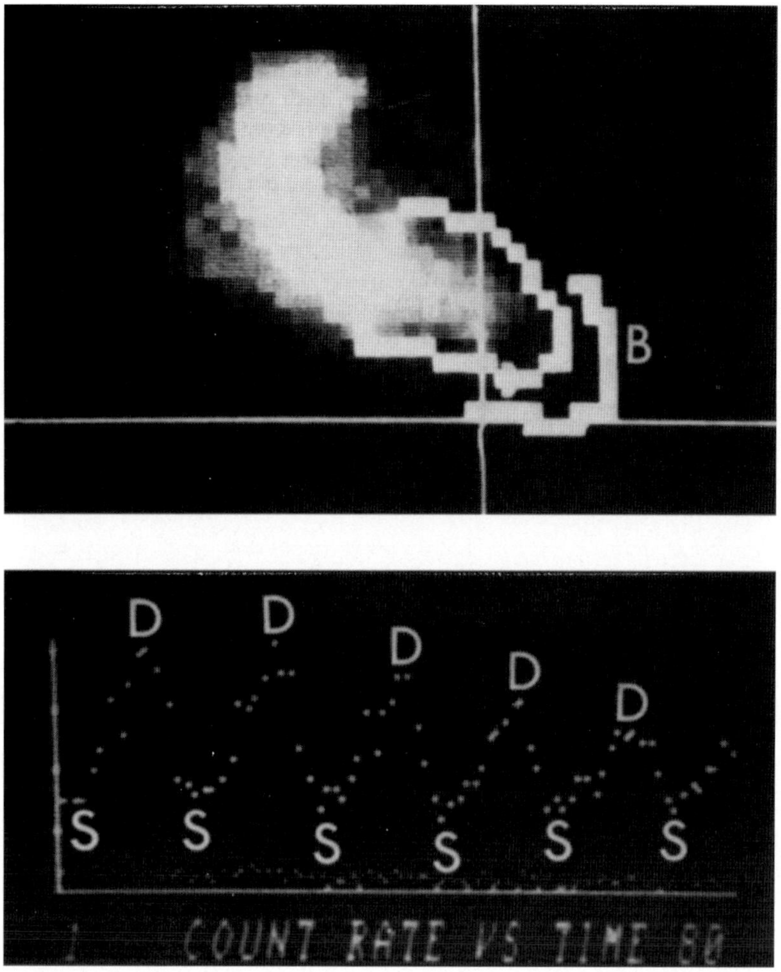

Figure 41 First-pass levophase analysis. Shown above is the levophase of a first-pass radioangiogram. A region of interest has localized the left ventricle. High-frequency analysis of the time-versus-radioactivity data in this region yields the curve below. Correcting for background, the peaks and valleys may be compared to calculate left ventricular ejection fraction. D = end-diastole; S = end-systole. (Reprinted with permission from Botvinick EH, Glazer H, Shosa D. What is the reliability and the utility of scintigraphic methods for the assessment of ventricular function? In: Rahimtoola S, ed. *Controversies in Coronary Artery Disease.* Philadelphia, PA: FA Davis;1983:65.)

The Effect of Sampling Rate. A limited sampling rate in gated images can also influence LVEF calculation. Here, slow heart rates are associated with a prolonged diastolic phase and contracted systole. In this situation, systole may be undersampled at low frame rates, increasing the possibility of missing true end-systole and so overestimating end-systolic volume and counts. This results in the underestimation of LVEF. This is a greater possibility at frame rates of 8 frames/min than at frame rates ≥16/cycle. The latter rate was established as the minimal required for accurate LVEF calculation using gated blood-pool studies (*241,243*). A compromise would apply 8 frames over the initial half of the cardiac cycle.

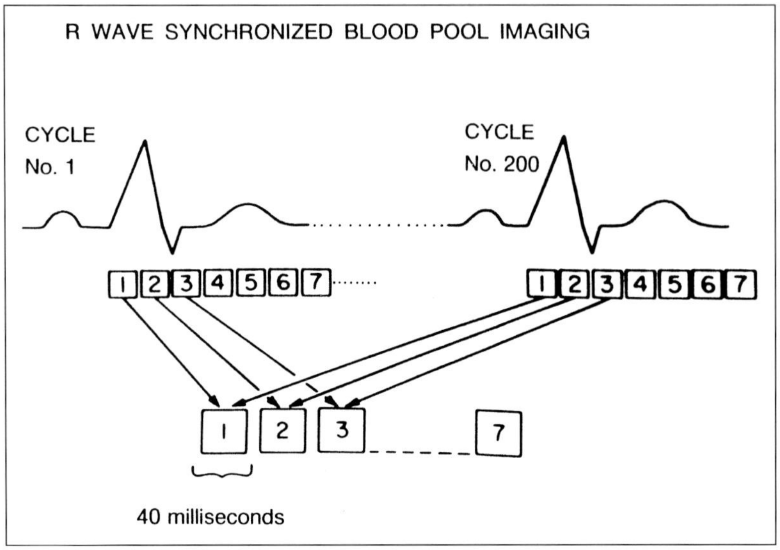

Figure 42 Electrocardiographic gating of blood-pool images. With frame mode acquisition, image data representing a preset fraction of the R-R interval, usually measuring 40 msec or less for equilibrium blood-pool imaging, but 1/16 to 1/8 of the cycle for myocardial perfusion scintigraphy (MPS), are collected during each cardiac cycle. These individual frames are pooled with the same frame of subsequent beats until summed frames (below) containing the sum of data representing all image intervals are displayed as an endless loop movie and analyzed for parameters of ventricular size and function. With gated MPS, 8 frames are usually in the resultant display. SPECT requires such 8-frame acquisition for each projection image, multiplying the required memory by the frame number, generally 32 or 64. Each of the 8–16 frames is then processed as a SPECT image, providing SPECT data sets in each and the potential for dynamic display of each SPECT slice in each axis. (Reprinted with permission from Strauss HW, Zaret BI, Hurley PJ, et al. A scintigraphic methods for measuring left ventricular ejection fraction in man without cardiac catheterization. *Am J Cardiol* 1971;28:575–583.)

The Influence of Gating Abnormalities. Acceptance of data over a spectrum of R–R intervals reduces the accuracy of LVEF calculation. Gating abnormalities also may produce perfusion abnormalities when an irregular rhythm is present during the acquisition. Gated SPECT studies usually take a little longer to acquire than ungated SPECT studies, because some beats are rejected when the R–R interval falls outside the acceptance window. This requires additional time to accumulate the appropriate counts and number of R–R cycles. A basic principle of SPECT requires that comparable data be acquired in each projection, so in the optimal situation the detector stays in a given projection until the prescribed acquisition time limit is reached. To fulfill these requirements, each projection requires image data for the same number of cardiac cycles or imaging time. Acquisition time plus the time lost as a result of bad beat rejection adds up to total elapsed time. If the heart rate is regular and R–R intervals are always within the acceptance window, the acquisition time will be the same for gated and ungated studies. Irregularities of cardiac rate bring a variable cycle rejection rate when a relatively narrow cardiac-cycle-length acceptance window is applied. This results in the acquisition of a varying number of cardiac cycles and variable related myocardial counts and intensities in different frames of the projection image set when projection images are taken to isotime. This brings apparent varying counts and intensities to different portions of the myocardium imaged at varying angles, which the SPECT backprojection reconstruction algorithm interprets as regional perfusion defects. This effect can be reduced by altering the "stop condition."

Gated SPECT can be set up to acquire for any 1 of 3 stop conditions in each projection: the number of seconds per projection, the number of cardiac cycles per projection or the number of counts per projection. When acquiring for a fixed time interval with an irregular cardiac rhythm, count data will likely vary in different projections. It is possible that no acceptable R–R interval may occur during some projection, resulting in no data being acquired in that projection. This will certainly cause problems in reconstruction and interpretation. If the acquisition time varies only slightly between projections, the counts in each image can be scaled to mimic constant acquisition time per projection. Acquiring data with a fixed number of counts per projection would be valid but could take excessive time. Using a fixed number of cardiac cycles in each projection is the method of choice and means that the actual acquisition time (the number of cycles × the cycle length) is the same for each projection. At least 1 vendor's product allows acquisition of all cycles during gated SPECT and puts all the rejected cycles into a separate image not used for gated SPECT reconstruction. These images are utilized during degated processing as an efficient way to increase the data density without additional acquisition time.

When acquiring gated MPS studies, perfusion data must never be sacrificed for function data. The counts (cycles or beats) in each projection frame must be constant. If beats fall outside a beat-length acceptance window and are rejected because of their length, counts per projection may vary if acquired to a fixed time. Acquisition should be to a fixed cycle number per projection frame, and the acquisition window should accept the widest possible range of cycle lengths. Beats rejected should be stored, if possible, and added to reconstruct the "ungated" images from which perfusion is read. However, rhythm irregularities may not bring the dramatic perfusion defects to SPECT reconstruction that might be expected (*244,245*).

STRESS TESTING PROTOCOLS

Dynamic (Treadmill or Bicycle) Exercise: An Indirect Test of Coronary Flow Reserve

Treadmill (bicycle) exercise is the most common mode of stress testing used in conjunction with MPS (*246–248*). Detection of CAD and evaluation of

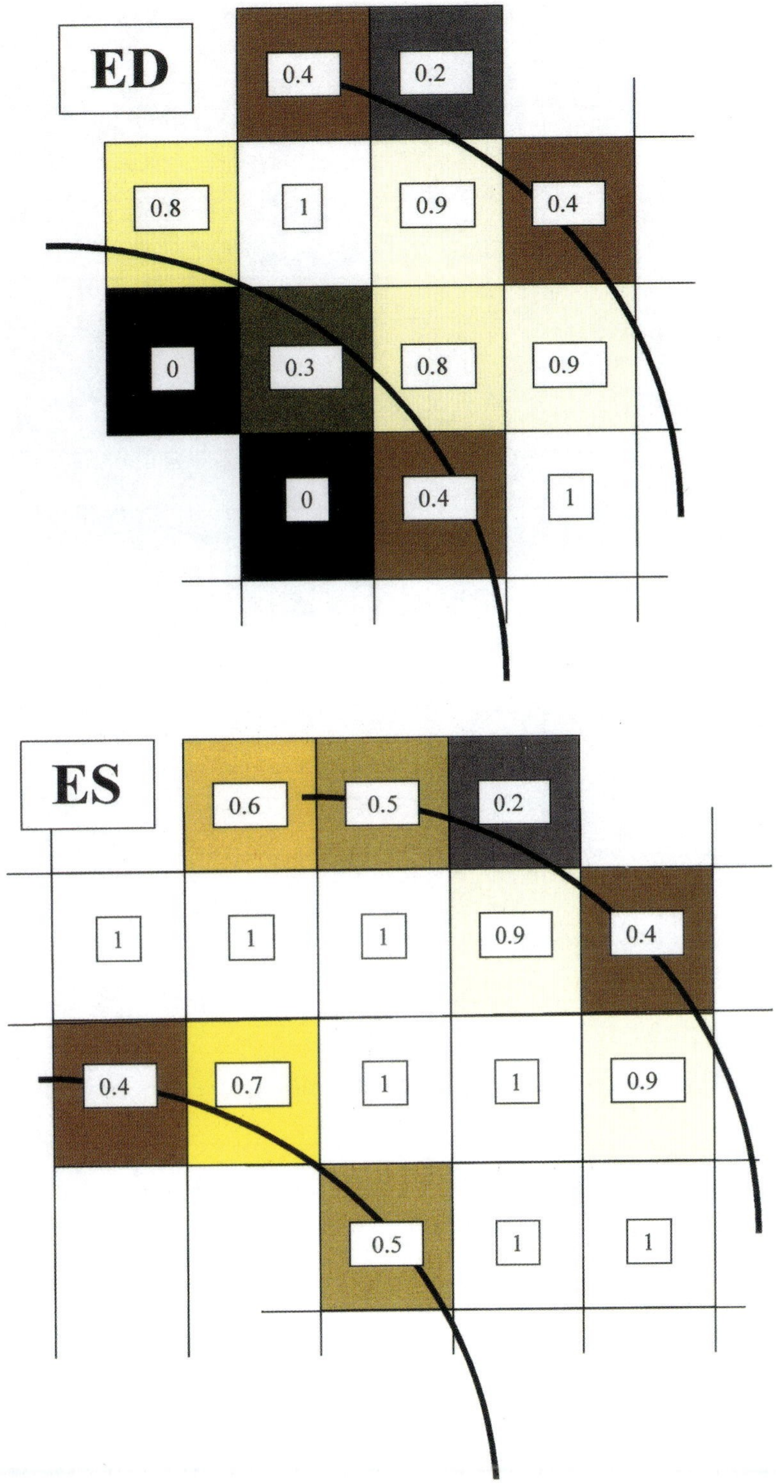

Figure 43 Brightening, wall thickening and the partial volume effect. Shown diagramatically is a myocardial region in end diastole (ED) and end systole (ES). The squares represent pixels that are color coded for and labeled with the percentage of the pixel occupied by the myocardium. Thickening fills pixels more completely by the myocardium and brings a brighter (lighter) intensity response. (Reprinted with permission from Cooke CD, Garcia EV, Cullom J, et al. Determining the accuracy of calculating systolic wall thickening using a fast Fourier transform approximation: a simulation study based on canine and patient data. *J Nucl Med* 35;1994:1185–1192.)

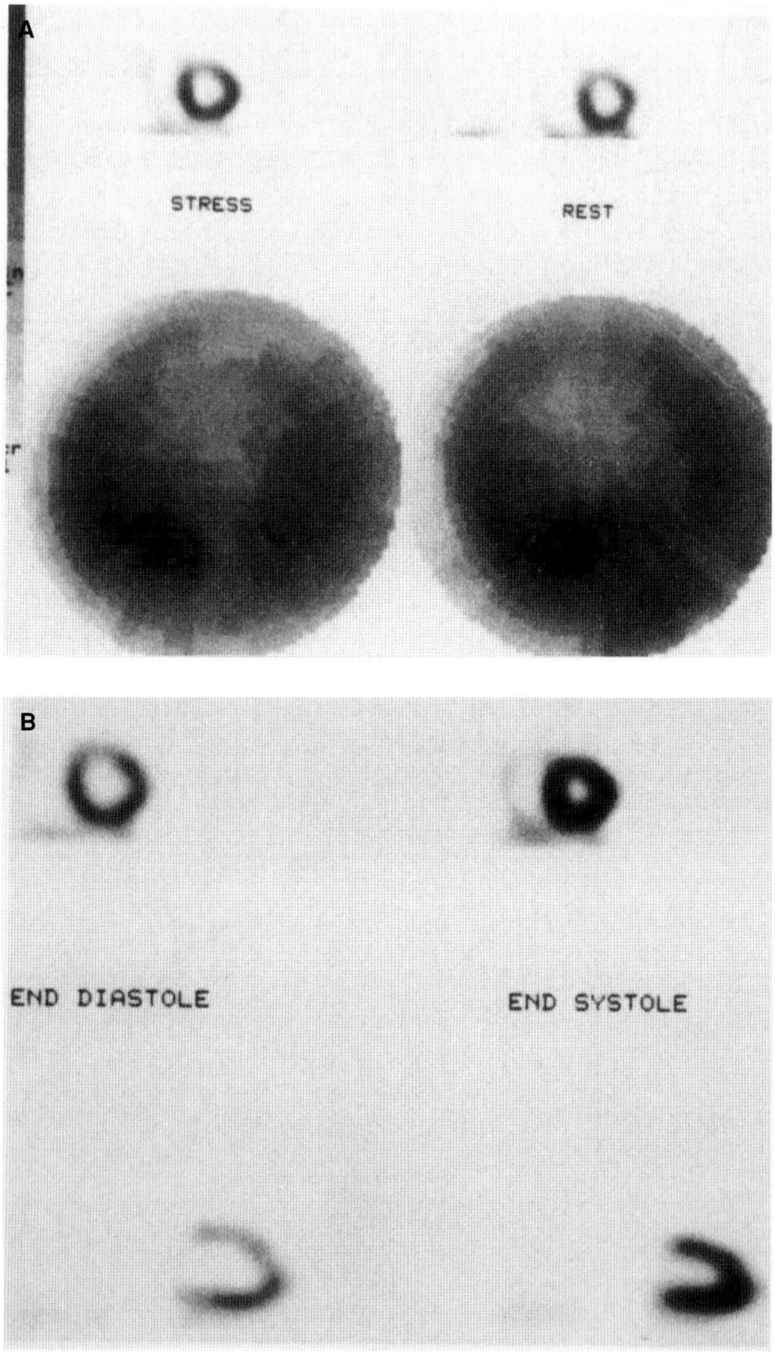

Figure 44 Wall motion clarifies potential attenuation artifact. (A) Shown are ungated short-axis slices and corresponding polar maps from myocardial perfusion scintigraphy performed in a female patient. Evidence of anterior breast attenuation (or infarction) can be seen well on both rest and stress studies. (B) Illustrates the end-diastolic and end-systolic mid-ventricular short-axis (top) and vertical long-axis (bottom) slices from the same patient with evident breast attenuation. Note normal wall motion and thickening (intensification) of the anterior defect, favoring attenuation artifact as its cause rather than scar. (Reprinted with permission from DePuey EG III. How to avoid myocardial perfusion SPECT artifacts. *J Nucl Med* 1994;35:699–702.)

the extent and severity of ischemia are enhanced when the disparity of regional coronary flow between normal and diseased arteries is large. Because induced myocardial hyperemia is related to exercise heart rate and to other determinants of myocardial flow demand, the disparity in regional flow is increasingly accentuated as achieved determinants increase in magnitude during exercise.

To assess perfusion in association with the peak rate response, it is recommended that beta blocker and calcium channel blocker medications be discontinued for 24–48 hr before exercise testing to facilitate this response and gain an evaluation of ischemia unaffected by antianginal treatment. Long-acting beta blockers should be discontinued for ~4 days before stress testing to allow for their effects to subside.

Long-acting nitrates increase baseline flow and should be discontinued for ~6 hr before exercise testing. Exercise may be performed, of course, without discontinuing medications, when the objective is to assess a patient's response to medical therapy rather than to assess the full extent of myocardium at ischemic risk and related prognosis.

The graded Bruce protocol is used most often for cooperative, vigorous patients, but more slowly graduated protocols, such as as the Modified Bruce or the Naughton protocols (*246–248*), may be employed to perform submaximal exercise testing in patients soon after myocardial infarction or in patients who are anxious, are at questionable risk or have limited exercise tolerance. With the low-level exercise protocols, exercise augmentation is more gradual and is more easily controlled and terminated at a preset heart rate. Exercise at peak achieved level is continued for ~60 sec after radionuclide injection, so that maximal myocardial blood flow is maintained during the period of major myocardial uptake of the radionuclide. Because ^{99m}Tc sestamibi and tetrofosmin extraction is somewhat lower than that of ^{201}Tl, a longer period of postinjection stress theoretically would be required to permit optimal extraction and maintain diagnostic sensitivity. Although this is desirable, a 1-min postinjection interval seems sufficient for these radiotracers, which may be accurately applied with both dynamic or pharmacologic stress testing.

Pharmacologic Stress Testing Using Coronary Vasodilators

Primary (or Direct) Coronary Dilators. Myocardial hyperemia induced by intravenous administration of dipyridamole or adenosine is an effective alternative form of stress testing to use with MPS (see Self Study Program III, *Nuclear Medicine: Cardiology, Topic 2: Pharmacologic Stress*). Dipyridamole and adenosine are coronary dilators that increase myocardial blood flow 3–5× the resting level in myocardial regions subtended by normal coronary arteries without increasing myocardial oxygen demand. In myocardial regions supplied by diseased coronary arteries, this hyperemic response is attenuated. Occasionally, after administration of coronary vasodilators, myocardial perfusion may actually decrease below the resting level in regions supplied by diseased coronary arteries, the result of a true "coronary steal" or other possible mechanism (*249–251*). In patients with CAD, infusion of these coronary vasodilators causes a disparity in regional myocardial perfusion in a manner similar to that achieved with exercise testing, even in the absence of induced ischemia. MPS will sensitively detect induced flow abnormalities regardless of whether or not true ischemia is produced. Because of this effect, pharmacologic stress testing with dipyridamole or adenosine infusion has been used in conjunction with MPS as an alternative to dynamic exercise perfusion scintigraphy for the detection and evaluation of CAD (*16,252,253*).

The main indications for pharmacologic stress perfusion scintigraphy are in patients who are unable to exercise because of peripheral vascular, musculoskeletal, pulmonary or neurologic diseases or other limitations (Table 6) (see Self-Study Program III, *Nuclear Medicine: Cardiology, Topic 2: Pharmacologic Stress*). Pharmacologic stress scintigraphy also may be used instead of exercise imaging in patients who are unable to achieve a high heart rate during exercise, such as those on beta-blocking medications and in whom discontinuation of medications before exercise testing is not considered to be safe, in poorly motivated patients and in those who are pacemaker dependent. A recent study suggests that the sensitivity of vasodilator pharmacologic stress may be somewhat reduced with concomitant use of beta blockers (*254*). However, the significance of this finding and its relationship to prior reports and general experience suggesting the contrary remain to be seen.

Table 6
INDICATIONS FOR PHARMACOLOGIC STRESS TESTING

The presence of limiting conditions, including excessive weight, that make it impossible to answer the clinical question with exercise testing.*
Coronary risk stratification before noncardiac surgery
Risk stratification early after uncomplicated infarction
Risk stratification in unstable angina
Coronary artery disease risk stratification on beta-blockers (see text)
Coronary artery disease diagnosis and prognosis in aortic stenosis, cerebrovascular disease, arteriovenous malformations and other high-risk conditions

*See Self-Study Program III, *Nuclear Medicine: Cardiology, Topic 2: Pharmacologic Stress*. Reston, VA: Society of Nuclear Medicine; 1998: Table 3.

Pharmacologic stress is not a substitute for dynamic exercise testing, nor does the achieved heart rate on exercise necessarily provide an indication for pharmacologic stress. Instead, the clinical question and the ability of the intervention to respond to that question should determine the method applied. Questions of exercise tolerance or exercise prescription, the relationship of symptoms to activities or the extent of induced ischemia on antianginal therapy may be resolved with dynamic exercise testing without medication adjustment. The assessment of coronary pathophysiology in uncooperative patients, of the full extent of coronary involvement for those on antianginal drugs or at risk for vigorous interventions (such as extensive noncardiac surgery) or with limited exercise tolerance or blunted heart rate response requires maximum pharmacologic stress evaluation (Table 6).

Indirect Coronary Dilators. Unlike dipyridamole and adenosine and more similar to dynamic exercise, the sympathomimetic agent dobutamine acts to augment contractility, heart rate and blood pressure, important determinants of myocardial oxygen demand. Because coronary flow demand is affected, an inadequate coronary supply results in a supply/demand imbalance and ischemia. This rarely occurs when primary or "direct" coronary dilators are used, because they usually do not produce augmented flow demands and only occasionally result in reduced supply.

Dobutamine infusion may be applied as a true ischemic stress to test CFR. This method may be used with echocardiography to assess the functional ischemic endpoint and has been said to be as accurate as exercise echocardiography (*255*). Alternatively, it may be applied with scintigraphy to assess the perfusion or functional endpoint. It is most valuable in instances in which the risk with dipyridamole or adenosine is increased by the presence of ongoing bronchospasm. Recently, this ischemic stress has been shown to have acceptable sensitivity for CAD detection with scintigraphy but to be less sensitive when applied with the echocardiographic functional endpoints (*256,257*). Not infrequently, it fails to provide the required increase in myocardial oxygen demands needed to test the CFR sufficiently and is not without risk, especially in the setting of acute coronary syndromes.

Induced perfusion heterogeneity (possibly but not necessarily related to ischemia) and induced regional ventricular dysfunction (a true ischemic endpoint) may be used to measure the adequacy of the CFR (*6*). MPS is the only clinical imaging modality currently available for the evaluation of the perfusion (ischemic) endpoint in the presence of perfusion heterogeneity induced by direct coronary dilators in the absence of induced ischemia. Either scintigraphic or echocardiographic methods may be used to assess the effect of true ischemia induced by indirect coronary dilators (dynamic exercise or dobutamine) or, rarely, by direct dilators, using either the functional ischemic endpoint or scintigraphy to assess the perfusion endpoint.

As noted, echocardiography may be applied to identify induced ischemic dysfunction with dynamic exercise or indirect pharmacologic dilators. Although reported by some to be the imaging modality of choice for this application, echocardiographic interpretation is entirely subjective, is limited to the functional endpoint, has a significant finite failure rate, a strong potential for abuse and has not been as thoroughly tested as MPS (*257*). A full examination of the mechanism, indications, performance and evaluation of methods of pharmacologic stress testing are described in Self-Study Program III, *Nuclear Medicine: Cardiology, Topic 2: Pharmacologic Stress.*

IMAGING PROTOCOLS

Overview

Each currently available perfusion imaging agent has been successfully applied with all forms of dynamic and pharmacologic stress testing. A full tabulation of guidelines for instrumentation quality assurance and quality control procedures, along with all myocardial stress perfusion protocols including the evaluation of left ventricular function, is available (*258*).

Thallium-201 Protocols

General Method. Administration of the radiotracer should be made near the end of and close to peak exercise or peak pharmacologic effect. The stress is continued for ~1 min for radionuclide extraction at peak stress or somewhat longer with pharmacologic stress; then the test is ended. After adequate postexercise monitoring and when the patient is at baseline, he or she is sent for imaging. A delay of 5–10 min is needed before imaging for radionuclide background and organ clearance, compared with sestamibi, which often requires more time to optimally clear from the adjacent gastrointestinal tract before imaging.

Imaging usually is begun 10–15 min after injection of ^{201}Tl, and planar images usually are acquired for a preset time of ~10 min/projection in the anterior, 45° left anterior oblique (LAO) and steep LAO or left lateral projection. Alternatively, the anterior projection is obtained to optimal counts and the subsequent images to isotime. The first 2 planar projections are obtained with the patient supine, but the steep LAO or left lateral projections are obtained with the patient in the right lateral decubitus position, with the left side of the chest against the collimator, because this diminishes the frequency of diaphragmatic attenuation of activity in the inferior left ventricular wall activity (*259*) (Fig. 45). To evaluate initial abnormalities, delayed redistribution images in identical projections are obtained 3–5 hr after injection of ^{201}Tl. If defect reversibility is not complete by the time of the redistribution study, a late redistribution study (18–72 hr after injection) is recommended to further assess reversibility of perfusion defects (*260*). For late imaging, 15 min/view are used for planar acquisition. Optimal normalization or redistribution of ^{201}Tl perfusion defects appears to require both time and agent availability.

Reinjection Technique. A second injection or reinjection appears to satisfy the requirement for availability (*261*) in instances in which ^{201}Tl may be otherwise sequestered in the gastrointestinal tract or skeletal muscle before resolution of the heterogeneous perfusion pattern. Time, however, often will allow ^{201}Tl to distribute into the K+ or viable intracellular space. This would permit ^{201}Tl localization in even chronically underperfused myocardium, serving as evidence of tissue viability. This is likely the basis for defect reversibility or imaging performed late after rest ^{201}Tl injection, an important scintigraphic method for viability assessment (*262,263*).

The reinjection technique has been applied widely to ^{201}Tl imaging. An additional 1.0–1.5 mCi of the agent is administered intravenously, shortly before acquisition of delayed (4-hr) imaging to optimize normalization of regional perfusion defects. Such normalization appears to equal or exceed that seen on 24-hr imaging and has been said to be the equal of PET metabolic evaluation of viability (*262*) (see Self-Study Program III, *Nuclear Medicine: Cardiology, Topic 3: Cardiac PET Imaging*). The method appears to augment regional radioactivity in segments that previously appeared not to redistribute. It does so either by a specific preferential increase to the deficient region or by generally increasing

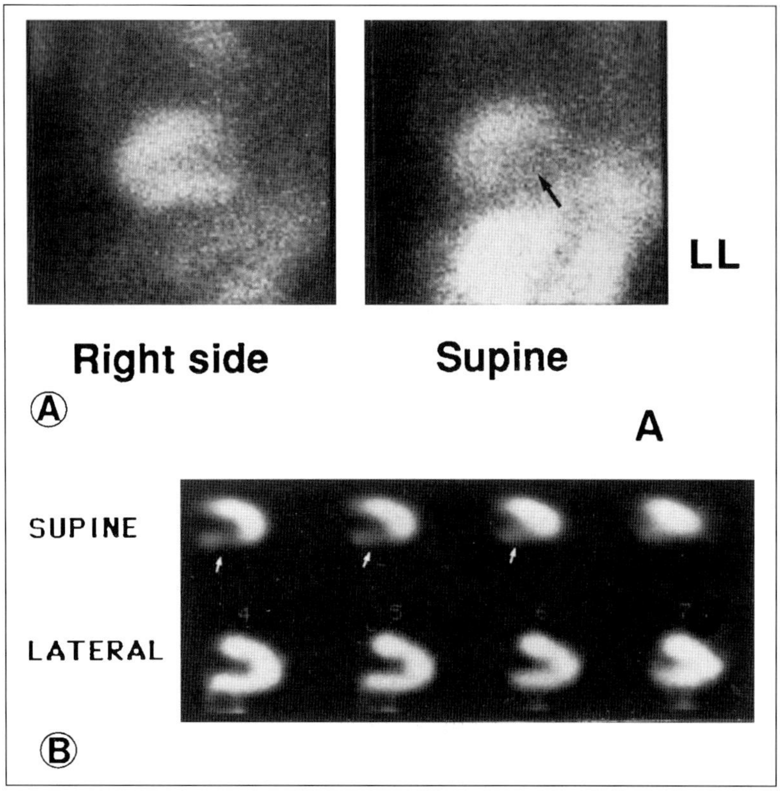

Figure 45 Overcoming diaphragmatic attenuation in planar/SPECT images. Shown in (A) are left lateral (LL) planar thallium-201 (^{201}Tl) images with the patient supine (right) and on his/her right side (left). The image acquired with the patient in the right decubitus position is normal, whereas the image in the supine position shows attenuation of the inferior wall (arrow) by the left hemidiaphragm. Shown in (B) are vertical long-axis ^{201}Tl SPECT images in a patient with a low likelihood of coronary artery disease and with normal planar images. SPECT images acquired in the supine position (above) suggest an inferior wall perfusion defect (arrow), whereas those associated with acquisition in a right lateral decubitus acquisition (below) are normal! The false-positive inferior wall defect was caused by attenuation by the left hemidiaphragm. Without attention to detail, the specificity of SPECT imaging will be reduced. More stable than right lateral is prone positioning. (Reprinted with permission from Wackers FJTh. Artifacts in planar and SPECT myocardial perfusion imaging. *Am J Cardiol Imaging* 1992;6:42–58.)

regional radioactivity in equal increments to all viable segments and thus reducing relative regional differences to produce the visual appearance of "redistribution" (Figs. 46,47). Many clinicians "reinject" all patients; others reinject those with defects after stress. Alternatively, an abbreviated planar image set at 4 hr will help identify those with persistent defects to target for reinjection. A variety of possible reinjection protocols have been developed (*264*), including poststress imaging followed immediately by imaging postreinjection. The optimal yield of redistributed or normalized segments after reinjection will occur with reinjection and imaging late (after ~4 hr) and not immediately after stress. Generally, a period of redistribution before reinjection imaging is additive and beneficial.

The simple reinjection of an additional 1–1.5 mCi ^{201}Tl would add to the regional distribution according to the then current distribution of myocardial perfusion, improving but not necessarily eliminating defects no longer based in perfusion abnormalities. However, regions with continued, ongoing ischemia at the time of reinjection would continue to reveal defects resulting from persistent underperfusion and could even be enhanced by this added reinjection dose, overcoming the effects of temporal redistribution (*265–267*). The postreinjection image could then bring back to visibility the ^{201}Tl defects that had resolved over time. For this reason, the immediate imaging of the postreinjection dose, if given after 4 hr and in the presence of a spontaneously reversible defect related to a chronically ischemic segment, may cause the defect to recur. Such "differential uptake" or "apparent washout" may cause image misinterpretation. If imaging is performed only after stress and after reinjection, such defects may appear fixed, although they may be seen to redistribute on imaging after 4 hr. It is thought that 5%–25% of segments that redistribute after 4 hr become abnormal again with reinjection (*267*), when such defects could recur. However, this frequency probably relates to the incidence of resting ischemia in the study population (Fig. 48). Because reappearance of defects after reinjection suggests the presence of ongoing ischemia, if there is a question about the nature of defects after reinjection, then 24-hr imaging can be performed with reclamation and redistribution of these same defects in

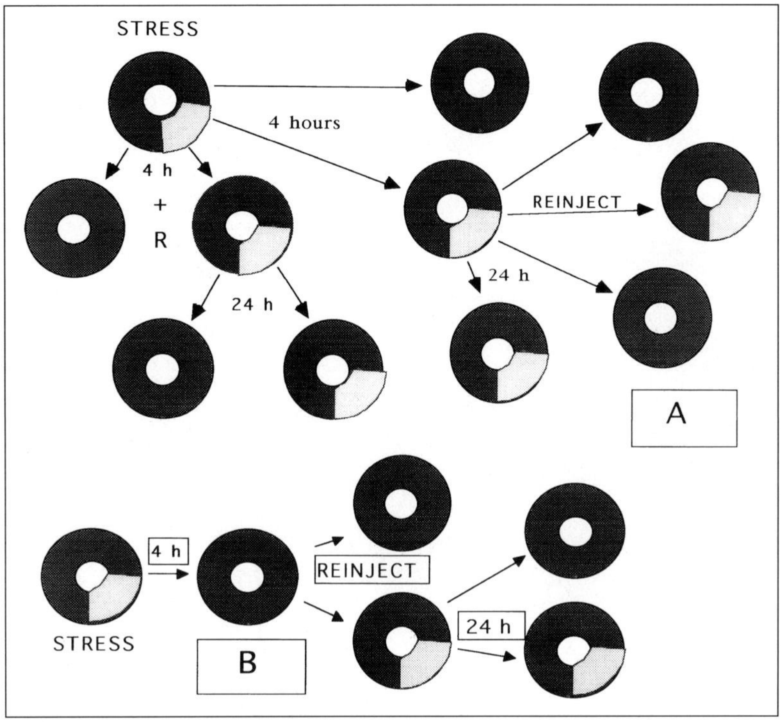

Figure 46 Redistribution and reinjection. (A) Shown diagrammatically are the possible image outcomes when delayed imaging is performed at 4 or 24 hr and the reinjection technique (R) is applied before (left) or after (right) acquisition of the 4-hr delayed thallium-201 image in the setting of an abnormal stress image. When reinjection is performed before 4-hr imaging, a 24-hr image may yet resolve apparently persistent defects. Similarly, reinjection or 24-hr imaging may resolve stress-related defects evident at 4 hr. (B) In this possible scenario, reinjection may actually restore a defect to an image that normalized after 4 hr. Here, the potential value of 24-hr imaging after reinjection is evident. The mechanism, described in the text, may explain some cases, like those shown in (A), of persistently abnormal images acquired after reinjection, after 4-hr poststress imaging.

roughly the same percentage (*268*) (Fig. 46). Although the performance of SPECT acquisition after stress, after 4 hr and again at 4 hr, after reinjection, would resolve this potential problem and was the protocol originally applied in the pivotal study by Bonow et al. (*265*), this requires 3 SPECT studies in a single day. Alternatively, imaging at 24 hr will again permit redistribution and regain identification of the viable segment. Although 24-hr imaging is rarely required after a reinjection dose, it occasionally results in normalization of a segment that appeared fixed after reinjection. Because the immediate postinjection ^{201}Tl image is a map of perfusion and because delayed imaging is an image of intracellular space, permitting access to viable yet underperfused cells, the 2 may differ in the setting of resting ischemia or hibernating myocardium. This rest–redistribution ^{201}Tl protocol may be an excellent alternative for identifying such viable myocardium (Fig. 49) (Table 7).

It has been suggested that thallium localization in viable myocardium may be aided by the concomitant infusion of glucose and the administration of insulin (*269*). Others have reported that washout analysis of a standard stress–redistribution study appears to be as accurate as the reinjection methods for viability evaluation and does not require a postreinjection image (*270*). Of course, the added reinjection dose removes the ability to assess washout and, if one were intent on performing reinjection analysis, washout analysis would require the acquisition of a prereinjection delayed image.

Technetium-99m Sestamibi and Tetrofosmin Protocols

Because current ^{99m}Tc-based agents do not redistribute significantly, their use in imaging perfusion to evaluate ischemia requires 2 injections, 1 at peak stress and 1 at rest. There is no demonstrated kinetic basis for delayed imaging beyond that required for optimal sestamibi or tetrofosmin cardiac visualization (Fig. 34). This time-dependent image normalization is a principle theoretical difference between ^{201}Tl and ^{99m}Tc sestamibi or tetrofosmin. It is such redistribution that appears to maximize the ability of ^{201}Tl to identify viable myocardium. Without this characteristic, viability evaluation for perfusion images simply relates to the

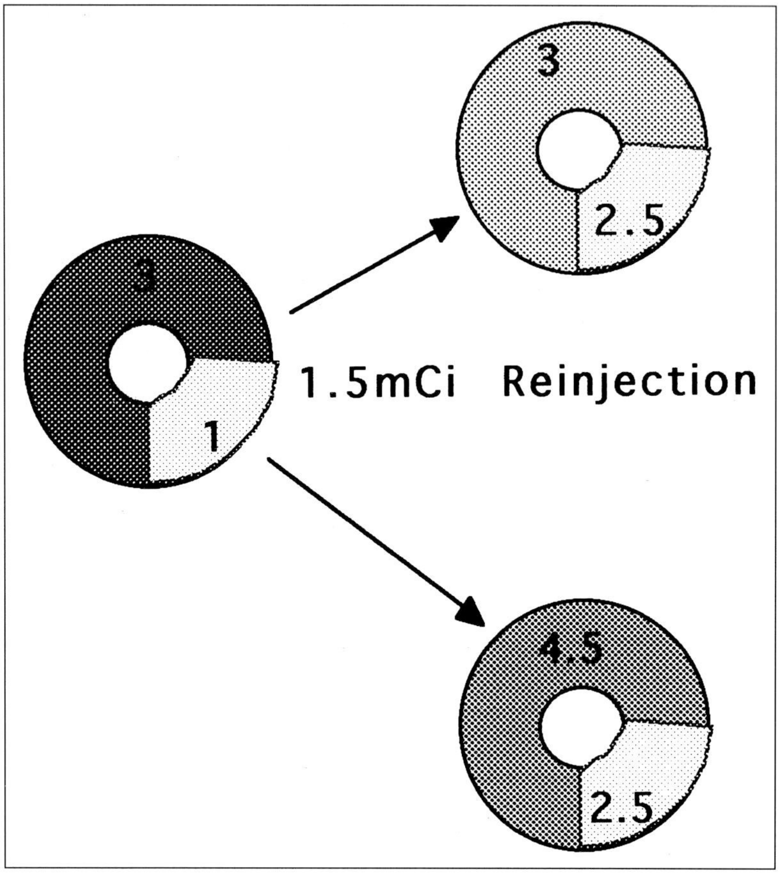

Figure 47 Mechanism of reinjection. Shown diagrammatically are 2 possible mechanisms of image improvement with thallium-201 reinjection. Either the added radionuclide localizes totally in the abnormal region (above), or, more likely, it adds equally to normal and abnormal regions (below). In either case, image homogeneity improves, and the image seems to normalize or "redistribute."

relative regional perfusion of viable cells. The viability assessment capability of ^{99m}Tc-based perfusion agents would appear to rest on this fact. Although relative regional perfusion also appears to be of importance for viability evaluation (*266*), the redistribution capability of ^{201}Tl suggests its possible superiority for this purpose. Although transmembrane ^{201}Tl transport is active and requires energy, that of sestamibi (and tetrofosmin) also requires viable membranes and intracellular elements for localization. The localization of each agent appears to relate to both perfusion and viability. However, does sestamibi and tetrofosmin distribution underestimate the extent of viable myocardium? Some studies suggest an actual difference in regional localization of ^{99m}Tc sestamibi and ^{201}Tl (*151,160,264*). Although the 2 agents appear to mark well the region of anatomic infarction, some studies on ischemic models or in patients show the sestamibi defects to vary, sometimes appearing smaller than those of ^{201}Tl, which seems to conform better to the area of ischemia. This difference may further jeopardize viability evaluation with sestamibi. Yet, surprisingly, some studies seem to support the ability of sestamibi to identify viable myocardium (*158,271*), noting that the initial localization of the agent parallels the delayed distribution of ^{201}Tl! Tetrofosmin has not been studied thoroughly but appears to share many of the characteristics of sestamibi. Technical factors would suggest that similar defects might be seen better with imaging the high-dose ^{99m}Tc 140-keV photon, which would display better contrast resolution.

After injection, the distribution of ^{99m}Tc sestamibi and tetrofosmin, like that of ^{201}Tl, has been reported to parallel regional myocardial blood flow (*110–124,134–136*). Like other agents, ^{99m}Tc appears to underestimate flow at high rates (*128,130–132*). In low flow areas, myocardial uptake of sestamibi is relatively greater than expected, compared with microsphere-determined flow in normal flow areas. This is the result of increased extraction at low flow rates, as is typical for diffusible and transported tracers, including ^{201}Tl (*136*). Sestamibi defect size correlates well with pathologic infarct size produced after 2-hr coronary occlusion in dogs, by both planar ($r = 0.85$) and SPECT ($r = 0.95$) methods (*272*) and is able to assess well the effects of thrombolytic therapy in humans (*273*). Evidence of increased extraction is not seen when flow is reduced and sustained at levels <10% of normal because of loss of viability. As with ^{201}Tl, evidence of increased ^{99m}Tc sestamibi extraction in low flow areas relates to viability (*179,274*). However, compared with ^{201}Tl, clearance is reduced and delayed redistribution is negligible (*129*). Although this is potentially disadvantageous for the assessment of myocardial viability with sestamibi, after 3 hr of coronary occlusion sestamibi defect size correlated well ($r = 0.94$) with the autoradiographic risk area in dogs (*159*). Moreover, the distribution of a second injection made 90 min after reperfusion (again, after 3 hr of occlusion) correlated well with postrevascularization infarct size ($r = 0.98$)! This again suggests that, after acute infarction, sestamibi distribution reflects both viable myocardium and regional perfusion, correlates with the area at ischemic risk after occlusion and identifies the area salvaged after reperfusion. This supports its use in assessing the results of thrombolytic therapy and other revascularization procedures applied in the acute postinfarction period (*275,276*). The application of sestamibi to viability evaluation may be enhanced with nitrate administration (*277–279*) or, reportedly, with quantitation of its minimal redistribution (*280,281*).

Because ^{99m}Tc-sestamibi and tetrofosmin require 2 separate injections, 1 at peak stress and the other at rest, 3 protocols may be followed. Rest and stress studies may be performed at least 24 hr apart to allow adequate decay of myocardial ^{99m}Tc sestamibi activity from the first to the second study. This 2-day protocol is not optimal for a rapid clinical response. However, as in ^{201}Tl studies, if the initial ^{99m}Tc study is performed with stress and found to be clearly normal, the study may be completed quickly, without rest evaluation. DePuey et al. (*282*) have demonstrated the efficacy of fast sestamibi acquisitions for the separate-day protocol using multihead detectors. Investigation has confirmed that a normal stress study rarely needs a rest study in patients without prior infarction, revascularization or ventricular dysfunction (*283*), but this stress-only protocol should be studied further.

Alternatively, the studies may be performed on the same day, with the rest study acquired first by injecting a low dose (7 mCi) of ^{99m}Tc sestamibi, followed 2–4 hr later by a higher dose (22 mCi) of the agent injected during stress (*179*). With this protocol, the ratio of exercise-related myocardial ^{99m}Tc sestamibi and the radioactivity from the previous rest injection is >5:1. This protocol is preferred to a 1-day stress-first protocol, which can result in an increased number of non-normalizing yet fully "reversible" ischemic segments on late rest imaging, with overestimation of fixed defects (*179*). This probably relates to the effects of the remnant heterogeneous stress-related agent lying in the background of the rest study. In any case, even the same-day protocol takes 3–5 hr and presents logistical difficulties, especially for in-patients. Alternatively, stress testing may be performed and imaged early after rest imaging, with some likely sacrifice in sensitivity. Again, stress-first imaging can still be employed in relatively low-likelihood patients as a 2-day protocol, with rest imaging performed only if the initial study is abnormal. Technetium-99m sestamibi studies are rarely performed as planar images, in which the higher energy of ^{99m}Tc permits transmission of deep myocardial radioactivity and

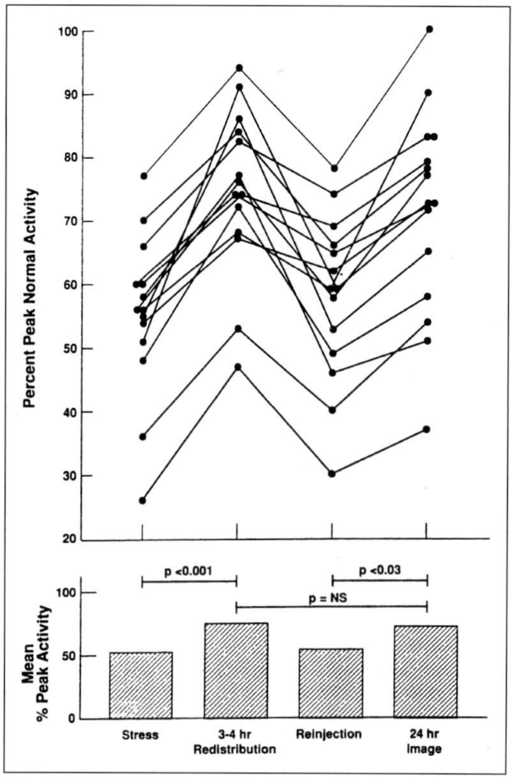

Figure 48 Reinjection compared with redistribution. Shown at left is the relative regional thallium-201 (^{201}Tl) activity (percentage of peak normal activity) in myocardial regions showing a persistent reduction in ^{201}Tl activity after stress study. The defect improves over time (redistribution) but worsens again after reinjection, which reinforces any persistence of resting underperfusion. On images acquired 24 hr after reinjection, redistribution is again apparent. If 3- to 4-hr redistribution images were not performed and only reinjection images were acquired at 4 hr, perfusion in these regions would be incorrectly determined to be fixed. However, the reversibility of the defect would be captured at 24-hr imaging. An unpalatable alternative is to perform both redistribution and reinjection imaging in the same sitting. The bottom panel represents the mean activity at the time of each imaging study. (Reprinted with permission from Dilsizian V, Bonow RO. Differential uptake and apparent Tl-201 washout after thallium reinjection. Options regarding early redistribution imaging before reinjection or late redistribution imaging after reinjection. *Circulation* 1992;85:1032–1038.)

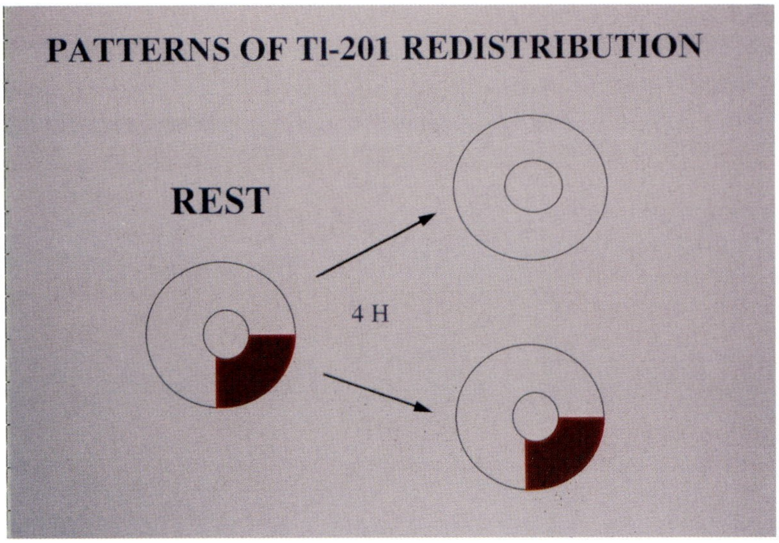

Figure 49 Rest-redistribution. Shown are patterns of perfusion with delayed imaging following the acquisition of an abnormal rest image. The immediate postinjection thallium-201 (^{201}Tl) image is a map of perfusion, whereas the pattern of uptake on delayed imaging is an image of intracellular space. Although generally identical, the 2 may differ in the setting of resting ischemia. Hibernating myocardium and the delayed normalization of a rest defect permit identification of viable yet underperfused cells. A rest-redistribution ^{201}Tl protocol may be an excellent alternative for identifying such viable myocardium.

Table 7
DELAYED 4- AND 24-HR IMAGES

Are not the same as, but are complementary to, rest or postreinjection images, whether performed at 4 or 24 hr

may obscure defects in walls located more superficially. Yet, diagnostic accuracy, here, too, appears to be maintained (*284*) in instances in which planar studies are applied in very obese or uncooperative patients.

Advantages of the Technetium-99m Sestamibi/Tetrofosmin Protocols. The 2-day protocol may be impractical if a rapid clinical response time is required but permits stress-first imaging without diagnostic loss. Here, both stress and rest studies can get a maximal dose, permitting gating, and late rest study need not be performed if the initial stress study is normal.

A rest image acquired after an abnormal stress image may still reveal apparent radiotracer heterogeneity deriving from the background distribution of the earlier stress image. A 1-day protocol should be employed with rest first to avoid overestimating infarction (*285,286*). Also, because a lower dose is injected with the first of the 1-day imaging studies, rest-first imaging employs the high dose for the more informative stress study. The results of this 1-day protocol agree well with results of the 2-day protocol and with conventional ^{201}Tl protocols (*285*).

Dual-Isotope Protocols

A dual-radionuclide sequential-acquisition imaging protocol combines the 2 agents in an efficient and accurate method, which involves imaging ^{201}Tl at rest, followed immediately by imaging with ^{99m}Tc sestamibi (or tetrofosmin) at stress (see Self-Study Program III. *Nuclear Medicine: Cardiology, Topic 6: Myocardial Perfusion Scintigraphy—Clinical Aspects*) (*286,287*) (Fig. 50). This is generally performed with SPECT technique. Although imaging with 2 different perfusion agents presents problems because of different energies, kinetics and possibly localizing characteristics, the method is efficient and has been shown to give reliable diagnostic results in a little more than 90 min (*4,287*) and somewhat longer in busy or less efficient labs. The dual-isotope study is made possible by modern cameras, which permit excellent energy resolution. When stress ^{99m}Tc sestamibi imaging is performed, there is little downscatter from the low-abundance, high-energy ^{201}Tl window. The differing physical and imaging characteristics of the radionuclides may present a minor difference in apparent left ventricular size on ^{201}Tl and sestamibi images, not to be confused with pathologic cavitary dilation (*98,287– 289*).

Advantages of the Dual-Isotope Protocol. The sequential, dual-isotope ^{201}Tl rest/^{99m}Tc sestamibi or tetrofosmin stress protocols employ the physical

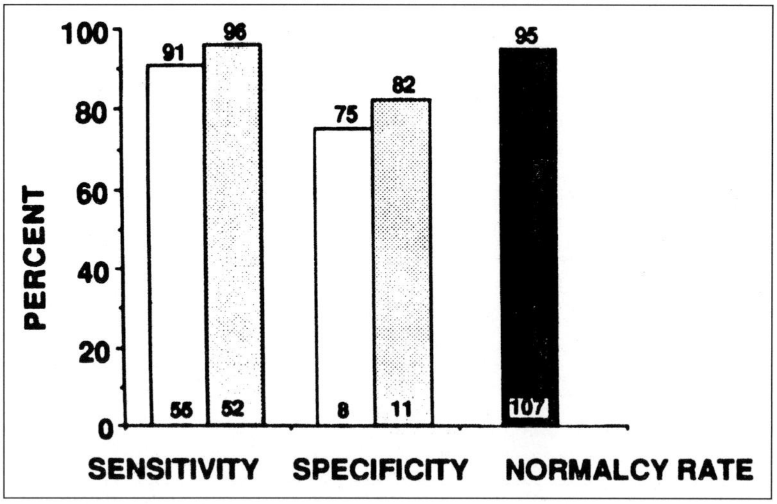

Figure 50 Accuracy of the dual-isotope protocol. Shown is the sensitivity, specificity and normalcy rate for the dual-isotope thallium-201 rest/technetium-99m sestamibi stress SPECT protocol, which considers as significant stenosis of 50% (open bars) or 70% (gray bars). (Reprinted with permission from Berman DS, Kiat H, Friedman JD, et al. Separate acquisition rest thallium-201/stress technetium-99m sestamibi dual isotope myocardial perfusion SPECT. A clinical validation study. *J Am Coll Cardiol* 1993;22:1455–1464.)

radionuclide differences to advantage. Although the 2 radionuclides have imaging differences, image acquisition parameters minimize these differences and permit efficient completion of the full rest–stress protocol. If sestamibi is fabricated from a single vial, the method cost equals that of a 2-injection sestamibi protocol, when performing >5 studies daily. Slightly more expensive than a straight ^{201}Tl protocol, the dual-isotope protocol provides other advantages, including increased throughput and rapid completion and reporting. Technologists love it (the editor reports from personal experience). However, it should not replace a stress-only protocol in patients who have relatively low likelihood of disease. Preserving the potential use of ^{201}Tl for viability evaluation, a full ^{201}Tl protocol may be preferred when viability is the primary test indication. A 24-hr image in the ^{201}Tl window will permit full ^{201}Tl viability evaluation with the dual-isotope protocol. The dual-radionuclide protocol provides the improved imaging capabilities of sestamibi or tetrofosmin imaging with stress and its increased data density for function analysis. Its high energy is especially valuable in patients who are large.

Because of the kinetics of sestamibi and tetrofosmin localization, this (like other ^{99m}Tc-based protocols) may not be optimal when viability determination is the primary test indication. However, when applying the dual-isotope method, delayed 24-hr ^{201}Tl imaging in its low-energy window provides a rest–redistribution ^{201}Tl image set when ^{99m}Tc is decayed, potentially permitting optimal viability evaluation. After 24 hr, downscatter from the higher ^{99m}Tc energy accounts for <7% of counts in the low-energy ^{201}Tl window (*286*). Inpatients may be injected with ^{201}Tl the night before the study (preinjected), providing a delayed ^{201}Tl image at the onset of the study.

A further potential advantage of the dual-isotope protocol relates to the possible assessment of the differential attenuation of the 2 radionuclides in the same myocardial region (Fig. 51). This may determine whether a relatively subtle "defect" seen with stress is, in fact, perfusion or attenuation related (*290*) (Fig. 52). If the defect appeared more severe on the rest ^{201}Tl than the stress ^{99m}Tc study, attenuation artifact may be the most likely cause. Although this differential attenuation may require a specific ^{99m}Tc perfusion-related defect to be more impressive and so potentially reduce diagnostic sensitivity, it will also reduce the likelihood of false-positive results, the most frequent problem in image interpretation. In addition, the improved contrast resolution of ^{99m}Tc images (*4,131,284, 290–295*) would be expected to counter the effects of attenuation, making defects appear more prominent on the poststress image and resulting in a possible overestimation of ischemia. Because of the improved

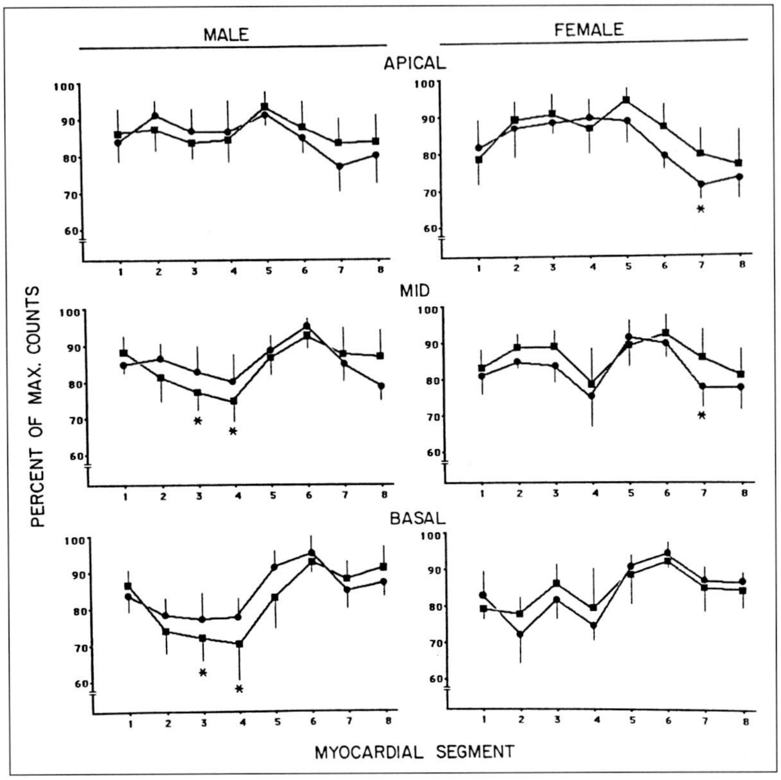

Figure 51 Circumferential profiles of differential attenuation. Shown are plots of circumferential thallium-201 (^{201}Tl) (square) and technetium-99m (^{99m}Tc) sestamibi (circle) activity for males and females. The curves represent the mean values from the 3 short-axis sections in normal subjects. Vertical lines represent 1 standard deviation. Note the significant reduction (*) in relative ^{201}Tl activity in the inferior wall segments in men, as a result of diaphragmatic attenuation, and in anterior wall segments in women, as a result of breast attenuation. This is a result of the greater attenuation of the lower energy of ^{201}Tl compared with that of ^{99m}Tc. (Reprinted with permission from Kahn JK, McGhie I, Akers MS, et al. Quantitative rotational tomography with Tl-201 and Tc-99m methoxy-isobutyl-isonitrile: a direct comparison in normal individuals and patients with coronary artery disease. *Circulation* 1989;79:1282–1293.)

resolution of the ^{99m}Tc-based study, a normal study may demonstrate normal image heterogeneity with greater prominence. The normal apical slit, related to normal apical thinning, may be seen better on the stress ^{99m}Tc than on the rest ^{201}Tl image and should not be confused with a reversible perfusion defect.

Reports indicate that diagnostic accuracy appears to be maintained well, compared with more established imaging protocols (*286,287,292*), and dual-isotope image sets show no diagnostically significant image differences in defect reversibility compared with full rest and stress sestamibi sets performed in the same patients (*286*). This dual-isotope procotol is most cost effective for high-volume laboratories with high incidences of abnormal studies. The protocol continues to evolve.

Simultaneous acquisition of such a dual-isotope protocol would confine acquisition of rest and stress studies to a single sitting (*293–295*)! Early reports on the development of a simultaneous dual-isotope ^{201}Tl rest/^{99m}Tc stress protocol are promising. If the photons of the 2 agents can be well separated, the protocol acquisition time will be halved and the throughput will double, with a 2-fold increase in cost effectiveness (*293–297*). Simultaneous acquisition of dual ^{99m}Tc sestamibi or tetrofosmin and fluorine-18 fluorodeoxyglucose (FDG) are other attractive protocols to gain perfusion and metabolism information in a single study (*298*).

The varied protocols should not add to the confusion over techniques. Instead, they represent an asset to MPS and will likely proliferate. Although the uniformity demanded in laboratory operations does not always permit such variation, specific protocols can be chosen for individual patient characteristics and test indications (Table 8). All protocols may be applied effectively with all conventional stress interventions.

Gating

High count rates available with imaging high-dose ^{99m}Tc perfusion agents also allow acquisition of high-quality gated studies. This permits the simultaneous assessment of regional myocardial perfusion and wall thickening (*207–211*), as well as left ventricular contraction pattern and LVEF (*212*). The Emory Toolbox software package also utilizes an epicardial edge to calculate left ventricular mass. The evaluation of systolic wall function on a gated study has added to the ability of the method to assess regional viability (*224*). Some authors suggest that scrutiny of systolic function on an abnormal initial poststress ^{201}Tl image could predict delayed defect reversibility and permit condensation of the entire evaluation to a single image acquisition, with only a gated stress perfusion and function evaluation (*224*). Beyond this, gated function often permits the objective identification of the cause of reduced regional radioactivity in attenuation artifact or areas of physiologic thinning (*236, 299*). Such function evaluation potentially would be available to both the ^{99m}Tc stress and ^{201}Tl rest aspects of the dual protocol. Evaluation of concomitant function with perfusion has already demonstrated added diagnostic and prognostic value, as has evidence of extracardiac localization (*236,300,301*).

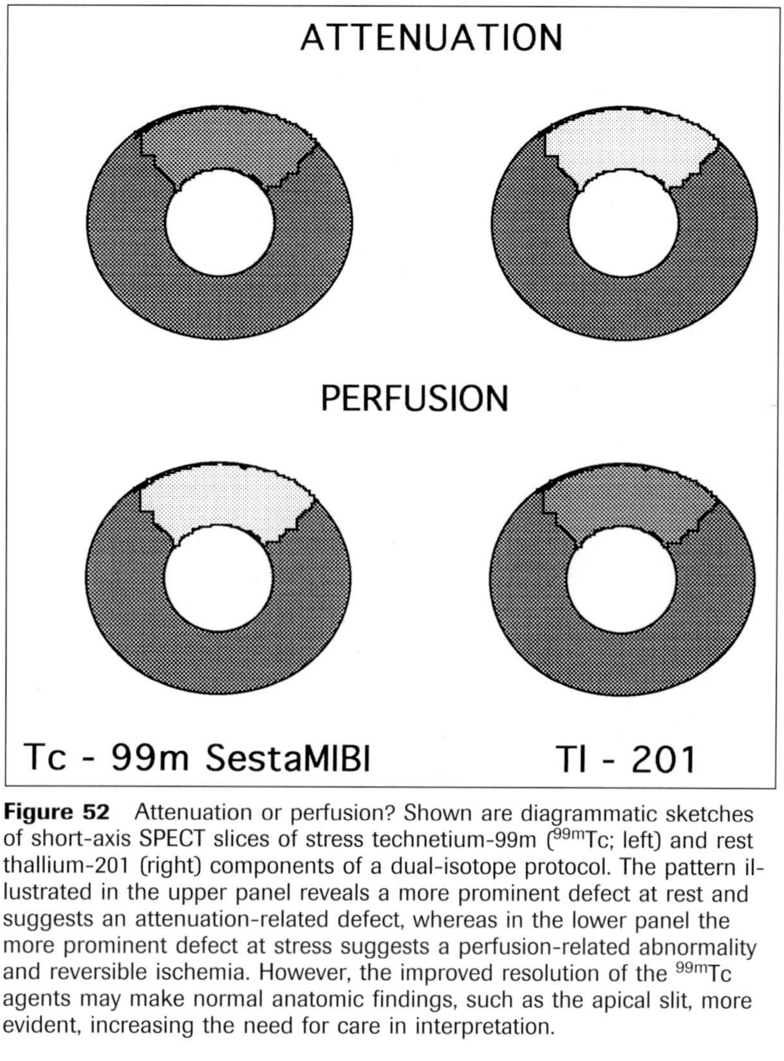

Figure 52 Attenuation or perfusion? Shown are diagrammatic sketches of short-axis SPECT slices of stress technetium-99m (^{99m}Tc; left) and rest thallium-201 (right) components of a dual-isotope protocol. The pattern illustrated in the upper panel reveals a more prominent defect at rest and suggests an attenuation-related defect, whereas in the lower panel the more prominent defect at stress suggests a perfusion-related abnormality and reversible ischemia. However, the improved resolution of the ^{99m}Tc agents may make normal anatomic findings, such as the apical slit, more evident, increasing the need for care in interpretation.

Care must be taken in the evaluation of images from gated studies. Gated planar images may be misleading, because these studies do not actually image the left ventricular cavity but the varying relative intensity of the overlying walls. No evidence suggests that diastolic, systolic or intermediate frames of the gated study provide more accurate image data than the ungated study itself. It is the "collapsed" ungated data derived from the gated study that are generally evaluated. Therefore, errors in gating that result in varying count and intensity levels in random projection images will lead to varying abnormalities in the processed SPECT images. Because SPECT images also derive from a larger planar set, SPECT assessment of the cavity, its size, intensity and even motion must also be incomplete and affected by factors similar to those for planar imaging (see Self Study Program III, *Nuclear Medicine: Cardiology, Topic 6: Myocardial Perfusion Scintigraphy—Clinical Aspects*).

IMAGE ACQUISITION

Planar Imaging

Camera and Collimator. For planar imaging, a standard or large-field-of-view camera with an all-purpose or high-resolution, parallel-hole collimator is employed. The preferred NaI crystal thickness is 1/4 or 3/8 in. The recommended energy windows for ^{201}Tl imaging are 20% centered on the 69–83-keV peak and 10% centered on the 167-keV peak. With ^{99m}Tc sestamibi or tetrofosmin, which

Table 8
A PRACTICAL COMPARISON OF ADVANTAGES AND DISADVANTAGES OF THE DIFFERENT IMAGING PROTOCOLS

Thallium-201 (^{201}Tl) stress–rest protocol
High half-life, low dose, low count density, not well gated, poor spatial resolution; low energy, greatest scatter, attenuation
Avoid application in large patients
Stress always first
Relatively inexpensive, because of single radionuclide dose
Probably optimal viability agent
Thallium-201 rest–redistribution protocol
Likely optimal and most cost-effective viability study
Technetium-99m (^{99m}Tc) sestamibi/tetrofosmin protocols
Employs agent with best imaging characteristics, highest resolution and least attenuation and that does not significantly redistribute, so image acquisition can be delayed if clinically necessary
Same-day: brings some degree of background to second acquisition
Two-day: Prolonged protocol but no interference from preceding dose
Dual-isotope ^{201}Tl rest/^{99m}Tc stress protocol
Brief with high throughput; each patient completed in 2 hr
Most cost effective in busy laboratories
Combines advantages of ^{99m}Tc with viability data from ^{201}Tl
24-hr ^{201}Tl imaging to maximize viability assessment
May "pre-inject" ^{201}Tl the night before study for viability evaluation
Difficulties in comparing ^{201}Tl and ^{99m}Tc images
Costly if performed in low-volume laboratories

has a higher count rate, a high-resolution collimator is preferable and a 20% symmetric window centered on the 140-keV peak is used. The recommended acquisition matrix for planar imaging is a 128 × 128, 8-bit matrix.

Timing. As conventionally performed, ^{201}Tl is imaged 10–15 min after administration, and ^{99m}Tc sestamibi is imaged 15–30 min after the exercise injection and 30–60 min after pharmacologic stress testing or with bowel clearance. Technetium-99m tetrofosmin has reduced hepatic clearance and can be imaged somewhat earlier in most cases, reportedly with reduced background interference.

Technical Developments. Because myocardial-to-background activity is maximum ~60 min after injection of ^{99m}Tc sestamibi (*179*), imaging initially was delayed for 1 hr. Recent practical experience, however, shows a frequent incidence of high background interference from excreted biliary activity in bowel loops at that remote time. For this reason and because of a theoretical temporal influence of limited ^{99m}Tc sestamibi redistribution, the delay to start of imaging may be reduced to 15–30 min for the postexercise study. The once compulsory ingestion of milk to clear the biliary tree has lost favor because of its tendency to fill the adjacent bowel and obscure or alter myocardial radioactivity. It may be apparent why such high background radioactivity would obscure underlying myocardial defects, most commonly corresponding to the inferior left ventricular wall. This may be the result of direct superimposition or the effects of scatter. The reason why such accumulation might create apparent SPECT defects in adjacent well-perfused myocardium is less clear. For this reason, dense myocardial defects adjacent to intense regions of background must be analyzed carefully.

SPECT Imaging

Camera and Collimator. Generally, for ^{201}Tl SPECT imaging, either a large-field-of-view camera, specially designed to rotate around the patient, or a specially designed dual-head cardiac SPECT camera with a more limited field of view is used. Special tables support imaging of heavy patients. Higher injected doses (3–4 mCi) of ^{201}Tl are recommended to achieve an adequate count rate. An all-purpose parallel-hole collimator is used for ^{201}Tl and a high-resolution collimator for ^{99m}Tc-based agents, with a 64 × 64, 16-bit matrix. Although some researchers initially preferred the 360° acquisition, artifacts were introduced when imaging through bony structures, little data were added when imaging from locations remote from the myocardium and studies have shown no loss in diagnostic information accuracy with the 180° acquisition (*302*). The most common SPECT protocol with a single-head camera employs 32 projections obtained over a semicircular 180° arc, from the 45° right anterior oblique (RAO) to the 45° left posterior oblique (LPO) projection, imaging for 40 sec/projection in the step-and-shoot mode. Alternatively, dual-head acquisition can utilize 64 20-sec projection images, 32 with each head, again over a 180° arc. Alternatively, rapid acquisition protocols may be performed with ^{99m}Tc-based agents, sacrificing plentiful counts to gain scarce time. Point sources may be placed above and below the heart to serve as guides to sense patient motion. Current commercial programs present the placement of horizontal lines adjacent to the myocardium for the same purpose.

Tomographic image acquisition should begin no earlier than 10–15 min after injection of ^{201}Tl to diminish the frequency of "upward creep" artifact (*303,304*). During the 10–15-min waiting period, a single 5-min anterior view and, optionally, 45° LAO planar images may be acquired. These planar images may be used to assess lung uptake of ^{201}Tl, as well as transient ischemic dilatation of the left ventricle and soft tissue attenuation, and also to serve as a guide for SPECT image abnormalities, helping in recognition of artifactual SPECT defects. Additional planar images optimally may follow after completion of SPECT imaging. With this protocol, an adequate sample of planar as well as SPECT images may be obtained in each patient. Planar images also are available from the projection image set. Although raw ^{201}Tl images are data poor, those of ^{99m}Tc may be adequate for use as the planar image guide to SPECT interpretation, and they add much more.

For the separate-acquisition, dual-isotope protocol, both the standard 3-mCi ^{201}Tl dose delivered at rest and the 25-mCi ^{99m}Tc dose delivered at peak stress are imaged with a high-resolution collimator. Both employ a conventional 180° circular orbit, with 32 or, preferably, 64 20-sec stops. For heavy patients, the dose may be tailored to 0.043 mCi/kg ^{201}Tl and 0.36 mCi/kg ^{99m}Tc agents. For ^{201}Tl, a 30% symmetric window is employed at the 68–80-keV photopeak and a 20% window at the 167-keV photopeak. Technetium-99m is imaged in a 15% window at the 140-keV photopeak.

Once acquired, images are processed and undergo visual qualitative and quantitative analysis.

IMAGE PROCESSING AND QUANTITATION

Planar Studies

Processing Software. The processing software for myocardial perfusion studies primarily directs SPECT reconstruction, although several of these techniques were first developed for planar perfusion images. SPECT reconstruction is the process of using the raw data of planar projection images, acquired at different angles, to create a 3-dimensional representation of the myocardium. The final "processing" step organizes the reconstructed images on the display screen. Processing changes the data values in the image, and display software does not. Processing and display software are so interdependent that they are frequently treated as a single unit (*305*).

Simple Image Processing and Image Enhancement. Several image processing methods predate SPECT by many years. They were developed for processing planar images but also can be included in SPECT processing (*306*).

Background Subtraction. This method is applied to separate left ventricular counts from superimposed extracardiac activity. Background counts originate from tissue near the heart. It is often assumed that the first effort in background subtraction measured the average pixel value from an area in the image adjacent to the heart and subtracted that value from every pixel in the image, with the assumption that background contributed from noncardiac tissue adjacent to the heart contributed equally to all parts of the myocardium. When the target-to-background ratio is poor, defects can be seen that would otherwise be hidden by the large contribution of noncardiac counts in the area of the myocardium. Early application of the method reported increased sensitivity of planar ^{201}Tl perfusion studies (*307*). However, the method also increases image heterogeneity from any cause and could reduce diagnostic specificity.

Background around the heart is heterogeneous, however, so the average sampled in 1 area is not a true measure of background for different regions of the myocardium. Interpolative background subtraction was developed to correct for this problem (*308*). A region is drawn around the periphery of the myocardium to generate a ring, square or rectangle of background pixels. A background value for each pixel inside the ring is calculated, based on the distance to and value of each peripheral pixel. Outer background pixels closer to the pixel analyzed are more heavily weighted and have more influence. This provides an approximate yet more accurate measure of background contribution to myocardial counts than that provided by a single global value. The subtraction grid is created in a known, contrived linear fashion based on values taken at the edge of the region of interest, but the cardiac background is clearly nonlinear. In addition, myocardial regions close to but not overlying a high sampled background region will suffer from excessive background subtraction with possible production of an artifactual defect. Koster et al. (*309*) reported that the interpolative background subtraction algorithm developed for ^{201}Tl images causes errors when used for ^{99m}Tc sestamibi, because the distribution of noncardiac activity differs greatly between the 2 radiopharmaceuticals. Excessive background subtraction is always a concern. In processed images lacking visible background, it is very difficult to discern whether defects are real or caused by background subtraction; and such images should be viewed with suspicion.

Smoothing. Smoothing is a type of image filtering and, like filtering, changes the data in an image (see Self Study Program III, *Nuclear Medicine: Cardiology, Topic 1: Physical and Technical Aspects of Nuclear Cardiology*). Myocardial images acquired using ^{201}Tl, with its low permissible dose, are comparatively noisy. This noise can be reduced by averaging adjacent pixels. An unweighted average is the mean of the central pixel and the 8 adjacent surrounding pixels in the matrix, whereas a weighted average alters the contribution of counts from nearby pixels as a function of their distance from the central pixel. For example, 4:2:1 smoothing multiplies the central pixel by 4, the 4 closest pixels touching it on a full side by 2, and the next 4 pixels touching only at the corners by 1. The sum of these factors is 16, so the sum of the 9 factored pixels is divided by the square root of 16 to get the value of the multiple of the smoothed central pixel. The weighting factors for different pixels can be changed, or contributing pixels can be expanded to include a larger area of nearby pixels.

Many other smoothing algorithms are common in general image processing but are rarely used in nuclear medicine. A median filter replaces the central pixel with the median, rather than the mean value of surrounding pixels. This is good for removing a few pixels with wildly aberrant values. Directional smoothing filters preserve sharp edges by smoothing only in the directions with no sharp changes in pixel values. This is not needed in cardiac image processing, because, with cardiac movement and low count density, unprocessed myocardial perfusion images have no sharp edges.

Image Interpolation. Interpolation is the same process, whether applied to graphs or images. The values of intermediate points can be estimated from the known values of nearby points. The methods of estimation vary. Image interpolation creates a larger matrix with smaller pixels. Each original pixel is divided into smaller pixels, and the counts are distributed into those pixels. The distribution methods vary and may or may not preserve the original counts. Simple methods use the linear or weighted average of the original adjacent pixels. More complicated methods may use spline fits of several pixels in multiple directions from the original pixel to determine the value of the resultant pixel.

Edge Enhancement. Edge enhancements include a variety of different methods to sharpen edges in images or establish regions of interest for further analysis. Edge enhancement can be applied to restore edges blurred during smoothing operations. They may also be used to set chamber boundaries to measure values related to volume in blood-pool or perfusion images or to quantitate perfusion image abnormalities and measure infarct size. Because myocardial perfusion images lack sharp edges, this process may be difficult. One way to enhance an edge is to increase the difference between nearby pixels only when that difference is larger than a given value in the raw image. Another way is to subtract a smoothed image from the raw image and then add this difference back to the raw image. Treating a line of pixels as a curve and determining the first or second derivative may create a boundary based on the spatial rate of count change, or a simple threshold value may be applied and subtracted from the image to establish an edge or boundary. Edges or boundaries must be differentiated from noise, which may be increased by edge enhancement processes themselves.

Image Contrast Transformation. The relative visual intensity of pixels in an image can be altered by changing the data values as described later in this section or by changing the display intensities as described later in the section on display software. The dynamic range of an image is the difference between the highest and lowest pixel values in that image. When the brightest pixels are so bright that lower-count pixels are difficult to see, some method of enhancing the low-count areas can be applied.

Logarithmic transformation is a common method and replaces each pixel value with the log of the original value. This reduces the high-count pixels by a much larger factor than the low-count pixels and makes the low-count pixels more visible. An almost identical method uses the square root instead of the logarithm. The opposite effect can be achieved by squaring each value or taking the exponential value of each pixel to minimize the visibility of low-count pixels and enhance higher-count pixels.

Histogram equalization is considerably more complicated. First, a histogram is created with the number of pixels (histogram Y axis) in the image for each pixel intensity value (histogram X axis). This histogram plots the distribution of gray levels in the image. The shape of the histogram is used to calculate a transformation factor for each pixel. The intent is to reduce the range of intensities allocated when only a few pixels fall into that value range and distribute the number of gray levels in proportion to the number of pixels with those counts. With an 8-bit screen depth, 256 levels of gray cover the dynamic range of the image. When the image has been histogram equalized, more gray levels are allocated to count levels that contain many pixels, providing finer discrimination among these intensity levels. Because noisy images are likely to have a few pixels that are much hotter or colder than most pixels in the image, this transformation will suppress noise and enhance the rest of the image. When the gall bladder is filled with ^{99m}Tc sestamibi, the rest of the image will gain in dynamic range for better differentiation of structures. This transformation is helpful only when there are many pixels with similar values in the area of interest, so that the number of gray levels is expanded for that organ.

Image reconstruction principles and methods, including backprojection, frequency filters and iterative reconstruction methods were considered in Self-Study Program III, *Nuclear Medicine: Cardiology, Topic 1: Physical and Technical Aspects of Nuclear Cardiology* and are discussed elsewhere in this volume.

Visual Image Analysis. In the anterior view, myocardial activity has a horseshoe pattern. As a result of normal apical thinning or other technical factors, radioactivity in the apex usually is less than that in the anterolateral and inferior regions. Furthermore, activity in the inferior wall is generally less than that in the anterolateral wall because of inferior wall attenuation by the overlying right ventricle or diaphragm. Depending on the cardiac orientation, the myocardial image in the 45° LAO projection may appear as a horseshoe in vertical hearts or as a complete doughnut in horizontal hearts. The steep LAO projection, like the anterior view, has a horseshoe pattern. In this view, however, the anteroseptum may have less activity than the inferior wall, because the right ventricle, chest musculature in men, or breast, most commonly in women, may overlie the anteroseptal wall. Alternatively, the inferior wall may be attenuated by the diaphragm, most commonly in obese men and may appear to have less radioactivity. One approach to visual analysis of segmental myocardial activity is to divide each view into 5 segments for a total of 15 segments/study and to score uptake in each segment by a scoring system in which 0 = normal uptake, 1 = equivocal or possibly reduced activity, 2 = mild (definite) reduction of activity, 3 = moderate reduction of activity clearly above background and 4 = severe reduction of activity to the point that myocardial uptake is equal to or slightly greater than the background activity. The same scoring system may be used for the 4- and 24-hr redistribution studies. A visual score of 2-4 in at least 1 segment of the stress images is required for that study to be considered abnormal, and reversibility usually requires improvement of ≥2 score grades. Depending on the differences between the stress and redistribution scores, different patterns of reversibility for each segment may be interpreted as follows: nonreversible = 3-3, 3-2, 2-2, 2-3; partially reversible = 4-2; reversible = 3-1, 3-0, 2-0; and reverse redistribution = 0-3, 1-3, 0-2, 1-2.

Because various myocardial regions are supplied by different coronary arteries, it is possible in studies of patients with single-vessel disease to infer the coronary artery that is responsible by assessing the distribution of a given myocardial perfusion defect (see Self-Study Program III, *Nuclear Medicine: Cardiology, Topic 6: Myocardial Perfusion Scintigraphy—Clinical Aspects*). This prediction, however, is associated with some error, because the size and distribution of coronary arteries, their branching pattern and the dominance between the left and right systems vary from patient to patient (Fig. 53). The anterior wall and apex in the anterior view are most commonly related to the left anterior descending coronary artery (LAD) distribution. In general, the anterolateral wall, seen best in LAO projections, is supplied by the diagonal branch of the LAD. In some instances, disease of a large marginal branch of the left circumflex coronary artery (LCX) may cause a perfusion defect in the distal anterolateral wall. This region between the lateral and septal walls may sometimes be perfused by a large ramus intermedius vessel. The latter, when present, originates between the LAD and LCX coronaries and usually subtends a lateral aspect of part of the LAD region. The inferior wall in the anterior view represents the portion that is closer to the septum and is usually supplied by the posterior descending branch (PDA) of the right coronary artery (RCA) with a right dominant system or the LCX coronary artery with a left dominant system. The interventricular septum in the 45° LAO projection is supplied by the LAD. It is of note that the more posterior portion of the interventricular septum represents the territory of the posterior descending branch, but this can be truly appreciated only with SPECT imaging. Depending on the orientation of the heart within the chest, the region termed the inferoapical area in the 45° LAO view may represent the true inferior wall in horizontal hearts or the apex in more vertical hearts. The coronary blood supply to this region, therefore, is variable. The posterolateral wall in the 45° LAO projection is supplied by the LCX. The anterior wall and the apex in the steep LAO projection are again supplied by the LAD. The inferior wall in the steep LAO projection represents a more lateral portion and usually is supplied by the PDA. The more basal portion of this wall may overlap somewhat the distribution of the LCX (*310*).

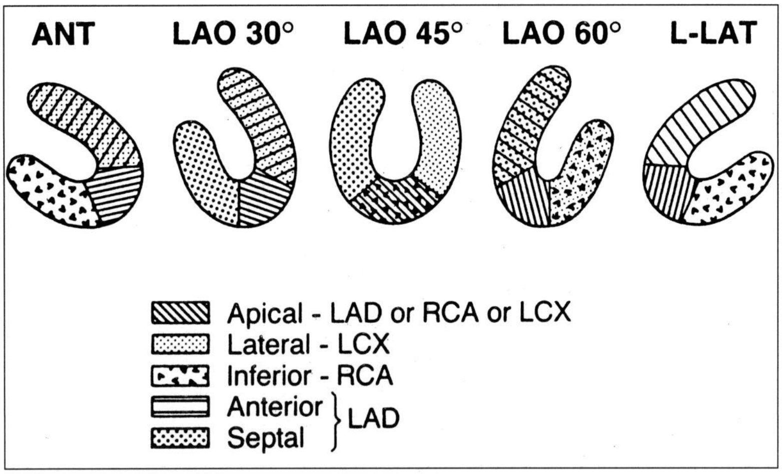

Figure 53 Coronary distribution. Shown is a diagram of the general anatomic distribution of coronary regions on the planar perfusion image. The distribution varies from subject to subject and is influenced by collateral vessels, cardiac rotation and other factors. Some regions may be perfused by a number of coronary arteries. (Reprinted with permission from Botvinick E, Dae M, O'Connell JW, Ortendahl D, Hattner RS. The scintigraphic evaluation of the cardiovascular system. In: Parmley WW, Chatterjee K, eds. *Cardiology.* Philadelphia, PA: JB Lippincott; 1991:1–121.)

Quantitative Image Analysis. Methods of perfusion image quantitation are reviewed in Table 9. The digital nature of nuclear cardiology data aids quantitation by permitting easy manipulation and analysis by computer, which can analyze some parameters, such as washout, that the eye cannot perceive. Perfusion images present a quantifiable continuum related to disease likelihood, prognosis and viability (*75*). Several approaches are used for the quantitation of the initial myocardial distribution and washout of ^{201}Tl, but, in general, similar steps are involved. Each image must be compensated for tissue crosstalk by performing background subtraction. The most commonly used method is the bilinear interpolative background subtraction, utilizing a rectangular boundary enclosing the heart, ~4 pixels away from the myocardium (*308*). The images are then smoothed, using a standard algorithm for 9-point weighted averaging. Several methods may be employed for myocardial sampling (*61,91,311*). Each permits quantitation of data, which is helpful in the scintigraphic method, provided that each planar and SPECT image is

Table 9
AN ANALYSIS OF METHODS OF PERFUSION IMAGE QUANTITATION

Operation	Method	Utilization
Sampling	Circumferential profile	
	Cylindrical	Standard
	Cylindrical and spherical	Optional
	Maximum count	Standard
	Average count	Optional
Normalization	Maximum count	Standard
	Average region	Optional
	Maximum count (%)	Optional
Analysis	Normal database	Standard
	Threshold	Optional
Variables	Extent	Standard
	Severity	Standard
	Reversibility	Standard
	Washout	Optional
	Transient dilation	Optional
	Lung washout	Optional
Display	Two-dimensional polar (bullseye) maps	Standard
	Circumferential profiles	Optional

*Adapted with permission from Garcia E, ed. Imaging guidelines for nuclear cardiology procedures. *J Nucl Cardiol* 1996;3:G3.

properly acquired and processed before such analysis (*299,312*). With the circumferential count profile method (*61,311*), the center of the left ventricle is assigned visually, and, from this center, 60 radii spaced in 60 arcs are generated through the myocardium. Along each radius, the maximum count per pixel is automatically determined and is intensity normalized to the maximum value observed in that projection. The profile is then constructed by the computer from the values of the 60 samples, which are plotted clockwise. The redistribution images are processed using the same approach.

The circumferential profiles then are aligned by visually identifying the location of the scintigraphic apex on the stress and redistribution profiles. The redistribution profiles are normalized to the maximum pixel value found on the stress images. In addition to initial and 4-hr redistribution circumferential count profiles, percent washout circumferential profiles are calculated as a percentage of washout from the initial to the 4-hr redistribution value (*96,97*). The results thus obtained are then compared with results generated from a normal database or images acquired in specific angulations when a specific myocardial contour is expected. Programs identify any points of the profile that fall below normal limits. These profiles are then interpreted with an anatomic and clinical reference. Alternatively, the planar images may be applied to the generation of functional color washout images (*288*) (Fig. 25). Of course, washout cannot be so assessed if reinjection has been performed first.

Sources of Error and Quality Control. Several potential sources of error warrant particular attention when undertaking planar imaging. Because orientation of the heart in the chest is variable from patient to patient, it is important that the appropriate imaging angles be determined in each individual patient for comparison with normal standards. For this purpose, a brief 2-min scout-view image is obtained in the 45° LAO view. The heart ideally should appear as a complete doughnut or an ellipse, with the counts-poor base located superiorly in this view. If the left ventricular myocardium does not form a doughnut or vertical eclipse, an adjustment should be made to the camera angle with respect to the patient's chest to secure a "best septal" image, in which perfusion is similar in septum and lateral wall. During redistribution imaging, angles identical to those of the initial images are used in a given patient. Such orientation and analysis of nonstandard projections is more important for quantitative analysis and comparison with a standard database that must be corrected for cardiac rotation. This angular method is problematic in the presence of an obvious septal or lateral wall defect. Alternatively, the "best septal" and other projections may be approximated, or images can be acquired in standard projections, interpreted with regard to angulation in a visual qualitative manner or submitted to circumferential profile analysis as the angle they most resemble. Similarly, specific angulation is not critical for washout calculation. Correct positioning of the region of interest for background subtraction is important. The right ventricular activity should be included within the background subtraction region, which should not cross the left ventricular myocardium or any "hot" extracardiac region, so as to avoid artifactual defects resulting from oversubtraction of myocardial activity.

For quantitative analysis and the generation of circumferential profiles, assignment of the center of the left ventricle must be accurate to avoid artifactual defects as a result of "fanning" of the radii. Care also should be taken to avoid a sampling error, by ensuring that the selected point of maximum radial counts corresponds to the myocardium. Proper alignment of the initial and delayed profiles requires careful attention to ventricular orientation and correct assignment of the apical region (Fig. 54). If the initial and delayed profiles are not aligned properly, the comparison of regional perfusion will be erroneous, as will conclusions about defect reversibility and washout.

SPECT Studies

General Considerations. The steps in SPECT processing are outlined in Table 10. Each of the 32 (or 64) projections is first corrected for nonuniformity with a 30×10^6-count flood field collected using a cobalt-57 (^{57}Co) source. The mechanical center of rotation (COR), determined from the projection images, is applied to align detector data with the reconstruction matrix. Raw ^{201}Tl data are

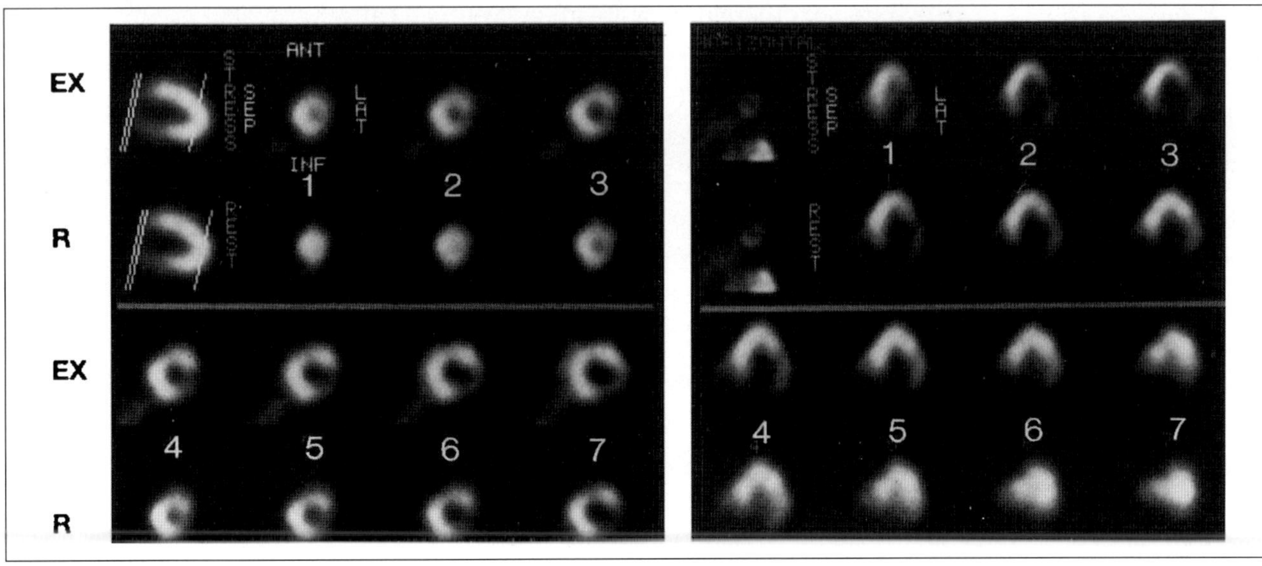

Figure 54 The importance of SPECT slice alignment. Apparent reversibility of defects caused by misalignment of slices in a patient with a fixed lateral defect. During processing, the short and horizontal long-axis slices were not lined up correctly. Stress short-axis slicc 1 corresponds to rest (R) slice 3. Exercise (EX) horizontal long-axis slice 3 corresponds to R slice 1. Because of erroneous selection of slices, these images could be interpreted as showing a reversible defect with cavitary dilation. (Reprinted with permission from Wackers FJTh. Artifacts in planar and SPECT myocardial perfusion imaging. *Am J Cardiol Imaging* 1992;6:42–58.)

Table 10
SPECT PROCESSING STEPS

	Process	Utilization
	Filtering	
Timing	Prereconstruction	Standard Mandatory
	With reconstruction	Optional
Types	Adaptive	Optional
	Conventional	Standard
	Reconstruction	
Transverse	Analytic (backprojection)	Standard
	Iterative	Optional
Oblique angle	Manual	Standard
	Automatic	Optional
	Display	
Cine review	Screen	Mandatory
Study review	Screen	Preferred
	Hard copy	Optional

*Adapted with permission from Garcia E, ed. Imaging guidelines for nuclear cardiology procedures. *J Nucl Cardiol* 1996;3:G3.

smoothed using a 9-point weighted averaging system. A Butterworth filter with a cutoff frequency of 0.2 cycles/pixel and order 5 (which has the highest efficiency) is used for filtering the images before reconstruction with the filtered backprojection technique (*313*). Different filters may be optimal with different camera–computer systems, protocols, radiopharmaceuticals, patient habitus and related data density (*13,314*) (Fig. 55). Three-dimensional axial data are reoriented in the short axis perpendicular to the long axis, as well as in vertical long-axis planes, whereas tomograms are reconstructed at 1 pixel/slice, representing a thickness of ~6.2 mm and displayed according to standard criteria (*315*). Generation of these slices involves the assignment of the long axis of the ventricle on midaxial and midvertical long-axis slices. No attenuation or scatter correction is used conventionally.

Gated images are acquired in ECG synchrony with 8–16 frames/cardiac cycle. Each projection image is acquired in gated mode to an equal number of cycles or to isotime. Although the 2 modes yield similar data with an absolutely regular cycle length, sinus arrhythmia or other limited rate irregularity can cause variability in counts per cycle, resulting in varying projection image intensities and potential image artifacts. Acquisition to isotime is preferred. In any case, marked gating irregularities should not be accepted and gating should not be performed if this is noted.

It should be noted that a gated ^{99m}Tc myocardial perfusion study, acquired with SPECT, usually is obtained within 30–60 min after injection of the agent at peak stress. For this reason, the findings usually represent regional myocardial perfusion at the time of exercise and regional myocardial function in the resting

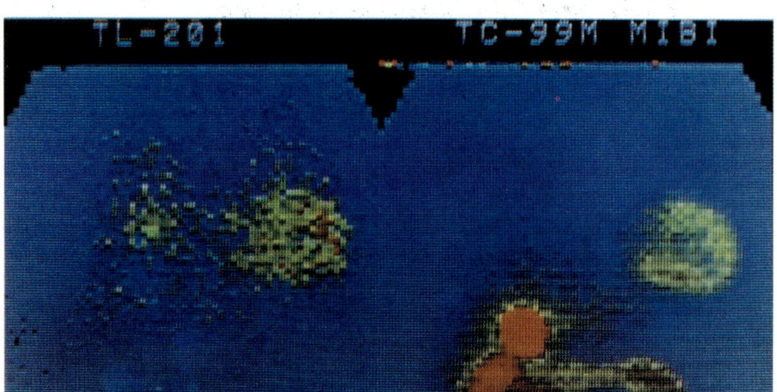

Figure 55 Planar projections, thallium-201 (^{201}Tl)/technetium-99m (^{99m}Tc). Representative planar projection images from tomographic acquisitions after exercise, with 3.0 mCi ^{201}Tl (left) and 30 mCi ^{99m}Tc sestamibi (right) in a patient with left anterior descending coronary artery disease. Image pixel counts have been normalized to equalize intensities. The ^{99m}Tc image has much greater data density and statistical reliability, permitting better edge detection for automated volume calculation, with low pulmonary and hepatic activity and high gallbladder and intestinal activity. A mild anterior defect is noted in the sestamibi image. (Reprinted with permission from Kahn JK, McGhie I, Akers MS, et al. Quantitative rotational tomography with Tl-201 and Tc-99m methoxy-isobutyl-isonitrile: a direct comparison in normal individuals and patients with coronary artery disease. *Circulation* 1989;79:1282–1293.)

state. Nevertheless, the presence of preserved wall motion in regions with reduced perfusion correlates with defect reversibility and is thus indicative of myocardial viability (*224,316*). If function evaluated with both gated rest and stress imaging demonstrates a decrement with stress, there is a strong possibility of stress-induced stunning. Perfusion in regions with significant wall-motion abnormalities indicates viability and stunned or, less likely, hibernating myocardium (*316,317*). A special, highly sensitive, multicrystal camera permits acquisition of first-pass blood-pool studies of the stress sestamibi dose. This permits a quantitative determination of the exercise left ventricular wall motion and LVEF, which may then be compared with stress regional perfusion and rest function. The method has been applied to the measurement of decremental function with balloon coronary occlusion (*318*), and limited studies suggest an added independent prognostic value of first-pass function evaluation performed with stress injection (*319,320*) (Fig. 56).

Quantitative Analysis of SPECT Perfusion Images: The Advantage of the Scintigraphic Method. One advantage of scintigraphic data is its digital nature, permitting amplification of the analysis and display of the data. Clinically relevant software for image acquisition, analysis and display has been developed and has added to the abilities and reliability of the scintigraphic method in portraying the coronary anatomy. This has added to the wide appeal of the technique. Early methods of graphic analysis were highly operator dependent and quite time consuming. However, the steps taken and outlined below are similar to those now performed in seconds with more automated equipment.

Visual Analysis. SPECT perfusion images may be analyzed with reference to the coronary anatomy (see Variants of Normal SPECT Analysis, p. 95) and present a quantifiable continuum related to disease likelihood, prognosis and viability (*75,321,322*) (Fig. 57). Scoring methods vary, but the summed segment score seems quite popular and easily automated (*14,322*). Similar to the evaluation of planar images, the SPECT slices can be analyzed on a segmental basis with 6 segments each from the basal, midventricular and apical short-axis slices. To avoid the partial volume effects related to the apex in the short axis, anterior and inferior apical segments are analyzed from the midventricular vertical long-axis slice. Each of these 20 segments is scored as for the planar segments listed, from 0–4, to gain quantitation of any defects. A possibly abnormal study has a score of 1–3, a mildly abnormal study has a score of 4–8, a moderately abnormal study has a score of 8–12 and a score ≥13 indicates a severely abnormal study. In current quantitative SPECT software, these scores are generated from an analysis of the segmental intensity and its standard deviation from that of the normal database.

To take full advantage of the graded quantitative image, the result must exclude artifacts. All defects scored must be analyzed to exclude artifacts. Readers must be obsessive in excluding artifacts (most often the result of motion and attenuation) with the numerous tools (polar maps, projection images, gated data) and methods (prone imaging) available to optimize diagnostic specificity without jeopardizing sensitivity (*236*). Of course, all such computer-derived methods are not themselves without potential artifacts (*323*).

Large patients, women (*237*), those with left bundle branch block (*324–326*), chronic obstructive pulmonary disease (*327*) and reduced left ventricular function (*328,329*) present special diagnostic challenges that can be successfully managed with proper choice of acquisition and interpretation methods, radiopharmaceuticals and stress methods (*95,312,330*). As with all forms of

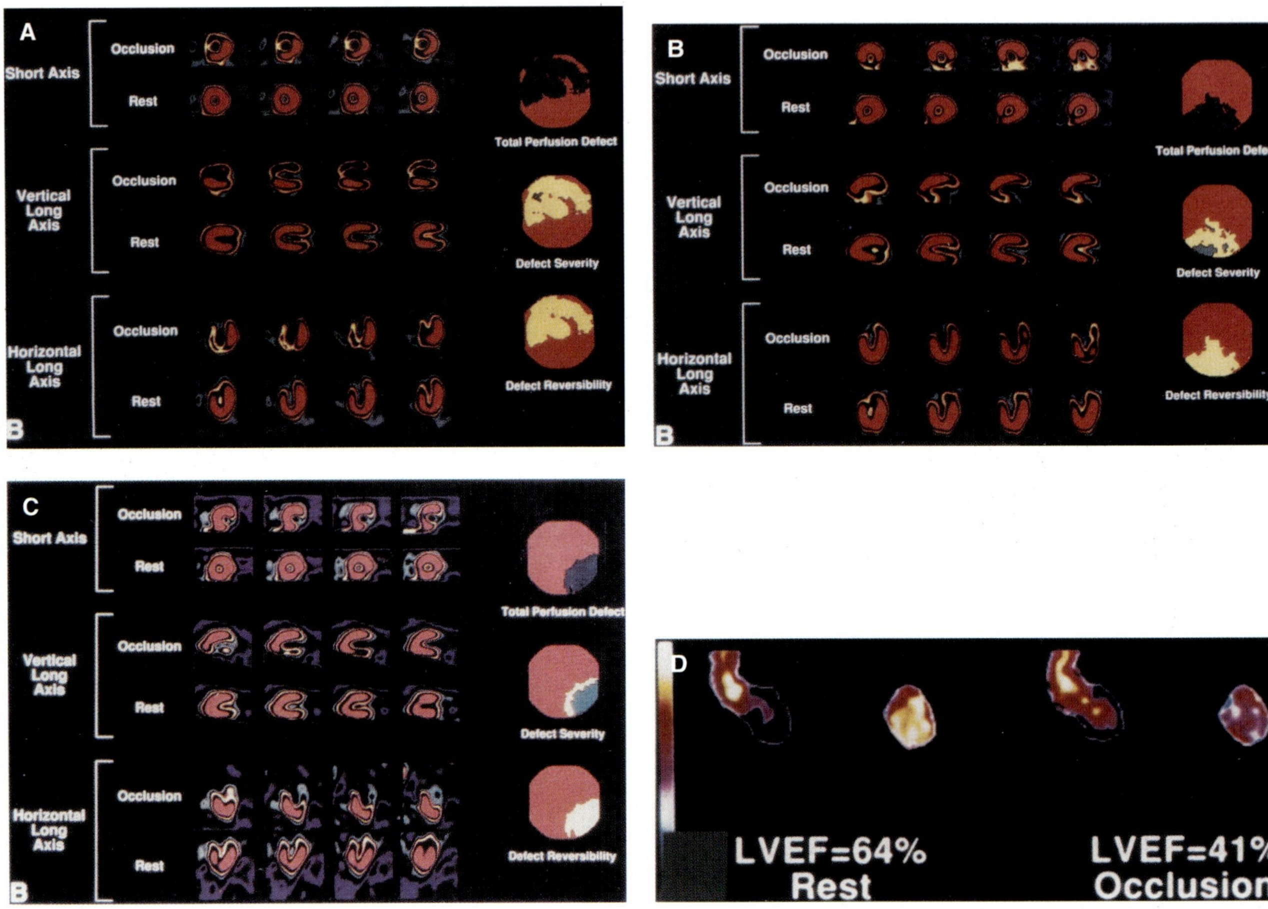

Figure 56 Effects of coronary occlusion evaluated by first-pass stress perfusion scintigraphy. The resultant perfusion defect is seen on SPECT perfusion imaging with clinically indicated angioplasty balloon occlusion of the (A) left anterior descending coronary artery (LAD), (B) the right coronary artery or (C) the left circumflex coronary artery in patients with single-vessel disease. The patterns of abnormality are typical for the involved vessel. Accompanying first-pass radioangiography performed with both rest and LAD occlusion demonstrated decremental function, as shown in (D). The functional abnormalities were resolved well by this sensitive method applied in the setting of absent perfusion. (Reprinted with permission from Gallik DM, Obermueller SD, Swarna US, et al. Simultaneous assessment of myocardial perfusion and left ventricular function during transient coronary occlusion. *J Am Coll Cardiol* 1995;25:1529–1538.)

stress testing, stress perfusion imaging may be problematic and is not generally recommended in asymptomatic patients who have a low risk of coronary disease (*330*).

Steps in SPECT Processing. All computer software uses the same sequence of SPECT reconstruction processing (Table 10). Transverse slices are created by filtered backprojection from the projection data, then the long and short axes of the heart are defined from the transverse slices and finally the images are arranged for interpretation. After the short-axis slices are created, they can be used to generate the polar map.

Axis Selection. The long axis of the heart is not parallel to the axis of the body, so the SPECT transverse slices of the heart do not lend themselves to easy identification or comparison of myocardial regions. The slices must be reoriented, in essence viewing the same 3-dimensional data set from a different angle, by rotating the heart to align the long axis of the left ventricle with 1 axis of the image-reconstruction, 3-dimensional coordinate system.

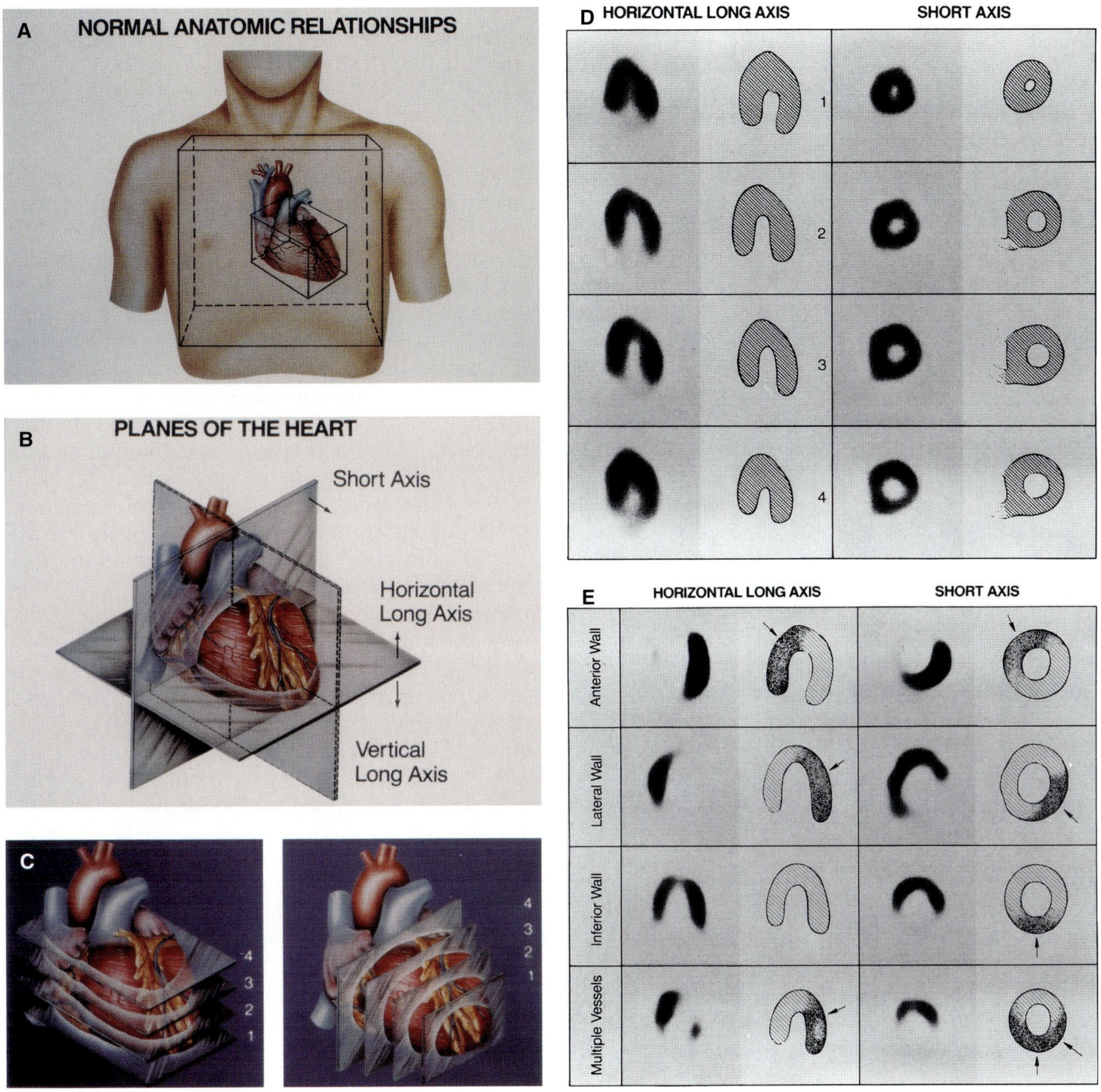

Figure 57 SPECT studies. (A) Diagram of the heart enclosed in a larger cube, as it lies in the chest, and after acquisition and initial phases of SPECT reconstruction in the smaller cube. The latter may be reoriented to conform with standard orientations and sliced along its 3 major axes, as shown in (B). Planes for standard horizontal and short-axis SPECT slices are shown in (C). (D) These are normal slices in these axes; whereas (E) shows typical perfusion defects with an accompanying interpretive sketch. (From the General Electric Co., Milwaukee, WI, commercial poster with permission.)

All computer systems require the user to first define or confirm the long axis of the left ventricle in the largest transverse slice of the myocardium. The axis may be defined by drawing a line through the center of the left ventricular cavity or by drawing lines parallel to the axis but outside the myocardium. Some computer-assisted axis definition programs are available, but the assumptions they must make about the shape of the heart are not always valid, especially when a large perfusion defect is present. The axis drawing routine needs to be performed twice, first in the transverse slice and then in the plane orthogonal to the transverse plane along the line defined by the first axis drawn. The original X, Y and Z axes are defined by the gamma camera. Cardiac axis selection defines a new set of XYZ axes, and the heart is reoriented so the long axis of the left ventricle lies along the Z axis.

Axis definitions (with respect to the left ventricle) should be identical for both parts of a stress and rest–redistribution study, so that corresponding parts of the myocardium can be aligned in the comparison images. The axis definitions can be compared by photographing the lines used to define the axis in both studies and comparing them. Some software allows the user to draw the lines for both studies on the screen at the same time. Some vendors even let the user apply the axes drawn for the first study to the second study, but this arrangement is only valid in the unlikely circumstance that patient position and cardiac axes are identical for both studies. A major ischemic area can make axis definition quite difficult by hiding the apex or an entire cardiac wall. It often helps to draw the rest–redistribution axes first, because the defect may have filled in and the myocardium will be easier to see. This knowledge of the conformation of the intact ventricle may be used to draw the axes on the stress study. Erroneous and/or varying ventricular axes are a common cause of image misinterpretation. Such errors can lead to the loss of image specificity, to an increase in apparently "reversible" defects and to errors in the polar display.

SPECT Circumferential Profiles. Objective analysis of myocardial perfusion studies began in the late 1970s with circumferential profiles of planar thallium images (*311*). Planar target-to-background ratio was poor, so quantitation was developed to improve accuracy and reproducibility and to reduce interobserver variability. The process is relatively simple: (1) the image is smoothed to reduce the noise; (2) background subtraction is applied to enhance the myocardial counts; (3) a reference point, such as the inferior right ventricular/left ventricular septal junction, is marked on the myocardium; (4) for each of 60 (or 30 or 120) equally spaced radii from the center of the myocardium, the hottest pixel is located along that radius; and (5) the resulting values are plotted as a curve representing sequential data points around the myocardium.

The length of the search radius is set by an observer-defined circle outside the heart. When a severe defect is present, the hottest pixel along the radius may not occur in the myocardial area. The operator must correct any choice of an extracardiac data point, but little additional operator interaction is required, so that the process is user independent and results are reproducible.

Each data point in the curve is expressed as a percentage of the hottest pixel value in the curve. This normalization produces only relative perfusion counts, so uniformly depressed perfusion in triple-vessel disease could be missed. This was a rare phenomenon in planar imaging, and it is seen even less frequently in the more sensitive SPECT study, because more regions of the myocardium can be differentiated. Similar stress and redistribution curves indicate normal perfusion with normal values or infarction with the same region of relative-counts depression in both curves. Significantly higher values in redistribution curves representing the same myocardial area indicate ischemia. Objective detection of defects is performed by specifying a percentage threshold compared with the normal sex-specific count distribution, below which the curve value indicates defects, whereas fluctuations above this threshold are not considered perfusion defects. This threshold was determined by averaging circumferential profiles in a large population of gender-matched normal patients.

Circumferential profiles were first applied to analyze planar images, as previously described, and were then used on slices produced from 7-pinhole and rotating slant-hole tomography. With current SPECT studies, circumferential profiles are still used in a modified fashion. Separate profiles are generated for each short-axis slice, resulting in multiple curves representing different areas of the heart. These are combined into a polar map image, as described later in this text. With the enhanced target-to-background ratio of SPECT images, the automatically selected myocardial points are usually within the myocardium, and operator interaction rarely is needed. Sestamibi can present problems near the apex when there is more activity in the jejunal loop than in the myocardium, but most programs do not allow the user to relocate these points into the heart.

Normal Databases. Because of the energy and other physical differences affecting attenuation and scatter, normal distributions are best determined by protocol- and radionuclide-specific normal databases. Normal myocardial distribution of ^{201}Tl in males is different from that in females, most likely because of differing attenuation patterns (*13,95,332,333*). With both sexes, activity is more attenuated in the basal inferior and septal regions of the left ventricle. However, in females, additional attenuation of anterolateral wall activity by breast tissue apparently balances the inferior and septal attenuation and results in more uniform apparent myocardial distribution. For these reasons, 2 separate sex-specific normal circumferential profile and polar map databases have been developed for reference. If the quantitative profiles of a male patient are compared with those in the female database, the normal male pattern of reduced inferior and inferoseptal activity may then be artifactually deemed to be a defect. Conversely, comparison of a female's quantitative circumferential profiles with those of the male results in an indication of artifactual anterolateral wall defect. Even with the gender-specific database, anterior wall attenuation may be greater than that observed in the normal female population in large subjects, resulting in false-positive studies. Polar maps may be similarly altered.

Image data on rest and stress polar maps and both planar and SPECT circumferential profiles are correlated separately to the range of sex-specific normal-counts distributions. These rest and stress distributions often are not compared, except by the reader. Therefore, distributions that differ widely but may each fall within their individual normal distributions, or, if compared with a normal "difference profile" or polar map, may fall within the large range of normal and will not appear as objective abnormalities on computer analysis, when, in fact, their difference may attest to redistribution. This may be a factor, although likely minor, in reduction in polar map sensitivity. Of course, the risk of reading such an image subtlety, not evident on polar maps, may again jeopardize specificity. Experience and judgment, with reference to the raw data and the distribution of image differences, will help resolve such issues. Defects at the periphery of the map, especially in the region of the basal septum, and nonsegmental defects should be treated with some skepticism and are most likely technical or artifactual in origin.

Polar Maps. A bullseye or polar map is basically a graphic display of a set of circumferential profiles of the short-axis slices. The hottest spot in the myocardium (the entire set of curves) is considered 100%, and all other areas are measured as fractions of this value. The concentric rings from center to periphery of the polar map are circumferential profiles of selected short-axis slices from the apex to the base. Three points must be chosen to create the polar map: the apex, the base and a reference point to ensure consistent rotational orientation between comparison polar maps. Edge definition and slice selection can be automated, but this is problematic in all but normal hearts (*334*).

The polar (coordinate) map may be compared with such a projection of the Earth. Here a polar map of the northern hemisphere would be a circular display, with the north pole at its center, the equator at it periphery and all intervening geography appropriately distributed between. The left ventricular perfusion polar map presents the apex at its center, the left ventricular base and atrioventricular groove at its periphery and all the regional myocardium distributed between. It is as if we were looking down at the Saturn moon rocket from its nose cone; here we are looking at the left ventricle from its apex. From the center (apex), the anterior wall is up, the inferior wall is down, the septum is left and the lateral wall is right.

Among short-axis slices, those extending from the subendocardial portion of the apex to the base of the heart are selected for quantitative analysis. The last 3 basal slices are not considered for quantitation because of significant dropout of activity in the inferior and septal regions. For the vertical long-axis slices, those extending from the subendocardial portion of the septum to the subendocardial portion of the lateral wall are selected for quantitation. The myocardial activity of the apex is analyzed from the apical portion of the vertical long-axis slices, and the myocardial activity of the remaining portions of the left ventricle is analyzed form the short-axis slices. Vertical long-axis, rather than short-axis, slices are used to assess the apex, because the apex is subject to partial volume effect on the short-axis slices. The center of the left ventricle, the left ventricular cavity and the radius of search are defined by the operator. From the center, 60 equidistant radii are computer generated, each 6° apart. Along each radius, the computer selects the maximum count value, which is normalized to the highest value found in each slice and plotted for each angular location on the myocardial periphery, thereby generating a circumferential count profile.

For proper comparison of stress and redistribution images and their normal profiles, a common anatomic landmark is defined at the inferior junction of the right and left ventricles in the short-axis slices. On the vertical long-axis slices, the most apical point is used for alignment. The center of the polar map is derived from the apical region of 1 of the long-axis slices, because a circumferential profile is difficult to generate without a distinct hole in the center of the myocardial ring. The slices through the apex in the short-axis set lack a ventricular cavity, but either long-axis view will show a ventricular cavity. The endocardial wall, marked at the apex in a long-axis slice, as described previously, defines the line in the polar map between data contributed from the short-axis image set and apical data from the long axis. The method used to generate circumferential profiles is similar to the method for apical profiles from long-axis slices. The main difference is that myocardial measurements are restricted to the apex of long-axis slices, so short, linear profiles are created. An alternative method of generating the center of the polar map is called spherical sampling and works in the 3-dimensional volume representing the apex. It uses the already defined long axis of the left ventricle to determine the center of the apex and draws radial profiles from that point to the apical limit already selected for circumferential profiles. This is equivalent to creating a series of long-axis slices at different angles around the left ventricular axis and then generating profiles from the apices of these slices.

The inferior septal junction of the right and left ventricles, the point where the right ventricle inserts into the septum, is another reference point. It is selected in a short-axis slice and used to rotate the polar maps from both stress and rest studies so that they line up with each other and with the normal database. The inferior junction of the right and left ventricle may be difficult to see in a ^{201}Tl image, because so little activity is in the right ventricle. Some basic knowledge of cardiac anatomy can guide the user to select a point in the correct general area. The junction is much more easily seen in ^{99m}Tc sestamibi and tetrofosmin studies, with their increased count density and better target-to-background ratio. To use the commercial normal databases, the rotational reference point must match that point used for the normal database. The normal database provides a polar map of usual coronary artery perfusion areas, and, if a different reference point is used, then the polar map will be rotated clockwise or counterclockwise. The comparison with normal values and the overlaid map of coronary artery perfusion territories will be incorrect. The role of these methods and their application is considered in Tables 10 and 11.

To account for individual variations in left ventricular size, the ventricle is divided into 5 regions of equal thickness representing the volume covered by the short-axis cuts and 5 equal thickness regions representing the volume covered by the apex. The mean value for each of the 60 angular locations of each of the 5 anatomical regions was determined from pooled data of 35 male and 20 females, each of whom had a $<5\%$ likelihood of CAD. In each of the 5 zones, representative circumferential profiles are averaged, resulting in 5 short-axis and 5 vertical long-axis mean normal profiles. The distribution of normal profile points around the mean is not Gaussian in all regions of the myocardium but is skewed in the anterolateral and inferoseptal regions. Therefore, the optimum method for developing normal limit profiles is to construct from the lowest observed value below the mean normal profiles (range approach) (*332,333,335*). These 5 short-axis profiles, with the apical section taken from the vertical long-axis projection, are compiled in a polar distribution format with the apex central and basal region placed peripherally. Such polar coordinate color maps can be applied to summarize radionuclide distribution after exercise and redistribution images and regional washout with simultaneous comparison with normal values.

Sometimes this image is referred to as a "bullseye" display, suggesting its direct origin from the successive circumferential display of larger slices around the central apical slice. However, although this term describes the pattern graphically, this is not its origin and, although it takes some explanation, "polar (coordinate) map" is a better descriptor.

In contrast to planar image quantitation and because of SPECT diagnostic accuracy, quantitative assessment of myocardial washout of ^{201}Tl with the SPECT technique has not been established as contributing to detection of disease in individual coronary arteries. For this reason, quantitation of SPECT images for detection and localization of CAD usually relies on quantitation of exercise and delayed or rest images for the presence and reversibility of perfusion defects. However, an assessment utilizing computer-generated composite exercise and redistribution ^{201}Tl SPECT short-axis slices and color coded for regional washout has demonstrated an

Table 11
FACTORS AFFECTING IMAGE DATA QUALITY

Energy window
Spatial resolution
Collimator
Detector sensitivity
Matrix size

advantage for CAD detection (*288*). Image abnormalities can be graded in terms of the involvement of coronary regions, as established and roughly applied in the analysis of commercially available polar map software, or in terms of their percentage left ventricular involvement. Guidelines may include a mildly abnormal study that involves defects including a limited part and certainly less than half of a single coronary region. A moderately abnormal study might demonstrate defects involving more than half of the designated right or left circumflex regions and up to half of the LAD region or a possible or minor abnormality in a second vascular area. A severely abnormal scan demonstrates obvious defects in multiple vascular areas or the full LAD region. More quantitative scores have been developed and are discussed later in this text.

Gated Processing. Gated SPECT processing is very similar to nongated processing. In fact, degating, or collapsing all the temporal frames in each projection into 1 static image, is often the first step. This new image set should be identical to what would have been acquired without gating and is processed the same way.

Because the time intervals of each projection can be collapsed into 1 image after acquisition, both gated and ungated data can be derived from the same study. To reconstruct a gated study, each time interval in all projections is treated mathematically as a separate SPECT study. The first time interval is treated as 1 study, the second time interval as a second study and so on. Processing takes 8–16× as long as ungated SPECT, because 8–16 images are in each projection instead of just 1 image. When finished, the standard myocardial slices can be viewed as a cine, showing wall motion and wall thickening (intensity) in each slice. Some display programs may show cines of selected slices, and other software may show all slices in motion. New programs quantify evaluation of regional brightening and wall motion, with calculation of wall thickening and LVEF values, and are influenced by acquisition protocols (*336*). Brightening has been shown to correlate with wall thickening, resulting from an interaction of partial volume effects and camera resolution properties (*337,338*). Shen et al. (*339*) developed a new computer algorithm for the objective quantitation of regional wall thickening from variations in regional count density changes during the cardiac cycle.

Other information may be gained from gated SPECT. If the endocardial wall can be defined in all short-axis slices, the total volume of the myocardial cavity could be calculated in each time frame, resulting in a volume curve showing absolute left ventricular volumes and LVEF. Reliable software for this purpose is available (*232*). Volumes also can be calculated from orthogonal long-axis slices following the same approach developed in cardiac angiography. Table 12 reviews the variety of technical factors related to the gated acquisition of SPECT perfusion images.

Principles of Display

Overview. The way images are displayed on the computer screen is critically important to the proper interpretation of data. The final presentation used for clinical interpretation should include as much relevant information as possible and exclude irrelevant and redundant information. Color, if used, should enhance and not obscure important information. Image enhancement can be performed as part of image processing or afterward as part of the display software or hardware. Image enhancement usually includes a combination of both steps. The basic principles of the display screen and a number of display-related features, such as color tables and scale, are described in Self-Study Program III,

Nuclear Medicine: Cardiology, Topic 1: Physical and Technical Aspects of Nuclear Cardiology. Some attributes of image display and common display formats are described later in this text. Table 11 lists a variety of factors that influence the quality of image data.

Image Enhancement. Image enhancement can be defined as the accentuation of some features of an image. Enhancement during processing changes the information in an image by changing the individual pixel values, whereas enhancement as part of the display changes only the appearance. Both methods change the way the image is perceived. The most common form of enhancement in nuclear medicine is the presentation of images in color, although the images are inherently gray-scale monochrome.

Table 12
TECHNICAL CONSIDERATIONS IN GATED SPECT PERFUSION IMAGING

Acquisition and reconstruction of a 16-frame gated SPECT study requires 16× as much random access memory (RAM) and takes 16× as long for reconstruction

For clinical utility, gated SPECT perfusion imaging needs a fast computer, with 8 Mb of RAM and 500 Mb of hard-disk space

Vendor software should:

- Permit acquisition of up to 16 frames SPECT
- Display time at each camera stop in seconds or in accepted beats within a user-defined R-R interval
- Permit collapse of the study to an ungated study or image including only specified frames, for example, an end-diastolic image
- Display of dynamic beating short-axis slices, selected long-axis slices and 3-dimensional rendering of the beating heart
- Calculate quantitative measures of regional perfusion, contraction and wall thickening

The dynamic range of an image is the difference between the highest- and lowest-count pixel values. Usually 256 gray levels are available to display a dynamic range from 0 to 65,535 counts/pixel in a word-mode image. The display hardware uses a lookup table to determine what brightness, gray scale, color or color brightness to show for each pixel as a function of the counts in the pixel. This association is a mapping between counts (the data range) and brightness (the display range). If a range of counts >256 needs to be displayed, some pixels with different numbers of counts will have the same intensity level. If the range of counts is <255, each count level gets a different intensity level and <256 intensity levels will be displayed. This all assumes that the gray scale covers the entire range of pixel counts. However, windowing (described later in this text) can limit the displayed range of counts data.

Contrast. Contrast is the relative brightness of different parts of an image. One of the major advantages of using a computer screen instead of film is the flexibility of control over contrast in images. High contrast means that some areas are very bright and some are very dim. Contrast can be increased or decreased in a display by windowing an image. Hardware usually can present 256 levels of gray, which is adequate for viewing any image, because this number of gray levels exceeds the number of intensity levels in human perception. The human eye adjusts to overall brightness in the visual field by changes in pupil size, concentration of light-sensitive chemicals in the rods and cones and neural signal output as a function of light intensity changes. If every pixel on the screen became twice as bright, after a brief adjustment period the eye could not detect any difference between the new and old states of the image. The eye is sensitive to relative intensities (contrast), especially at object edges with large differences in intensity over small visual angles.

Windowing. Windowing an image refers to changing the limits of display intensities for the range of pixel values in an image. The window spreads the gray scale over any limited range of the total pixel count range, and the range can be compressed or expanded as desired. If the highest-count pixels are shown as white, all pixels with counts equal to or above the upper threshold will be displayed at the highest intensity level, white. All pixels with counts equal to or below the lower threshold will be displayed at the lowest intensity level, black. A narrow display window range has few intensity levels, so it will result in images that show abrupt intensity changes and high contrast. The extreme case contains only 2 gray levels, black and white, so the image appears as a silhouette. Windowing is primarily used to concentrate the displayed intensity range so that the area of interest has the maximum contrast range. Myocardial ^{99m}Tc sestamibi perfusion images are excellent examples, because pixel counts in the gall bladder or small bowel often are so much higher than myocardial pixel counts. This makes the relatively low intensity myocardium difficult to see and also makes it difficult to compare with an image set in which the maximum counts occur in the myocardium. Bringing the upper threshold down to the maximum myocardial counts places the maximum image intensity in the myocardium and spreads the visual intensity range over the myocardium, emphasizing the clinically important area. This also aids comparison of images, all normalized to the maximum myocardial count value.

Normalization refers to the way the maximum brightness is chosen in sets of images. This can be performed as part of processing, by setting a maximum pixel value in the images and reducing any higher pixel values to that selected value. It also can be performed during display, by windowing the images. Perfusion images should be normalized to the full 3-dimensional data set, not to individual SPECT slices, so that the same region of myocardium will have the same appearance in all axes. When each SPECT image slice is normalized to itself, each image will have at least 1 pixel of maximal display intensity, regardless of relative pixel values between images. This makes each image equally bright. When an underperfused area encompasses an entire slice of myocardium, it would appear normal, because the image has been brightened without regard to other images. To detect relative defect intensity between slices, the mapping from pixel values to display intensities must be the same in all slices. When each image set is normalized as a unit, the relative brightness between images is maintained and the ability to identify relative perfusion defects preserved.

In nuclear medicine, the phrase "brighten an image" usually means to enhance the visual intensity of pixels by lowering the upper threshold. This will have more effect on low-count pixels than high-count pixels, because more of the lower-count pixels will become visible, whereas highest-count pixels simply maintain their brightness. Window brightening can be achieved in 2 ways. One is to spread the same number of intensity levels over a smaller data range, showing better resolution of differences in pixel values and changing the ratio of data values to intensities. Alternatively, the data can be kept to a gray-scale ratio constant, so that lowering the upper threshold reduces the number of intensity levels displayed. The first method provides more visual information and is usually applied.

The mathematical equation to calculate the appropriate display intensity level from the pixel values is:

$$\text{lookup table index} = \frac{(\text{pixel counts} - \text{lower threshold}) \times 256}{(\text{upper threshold} - \text{lower threshold})}.$$

Simply, the index into the lookup table is the pixel count relative to the window display range. For color displays, each lookup table entry will contain brightness levels for each of the 3 colors. For example, a table index of 170 might show red at 70%, green at 40% and blue at 90% of their individual maximum brightness levels.

Cine. Cine is another word for movie. It was originally applied to dynamic images that could be viewed on the screen to show the changing distribution of activity over time. The term has become more loosely used and now is also applied to the viewing of any image set when rapidly stepping through the images. For instance, a cine of the projection images will show what the gamma camera detected in each view as it moved around the body. A cine of the short-axis slices will show the progression of slices from the apex to the base of the heart. The final product of SPECT reconstruction is a 3-dimensional representation that can be rotated as a cine or viewed from any angle as a static image. A gated SPECT image can show the contraction cycle from any angle in any slice, or it can show the entire 3-dimensional myocardium as it repeats the cardiac contraction cycle.

Color Tables. Because each pixel is simply a number of counted photons, all nuclear medicine images are inherently monochrome in shades of gray, from black to white or vice versa. The images can be displayed in color by assigning different colors to specific pixel counts. A color table, or lookup table, defines the color to be displayed for each possible number of counts in a pixel. A rainbow color table, following the sequence of colors in a rainbow, would show low-count pixels as red and, as count levels increase, the colors would move through orange, yellow, green and blue. A monochrome color table using only 1 color is possible but is less interesting to the eye; so these are rarely used. All nuclear medicine computers let users design custom color tables. A good color table is designed to emphasize specific physiologically or clinically relevant ranges of contrast.

Any finding derived from a color image should be validated from a monochrome image. However, a color scale that seeks to highlight critical relative perfusion levels or ranges may make the visual interpretation easier. For example, if myocardial viability and a strong potential for functional improvement postrevascularization are said to be present when perfusion exceeds 50% of the peak (presumably normal) myocardial perfusion (*265*), setting a color threshold at this 50% level would simplify the image interpretation of viability. This may not correspond to a significant change in counts nor be visible as an edge in a monochrome image, and care must be given to the clinical interpretation of all color images. Of course, a 50% color threshold will make a 49% value appear very different and abnormal, in contrast to the probable clinical reality. Color can be used to display functional or kinetic data in ways that cannot be seen in monochrome images, but all anatomic images are inherently monochrome. Color can be used to simultaneously display stress thallium perfusion data and regional washout in a single image or to compare the distribution of different radionuclides in the same study.

Although hard copy may be needed for archiving, to carry elsewhere or for ready documentation, the computer display screen is the recommended vehicle for image review and reading. The intensity and contrast levels on film formatters drift over time, and film distorts the image contrast because of its characteristic sensitivity curves. The screen output is both stable and versatile, assuring consistent and optimal exposure, and presenting the possibilities of instantaneous adjustments of image parameters and color. In addition, a cine display of the projection images is important for the assessment of motion artifact and to more easily assess the nature and effects of background and attenuation. This cine display should be reviewed by the technologist after acquisition but before processing, and again by the reader before interpretation.

Standard Software Displays

Myocardial Slices. Once the SPECT reconstruction process is complete, the images must be displayed on the computer screen for interpretation. The standard method is to arrange 2 parallel rows of images for each orientation: short-axis, vertical long-axis and horizontal long-axis images. In the short axis, the slices are perpendicular to the long axis of the left ventricle and appear as flat doughnuts. Vertical and horizontal long-axis–oriented slices are parallel to the long axis at right angles to each other. The upper row of each pair usually includes the stress image slices, and the lower row includes the rest or redistribution slices. The images in each row are aligned so that the slice of myocardium in the stress state is directly above the equivalent slice of myocardium in the rest state. This allows easy comparison of identical or nearly identical anatomical areas. All programs that display the slices require the user to shift the upper and lower rows in relation to each other to align the slices. Clinicians should always be mindful of the comparison being made in the image interpretation and always compare corresponding slices. In the short-axis slices, either the base of the ventricle or the most apical slice showing a cavity may be used as a reference point for slice alignment. The base is more reliable and is easier to match when viewed in color. Poorly visualized structures with perfusion defects are poor choices. Correct slice alignments in the long axes are usually easy to see.

Because the 3 orientations are all slices from the same 3-dimensional matrix, any point in 1 orientation has a corresponding point in each of the other 2 orientations. Triangulation software can be used to indicate the same point in each orientation, usually by a mouse click on a pixel. This helps to ensure that the same area in different orientations is being evaluated for a perfusion abnormality. This does not aid in the elimination of image artifacts, because artifacts will triangulate just as do true perfusion defects.

Circumferential Profiles and Polar Maps. Polar maps of normal sestamibi and thallium distributions, matched to gender, have been created and incorporated into myocardial perfusion analysis programs (*340*). Because they are derived from limited sampling of circumferential profiles of SPECT slices, the term "polar maps" is used. Individuals with normal hearts were studied and their polar images averaged to create normal regional ranges of relative perfusion in different areas of the myocardium. Separate normal comparison polar maps were developed for each gender. As new myocardial perfusion agents are developed, new normal databases must be developed for them. Databases are currently available for most ^{201}Tl- and ^{99m}Tc-based protocols and for the dual-isotope ^{201}Tl rest/^{99m}Tc sestamibi stress protocol. These unique databases are made necessary by the varying physical properties and by the potentially different physiological distributions of each radiopharmaceutical. The proper database must be applied to each acquisition protocol.

The patient polar map is compared with the normal range, based on a "normal database" for each segment of the myocardium, so that abnormal segments can be displayed in different colors based on their standard deviation from normal. Any regional value outside 2 standard deviations from the normal image values in that area is considered abnormal. The magnitude of severity of this deviation serves as the basis for the segmental score.

The final display usually has multiple polar maps, including the patient's raw stress and rest polar maps and those comparing the patient's polar maps with the normal database. It may also include maps created by subtracting the stress from the rest images to produce a map of redistribution, or a "reversibility difference" map, and an "abnormality map," which marks abnormal pixels in the stress image. Polar plots of myocardial perfusion distort the image of the heart and the distribution of perfusion in the same way that a flat projection map or polar map distorts the shape of the earth and the representation of its features. This distortion varies with each individual study and the distribution of parameters mapped but generally exaggerates basal segments and underestimates distal or apical segments. To minimize this problem, polar plots of the myocardium can be generated based on geometric considerations (distance weighted) or area (volume weighted). Distance-weighted polar maps create every polar ring with equal width. Volume-weighted polar maps create rings with areas proportional to the myocardial volumes they represent. This provides a more accurate picture of the actual volume of the perfusion defect. However, any defect that is evident only at the outer edge of the polar map may not be a true perfusion defect, because the basal slice of the myocardium, especially in anterior and septal regions, is often difficult to define and would represent an unusual distribution for coronary disease.

Polar maps are the primary objective computer-based method of perfusion image quantitation, and both extent and depth (% reduction in perfusion) of defects can be quantified. A numeric report usually accompanies the reversibility polar map, including the extent (number of pixels) of both the stress defect and the area of improvement on a delayed or rest study, in which a 15% area improvement has been accepted as significant. The threshold method compares relative segmental count data with a database that takes into account normal variations in relative perfusion to generate a standard deviation from the normal segmental intensity. This value can then be plotted on a polar map, color coded and serve as the basis for a multisegment ($n = 20$) quantitative model in which each segment is graded from 0–4 for its intensity of abnormality. The resultant product (the number of segments × the segment score) for the rest image (the rest segmental score [RSS]) and for the stress image (the summed stress score [SSS]) quantitates the perfusion abnormality. These quantitative methods are valuable, adding objectivity, sensitivity and reproducibility. They should be used along with other available guides in interpretation and as a basis for quantitation of serial studies and the assessment of coronary risk. However, given their complexity and the opportunity for a multitude of computer- and operator-derived errors, the validity of the polar map must be established and errors in its generation recognized before data are applied. Such data certainly should be used only after careful comparison with the image data from which it was generated, and the image data, not the polar plot, should be the final arbiter of all interpretive decisions.

Although valuable and contributing to objectivity in image reading, the wide range of normal perfusion values means that stress image heterogeneity may appear abnormal in any given study yet fall within the range of normal when related to the normal database. This can be objectified with reference to the redistribution or rest image and also may be appreciated on the difference map. Interpretation must not rely entirely on the comparison of polar data with a normal database but must use this simply as an objective tool to guide interpretation and aid quantitation. This is acknowledged by the practice of reading a polar display as normal as long as regional abnormalities are within the bounds of established normal for each vascular area (*341*). Similarly, judgment must be applied, as apparent polar map abnormalities may result from normal regional count variation at the septal base or from attenuation or artifact. The reader must recognize these variations and not read image polar map defects automatically but inquire about and evaluate their cause with the many aids available.

Yet another potential application for polar images is to help indicate attenuation artifact in ^{201}Tl studies when using a rest ^{201}Tl/stress ^{99m}Tc sestamibi or tetrofosmin protocol, where defects will appear more severe in the low-energy rest ^{201}Tl images. The difference polar map, showing the difference between the rest and stress polar map, will show excess ^{201}Tl in areas of stress-induced ischemia but will show excess sestamibi in areas in which there is more attenuation of ^{201}Tl than of ^{99m}Tc (*342*). Again, care must be taken, as normal regional variations in activity, such as reduced apical activity, may be more clearly seen on the better-resolved images.

Gated SPECT. Gated images are a combination of planar multigated techniques, originally applied to blood-pool images, imposed on a standard myocardial SPECT acquisition to create a 3-dimensional dynamic image set. This allows any slice in any axis to be viewed as a movie of the cardiac cycle or examined as a static image at selected points in the cycle. The most helpful slices are the central vertical and horizontal long-axis slices and the entire set of short-axis slices. The long-axis slices can show apical motion and thickening that is not visible in the short-axis slices. Basal motion may also be better visualized in long-axis slices. The apex and base also appear to move toward each other, and this is not evident on the screen when watching a set of short-axis slices in motion. In a normal heart, the most apical slice containing myocardium in end diastole will be empty of myocardium at end systole. Peripheral long-axis slices may be misleading, because their apparent motion is not in the direction of the center of contraction of the heart but toward a line parallel to that center. All short-axis slices contract toward the center long axis of the left ventricle, visible on the display.

Methods for quantitative analysis of wall motion and thickening on MPS are established and also represent an important area of research today. These should be able to provide significant clinical information about myocardial function and viability that is not currently obtainable in any other way (*212,325*). The spatial resolution of gamma cameras does not allow accurate measurement of wall thickness or even changes in thickness. However, wall thickening does correlate very well with increases in myocardial intensity seen in gated SPECT cines (*211,212,338*).

Three-Dimensional Images. Rather than slice the myocardium up in different planes, the 3-dimensional image matrix can be viewed as a 3-dimensional object. Two basic methods can achieve this. In surface rendering, only the outside surface can be seen. This treats the heart as a solid object. The other method is volume rendering, in which semitransparent images indicate the complete radioactive distribution throughout the heart rather than just on the surface. This is similar to producing what the gamma camera would see as a planar view from any desired angle but with greater depth and internal detail. A variation for either method is called "cheese brick," in which slices of the heart can be removed from the front of the image just as slices of cheese are removed from a brick of cheese. A cross-section of the myocardium is visible along with the surface of the myocardial tissue behind the cross-section (*343*). Three-dimensional display methods have the potential to condense the data and make it more legible to the inexperienced viewer. The 3-dimensional data also can be applied in more direct comparison with other 3-dimensional data sets of other modalities and may be correlated well with the coronary angiogram. The 2 image sets can be directly superimposed for the best anatomic–physiologic comparison, in effect painting the coronary arteries onto the surface of the perfusion map. Three-dimensional imaging has been applied to view wall motion in a left ventriculogram derived from the gated perfusion study. From this data, LV end-diastolic and end-systolic volumes and LV mass can be calculated accurately.

Current Software

Commercial software has been developed with the collaboration of major research and clinical centers and implemented on fast computers with extensive memory and graphics capabilities (*235*). These programs have made it possible to isolate and reorient the left ventricle, automate SPECT reconstruction, automate the calculation of LVEF and other anatomic and functional parameters, generate 3-dimensional images of the left ventricular myocardium, display perfusion defects compared with normal databases and develop artificial intelligence or other systems to assist and standardize the interpretation of image data. Current nuclear medicine computer software performs these tasks. Parametric and polar maps plotting aspects of regional left ventricular function have not yet been thoroughly evaluated.

Transverse or axial image data oriented as the heart lies in the chest are reoriented along the ventricular long axis to produce slices in short, vertical and horizontal long axes, using spatial cues that are recognized by the reconstruction algorithm and applied by the operator. These tasks have become fully automated and rapid (*312,345*). Two automated methods generate slice data based on intensity thresholds to locate and extract the left ventricular myocardium. The method of Germano et al. (*335*) employs an ellipsoid of myocardial activity to fit myocardial edges. The method failed to localize the ventricular borders in only 6 of 400 studies. The method by Mullick et al. (*344*) applies a more complex algorithm to locate and orient the left ventricular myocardium and identify its boundaries, with a success rate of 116 out of 124 studies (*344*). A variation of the method of Germano et al. (*345,346*) applies an algorithm for the 3-dimensional quantitation of myocardial perfusion.

Commercial databases of normal male and female counts distributions were derived from the results of stress imaging in patients with a low likelihood of CAD. These databases have been analyzed and graphically presented as polar maps to serve as an objective guide beyond the visual analysis for the identification of perfusion defects. The maps have been well validated and add objectivity, while permitting a quantitative assessment of individual and serial studies. Yet, until recently, these maps were highly imperfect and suffered at least 5 serious limitations, including (*232*): (1) Significant operator choice and involvement, resulting in a potential loss of objectivity and reproducibility. This has been overcome by automation of the process in new software versions. (2) An inability to sample counts perpendicular to the ventricular walls, which artifactually increased apparent apical counts. New software addresses this problem. (3) Databases were available only for ^{201}Tl distribution with a stress and delayed-image protocol. Physical and biological differences exist between radionuclides, and different protocols yield different counts distributions. The application of a different (^{201}Tl) database to a stress sestamibi or tetrofosmin database will surely lead to errors. New methods are database specific. (4) The fact that the method has no intrinsic ability to correct for attenuation and scatter. Because of the wide range of body habitus, even within the same sex, variability in these physical parameters exceeds that represented in the normal database, resulting in apparent abnormalities unrelated to the perfusion pattern but more related to attenuation, exceeding the database limits. Current attempts to correct images for attenuation artifacts are only a developing approach to this problem. (5) Distortion of data presentation because of the nature of polar plots, expanding from center to periphery, apex to base, in which 3-dimensional data are warped to fit 2-dimensional coordinates. This results in the underestimation of apical defects, represented in the polar display with fewer pixels, and the overestimation of basal defects, represented by more pixels. Attempts to resolve or improve this distortion have been made in the form of maps weighted for volume or other appropriate measures (*312*).

A collaborative effort has developed a now widely disseminated data-based quantitative program called CEQual (for Cedars-Emory Quantitative Analysis), designed to overcome many of the disadvantages noted previously and with integrated software that permits almost total automation of the processing phase (*312,347*). Better, but not perfect, this new method does not resolve all problems and still needs a critical reader. The Emory Toolbox and the Autoquant software have improved on the method, adding objective and generally automated quantitation and function evaluation with polar maps and an elegant and clinically valuable 3-dimensional display (Fig. 58). Values related to defect size and LVEF are correlated with prognosis via studies in the literature. The trained reader, of course, remains indispensable.

A series of databases have been generated and others are under development to fit multiple protocols. Protocol- and agent-specific databases are needed, because agents differ in their physical parameters and resultant image findings differ when applied in a different sequence and with varying background activity. Each database was generated by the analysis of images studied with the CEQual method in a group of gender-matched patients with $<5\%$ likelihood of CAD, to define normal limits of myocardial perfusion or counts and intensity distribution. Normal databases have been validated for the: low-dose rest/high-dose stress 1-day ^{99m}Tc sestamibi protocol; high-dose stress and rest 2-day sestamibi protocol; stress–redistribution ^{201}Tl protocols; rest ^{201}Tl/stress sestamibi protocol; and low-dose stress/high-dose rest 1-day ^{99m}Tc tetrofosmin protocol. Other protocols are being generated.

Polar map displays are based on circumferential profiles similar to those applied earlier to planar images and present complex SPECT slice data for the entire left ventricle in a single, rapidly generated quantifiable image. Three-dimensional displays of the left ventricle have been adapted by many commercial camera manufacturers and software developers.

The polar map presents a quick and complete condensed image summary of the data contained in the slice circumferential profiles. The sampled points of each circumferential profile are color coded for relative local counts or intensity and displayed in concentric rings, in which the most distal slice is placed at the center, representing the apex, and the most proximal slice, at the atrioventricular groove, is placed peripherally, at the left ventricular base. Another polar map, the "abnormality map," is derived by blacking out pixels with a given level of diminished activity in the stress image. When highlighted in terms of the standard deviation of each pixel from the database mean, this "standard deviation map," is another method to plot defect severity. Areas that normalize at rest may then be highlighted in white, creating a "reversibility map." However, like polar maps of the Earth, these polar maps distort the size and shape of regional defects. To correct this, "distance-weighted" maps provide improved localization, whereas "volume-weighted" maps provide more accurate defect size. Three-dimensional graphics, derived from points on the endocardial and epicardial surface, provide a more accurate representation of the myocardium and related abnormalities. Surface points are connected by lines, and derived shapes

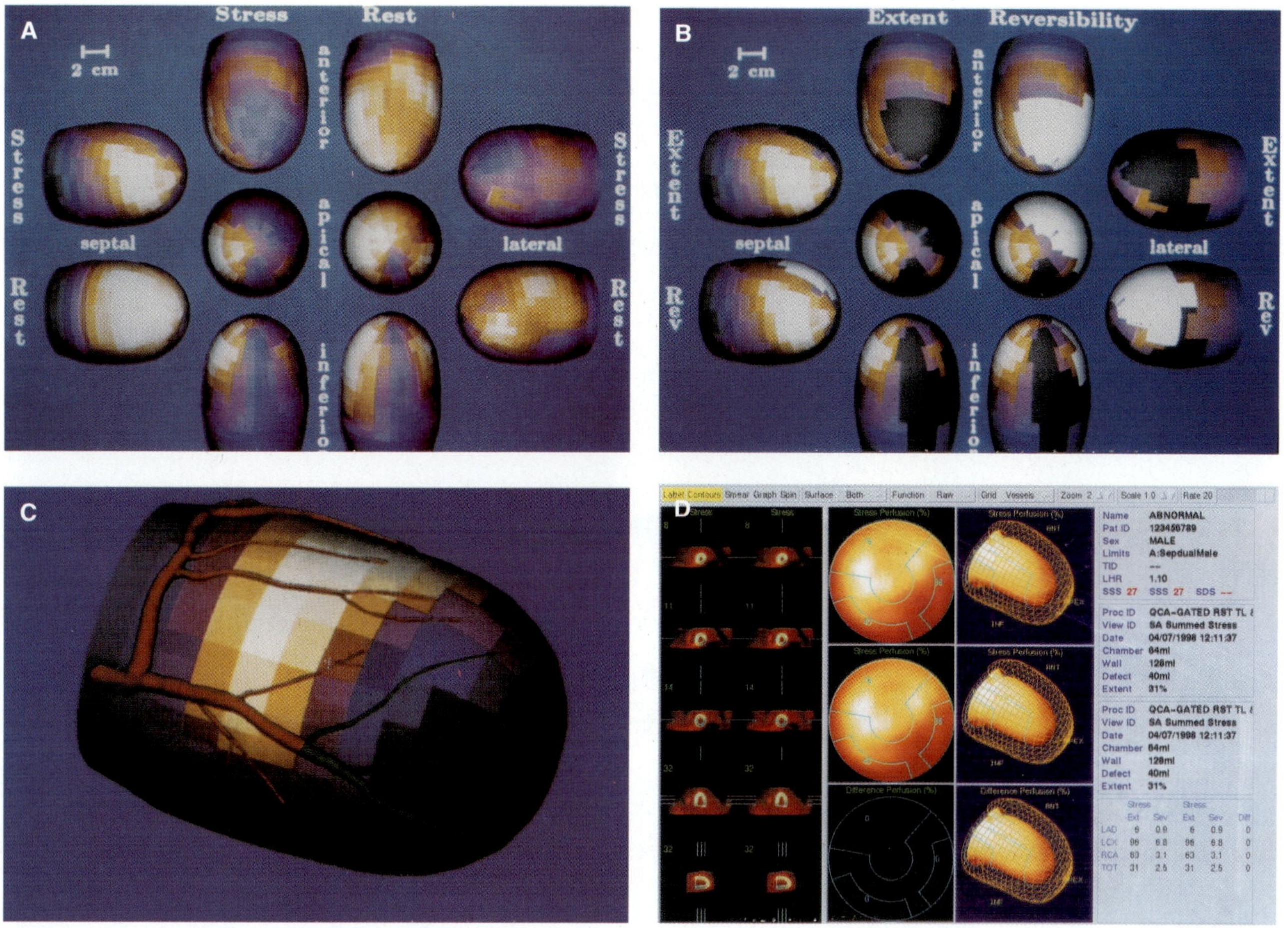

Figure 58 Three-dimensional advanced displays of perfusion abnormalities. (A) Current 3-dimensional display of regional left ventricular perfusion using the widely available Emory Tool Box software. Reversible anterior and inferior defects are evident. (B) The "blackout map," which highlights regional image heterogeneity (underperfusion) that differs by ≥3 or a preset threshold of standard deviations from the normal sex-matched database. (C) Patient-specific coronary anatomy superimposed on the 3-dimensional perfusion map. Although this display is still under development, it promises the ultimate clinically important display capability. (D) "Demo" page from the QGS Autoquant display of gated ventricular function. The actual clinical presentation contains (left to right) a selection of gated SPECT slices, perfusion polar maps (stress, above; rest, center; difference, below), wire mesh displays of diastolic and systolic surfaces that can be displayed at all angles, with quantitative measures of left ventricular perfusion and function. (Figure 58A–C, courtesy of El-Scint, Inc., TelAviv, Israel; Figure 58D, courtesy of ADAC, Inc., Milpitas, CA).

are colored for regional uptake. Boundaries can be smoothed to make a rounded rendition of the surface. The model can then be highlighted to provide apparent depth and rotated to view any wall from any angle. Once the epicardial surface is smoothed and painted with quantifiable perfusion data, it may be superimposed with actual angiographic anatomy, when known.

Correct alignment of the myocardium is important to ensure that the same parts of the patient's myocardial profiles are compared with the corresponding normal-limit database for presentation as circumferential profiles. It should also be kept in mind that the circumferential profile or polar maps are an objective guide to interpretation and quantitation. They must not be interpreted without evaluation of the raw data. Also, these methods relate stress and rest data to the normal population but do not compare the differences in these profiles, which may be viewed and annotated to add clinically important information as needed.

Table 13
CAUSES OF SPECT ARTIFACTS

Acquisition artifacts
Attenuation: breast, diaphragm, pectoral muscles, adipose of lateral wall, overlying right ventricular blood pool, self-attenuation at inferior base
Center of rotation correction
Point-spread function as a function of distance
Circular versus noncircular orbit
Field nonuniformity; uniformity correction
Changing distribution during acquisition
Patient movement
Physiologically changing biodistribution
Truncation: activity in/out of field of view
Artifacts related to thallium-201 (^{201}Tl)/technetium-99m (^{99m}Tc) differences
Differential attenuation of ^{201}Tl and ^{99m}Tc
Point-spread function for ^{201}Tl and ^{99m}Tc
Overlying or adjacent extracardiac activity
Tilted camera head
Anatomic and clinical variants
Apical slit
Noncoronary heart disease
Noncoronary cardiomyopathy
Left bundle branch block
Left ventricular hypertrophy
Processing (reconstruction) and display artifacts
Color table
Gray scale
Normalization to each image or over the entire image set
Background subtraction
Misalignment of comparative slices
Inconsistent wall definition for polar map creation
Incorrect inferior junction definition for polar map creation
Incorrect axis selection for short-axis definition
Incorrect filter selection for image reconstruction

A debate is ongoing currently regarding the most appropriate quantitative method to apply in the serial evaluation of myocardial perfusion before and after interventions. With the increasing use of MPS to assess important new therapies, this is not a trivial decision. Although segmental analysis is the most subjective method, circumferential profiles simply analyze the distribution of activity presented to them, cannot exclude artifacts intrinsic to the SPECT method and may be subject to artifacts of their own.

Sources of Error and Quality Control

In all aspects of the study, SPECT imaging is technically demanding and requires far more attention to quality control than does planar imaging (*315,348–350*) (Table 13) (see Self-Study Program III, *Nuclear Medicine: Cardiology, Topic 1: Physical and Technical Aspects of Nuclear Cardiology*). Many properties of gamma cameras affect the accuracy and quality of SPECT images (Figs. 59–68). Without attention to these issues, the image interpretation is inevitably flawed. The method is also victimized more than planar imaging by artifacts of technique and patient motion. However, the effort to correct errors is rewarded by increased image contrast and anatomic definition, with increased clarity of regional ischemia. A certain amount of inhomogeneity usually is evident as a result of currently unavoidable physical factors (*348,350–352*). Before patient imaging by SPECT, specific quality control steps are required.

Nonuniformity. The first step is correction for nonuniformity. The presence of uniform sensitivity across the entire detector field of view is critically important (*353,354*). Nonuniformities are magnified by the SPECT reconstruction process, so minor irregularities that would not affect planar images can be very misleading in SPECT studies. Acquired images must be corrected for detector uniformity, and this may be accomplished during acquisition or after the acquisition is complete. Nonuniformities have many causes. An imperfection, especially a dent in a collimator, can cause dramatic artifacts in reconstructed images. Variations in sensitivity between photomultiplier tubes (PMTs), poor linearity in the analog-to-digital converters (ADCs) that decide which pixel gets the detected count and variations in the way each PMT responds to different photon energies are 3 more factors that can degrade uniformity. This last factor is the reason that vendors recommend acquisition of nuclide-specific flood fields or floods, so the energy correction is accurate for each nuclide. For this purpose, a 30-million–count image is obtained weekly from a uniform ^{57}Co flat flood source. This image is then used to correct each of the projection images for nonuniformity. Failure to correct for nonuniformity may result in tomographic images with a rather patchy uptake appearance. If such images are subjected to quantitative analysis, scattered defects may be noted on the polar map display.

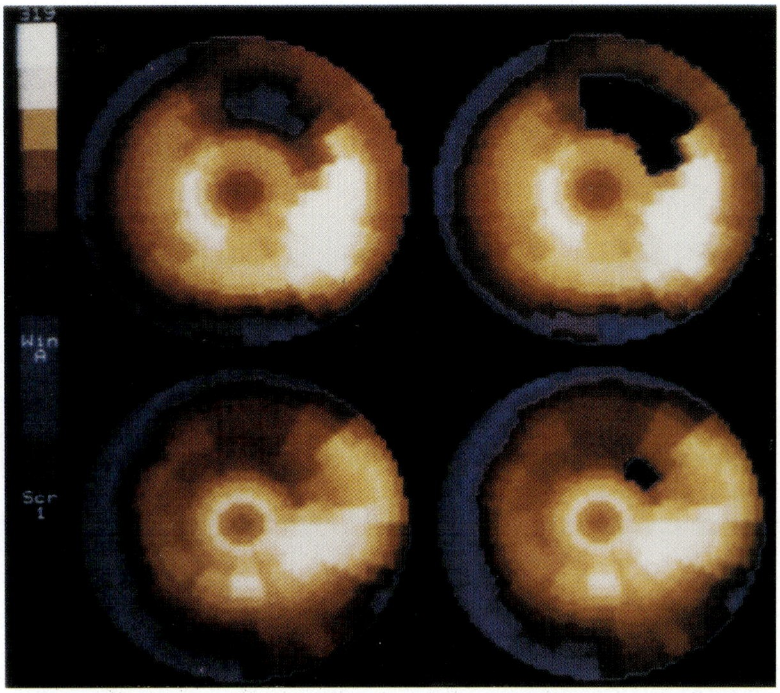

Figure 59 Breast attenuation: bra on/bra off. Polar coordinate map reconstructed from thallium-201 SPECT images obtained 3 hr postexercise in a woman with a 42-in chest circumference with bra on (top left) and, immediately after, with bra off (bottom left). Polar maps in which pixels >2.5 standard deviations below mean normal limits are blackened are displayed to the right. Defects related to breast attenuation vary with breast position and density. In a bra, the attenuating structure is generally more compact and more anteriorly located. Defects will be less dense and the impact of attenuation reduced without the bra. However, reproducible patient positioning on serial imaging is critical for accurate results. (Reprinted with permission from DePuey EG, Garcia EV. Optimal specificity of thallium-201 SPECT through recognition of imaging artifacts. *J Nucl Med* 1989;30:441–449.)

A basic assumption of SPECT reconstruction is that all areas of the field of view will have the same count response to the same amount of activity. Otherwise, projections of a uniform object registering in varying locations on the camera face will not be detected as identical in the different projections. Because photons from any 1 spot in the body tend to be detected in different field locations in different projections, periodic uniformity correction measurements must be performed. Flood correction is performed by filling the entire field of view with a uniform distribution of modest activity and then measuring the detector response. This is done by acquiring a high-count flood (The National Electrical Manufacturers Association [NEMA] specifies 10,000 counts/pixel), calculating the percentage change of each pixel from the average and multiplying each pixel in each projection image by the corresponding correction factor. This corrects the actual detector sensitivity to what it would be in each pixel if the detector sensitivity were truly uniform. A 64×64 matrix has 4096 pixels, so 41×10^6 counts should be acquired for a square detector. A round detector has about 3000 pixels in the field of view, so 30×106 counts are appropriate. A 128×128 matrix has 4× as many pixels, so it needs 4× as many counts. Some method of checking the uniformity should be used every time a new uniformity study is performed. NEMA specifications include a standard way to measure the maximum nonuniformity in a small area (differential uniformity) and over most of the field of view (integral uniformity). More backprojection rays intersect near the center of the field of view than near the periphery, so any slight nonuniformity near the center of the field of view will be multiply reinforced. This will cause ring artifacts, light and dark, around the COR of the camera.

The source used to acquire the uniformity flood on the computer may be a solid sheet containing ^{57}Co or a refillable liquid sheet source that might contain any nuclide used in nuclear medicine. The ^{57}Co flood is quite easy to use but is much more expensive, eventually decays and cannot be used when energy-specific uniformity floods ssare required. The liquid sheet source is reusable, inexpensive and can be filled with the nuclide needed at the time, but it is much more difficult to use. It must be filled very carefully to the correct volume to

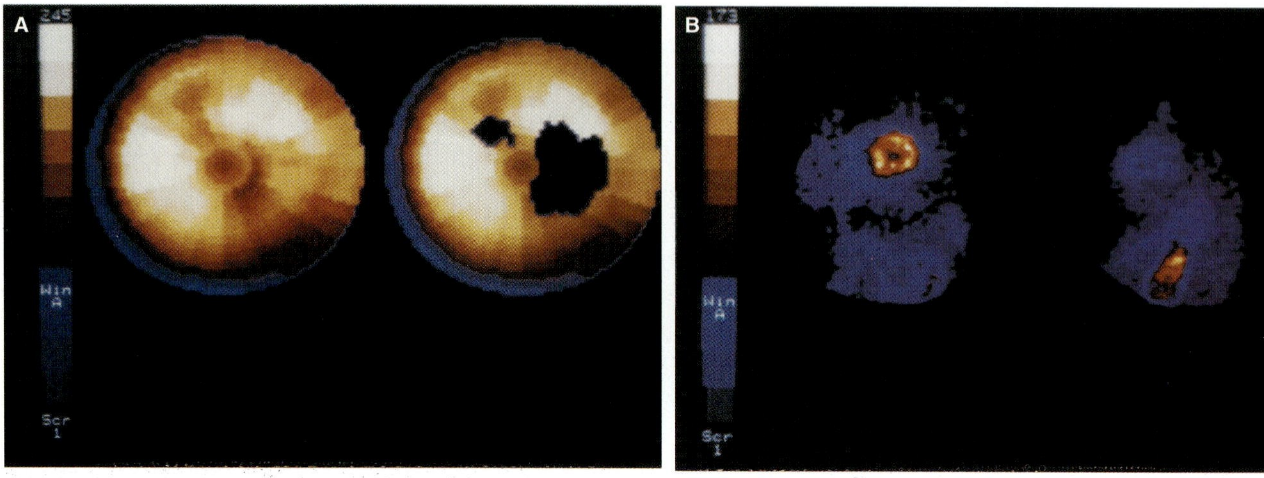

Figure 60 Attenuation by the lateral chest wall. (A) Immediate postexercise polar map (left) and standard deviation blackout plot (right) in an obese male patient with normal coronary arteries. His chest circumference is 50 in, with considerable accumulation of adipose tissue in the chest wall. (B) The 45° left anterior oblique (left) and left lateral (right) polar images obtained from the rotating planar projection image display. In the left lateral view there is marked attenuation of myocardial cavity by lateral chest wall soft tissue. The polar map defect is the result of attenuation by soft tissue in the lateral chest wall of this large patient. (Reprinted with permission from DePuey EG, Garcia EV. Optimal specificity of thallium-201 SPECT through recognition of imaging artifacts. *J Nucl Med* 1989;30:441–449.)

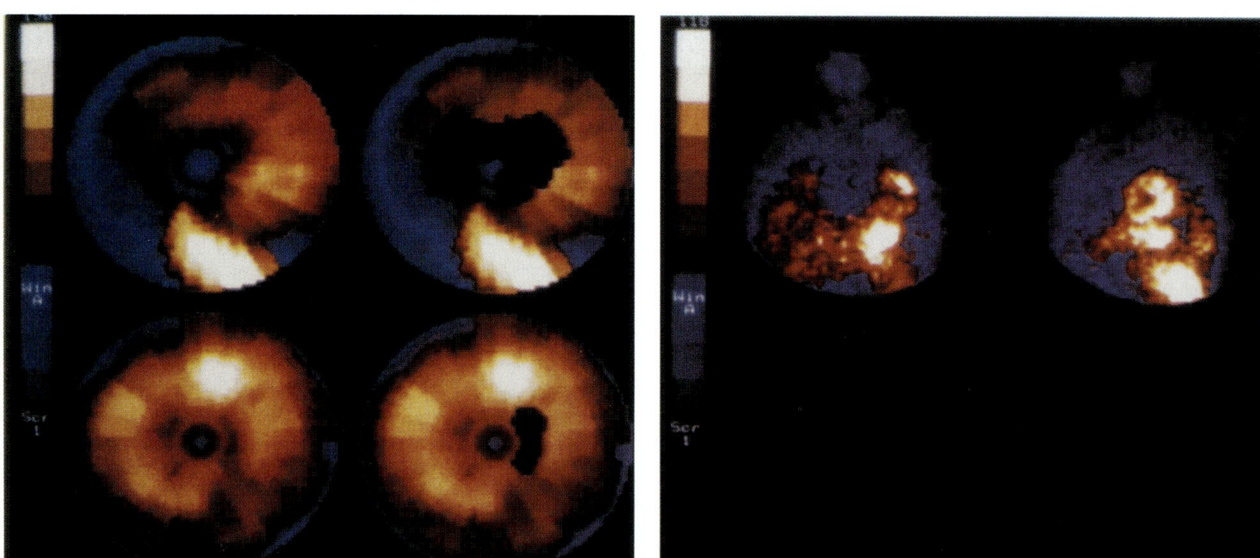

Figure 61 Effect of extracardiac activity. In the left panel are polar plots (left) and standard deviation blackout plots (right) obtained immediately after intravenous dipyridamole infusion (top) and at 4-hr delay (bottom). In the immediate images, high tracer concentration is apparent in the inferior wall of the left ventricle as a result of superimposition of splanchnic activity. Because the image is normalized to the area of greatest tracer concentration, the rest of the ventricle remains counts poor and is identified as abnormal in the standard deviation blackout plot. At 4 hr, after tracer washed out of the splanchnic bed, the inferior artifact is no longer present, and the image appears normal. The artifact mimics extensive ischemia of the septum, anterior and lateral walls. At right are anterior (left) and 60° left anterior oblique (right) planar images obtained from the rotating planar projection image display early after radionuclide administration. Marked splenic tracer concentration is present below the heart and contiguous with the inferior wall of the left ventricle. (Reprinted with permission from DePuey EG, Garcia EV. Optimal specificity of thallium-201 SPECT through recognition of imaging artifacts. *J Nucl Med* 1989; 30:441–449.)

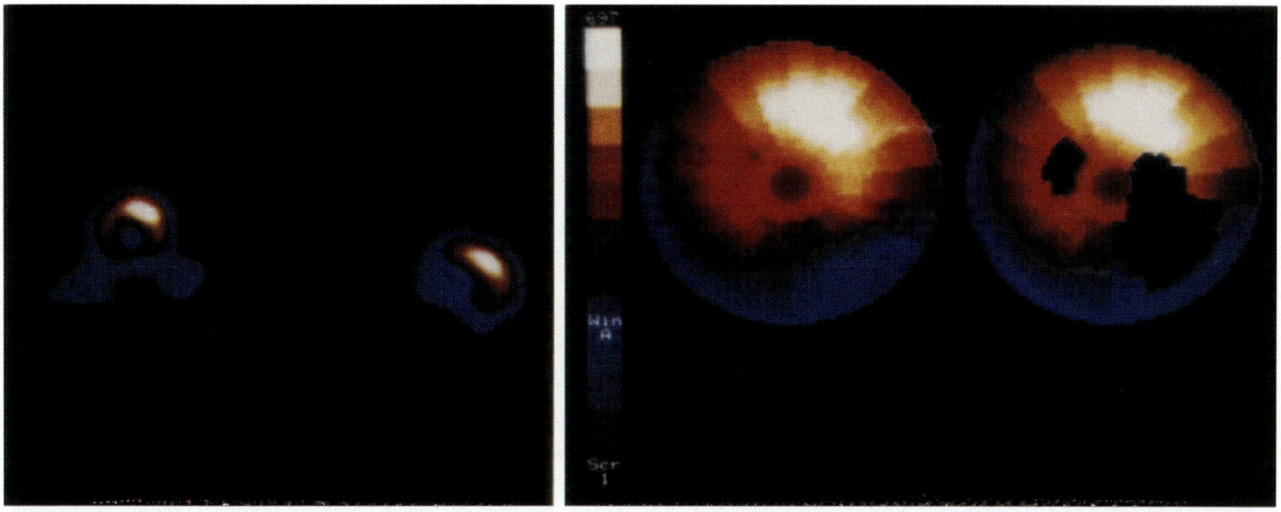

Figure 62 "Hot spot" in the myocardium. The left panel shows midventricular short-axis (left) and vertical long-axis (right) oblique tomographic slices demonstrating increased tracer concentration in the anterior wall of the left ventricle in the region of the anterior papillary muscle. The remainder of the myocardium appears relatively counts poor, because the images are each normalized to the area of greatest count density. The right panel presents the corresponding polar plot (left) and standard deviation blackout plot (right), which also show relatively increased tracer concentration in the anterior wall (11–2 o'clock). Because the polar plot is normalized to the area of greatest count density in the anterior wall, the remainder of the ventricle again appears abnormal. The finding misleads the reader toward a diagnosis of coronary artery disease. (Reprinted with permission from DePuey EG, Garcia EV. Optimal specificity of thallium-201 SPECT through recognition of imaging artifacts. *J Nucl Med* 1989;30:441–449.)

maintain a disk of uniform width, air bubbles must be avoided and there is a risk of contamination. It must be positioned on the collimator so that the plastic sides do not bulge in or out. If a long-lived radionuclide is used, the flood must either be decayed for many half-lives or drained and thoroughly rinsed and the solution stored for decay.

Either type of flood source should be positioned a few inches away from the collimator to reduce the percentage of detected photons that pass through the lead collimator septa. Photons that hit the lead at a steeper incident angle have less lead to pass through than photons closer to the collimator perpendicular. When the flood is farther from the collimator, more of the photons at steeper angles will miss the detector entirely, with little reduction in the number of photons that properly pass through the holes in the collimator. This will produce a more accurate map of detector sensitivity for uniformity correction.

Center of Rotation. Second, the mechanical COR must be determined (Figs. 69,70). Each camera gantry has a mechanical and electronic COR, which will vary over time. Ideally, the COR would be exactly in the center of the field of view, between pixels 32 and 33 in a 64 × 64 matrix. Because this rarely happens, images must be shifted so that the center of the acquisition matrix matches the COR (*355,356*). This COR is then used to align the detector data with respect to the reconstruction matrix. Failure to correct for the COR causes misregistration of pixels during the reconstruction process, which causes artifactual myocardial perfusion defects (see Self-Study Program III, *Nuclear Medicine: Cardiology, Topic 1: Physical and Technical Aspects of Nuclear Cardiology*).

Circuitry inside the camera can (and does) shift detected count locations before sending the location to the computer. Changes in tuning and gains of the PMTs shift the detected location of counts. The movement of the camera detectors does not maintain the same path, because mechanical components wear over prolonged use. This violates the assumption of SPECT reconstruction that all projections detect the same point in space at the same place. Consider a simple case of a hot point seen in 2 projections 180° apart. If the COR is incorrect, this will be seen as 2 different points instead of 1 and the reconstruction process will generate a false representation of that point.

To account for this instability, periodic COR correction measurements must be performed on the camera and acquired on the computer. The frequency of this adjustment may vary from daily to weekly to monthly with different cameras, and the manufacturer's recommendations should be followed. These COR measurements are used to shift each projection a small amount in the X direction, so that the center point of each image set matches the actual center point of the camera movement. This corrects the theoretical COR to match the actual mechanical and electronic COR.

The validity of the COR measurement should be checked every time a new COR study is performed. One simple method involves acquisition of a point source or line source parallel to the axis of rotation. When properly reconstructed, the transaxial image should appear as a round dot. A very-high-frequency cutoff is used for the reconstruction filter, because a smooth filter will blur the dot beyond the ability

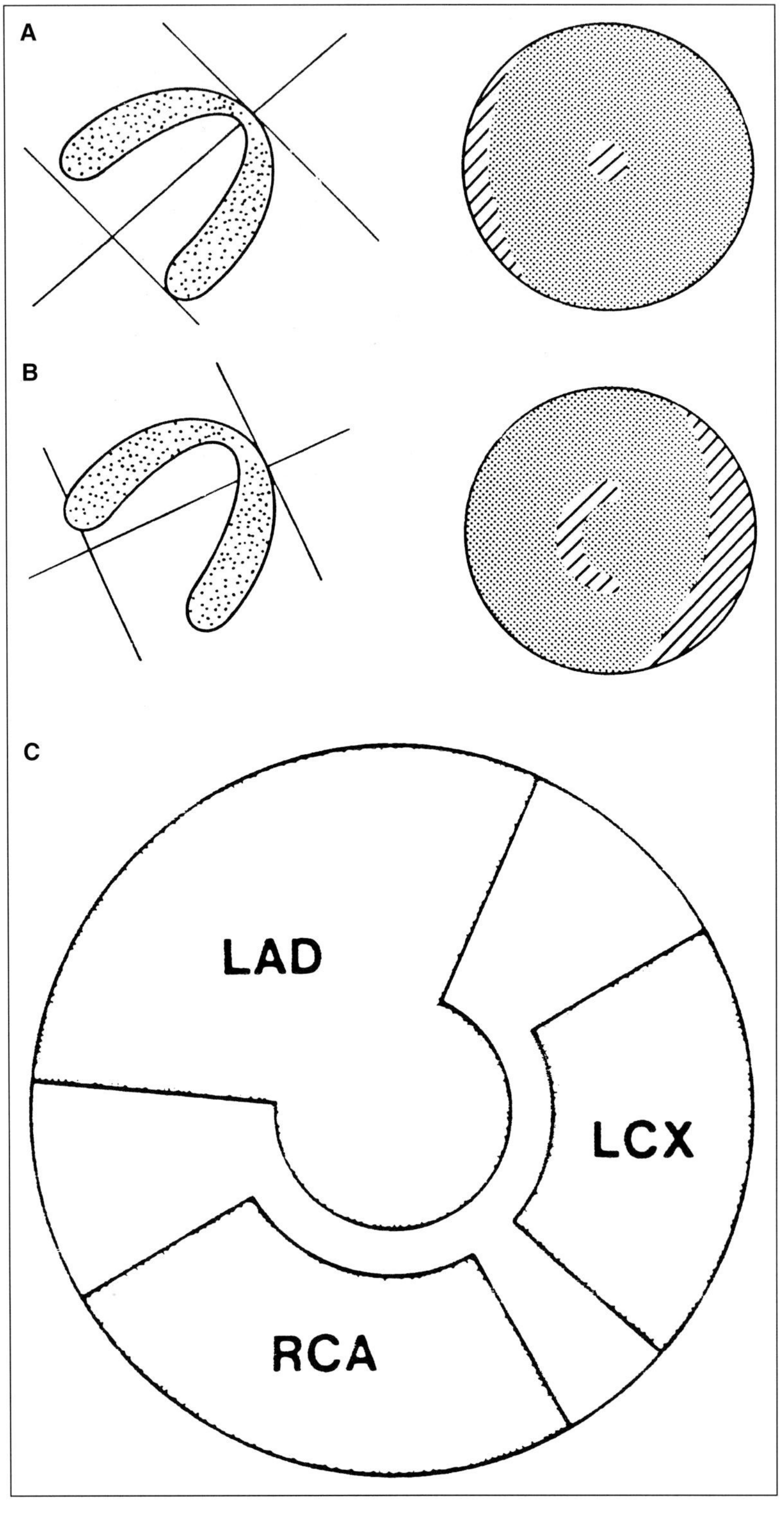

Figure 63 SPECT reconstruction. (A) The correct long-axis selection from the diagrammed transaxial tomographic slice, resulting in a polar image with regions of physiologically decreased count density (cross-hatched areas) at the base of the septum, as a result of the membranous septum, and at the apex, as a result of anatomic thinning. (B) Incorrect long-axis selection with the generation of a semilunar artifact at the periphery of the lateral wall. The apex is shifted anteriorly, creating a comma-shaped artifact in the septum, corresponding to the region of physiologic apical thinning. (C) The areas assigned to regional coronary distributions quantitated by the initial quantitative CEQUAL program (Cedars-Sinai, Los Angeles, CA). (Figures 63A and B were reprinted with permission from DePuey EG, Garcia EV. Optimal specificity of thallium-201 SPECT through recognition of imaging artifacts. *J Nucl Med* 1989;30:441–449.)

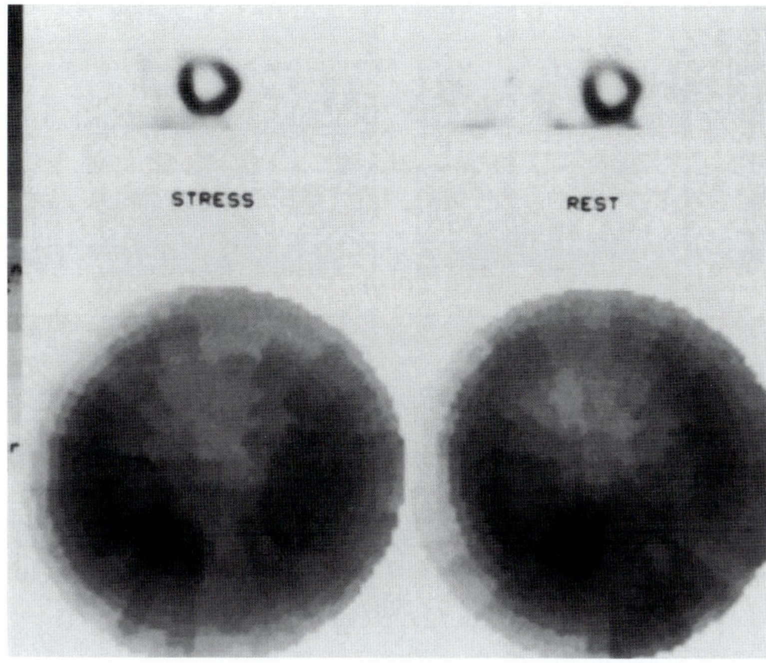

Figure 64 Breast attenuation; slices and polar map. Tomographic short-axis stress and rest slices (top) and polar maps (bottom) from a female patient with large breasts. Fixed breast attenuation artifacts are present in the anterior wall. (Reprinted with permission from DePuey EG. How to detect and avoid myocardial perfusion SPECT artifacts. *J Nucl Med* 1994;35: 699–702.)

to detect an aberration and recognize that the COR has drifted more than should be permitted. Visually, when the COR is starting to drift, the resultant dot will become slightly triangular or curvilinear. A very bad COR will exaggerate this distortion of the point source into a tuning fork artifact, but it should never be allowed to progress to this point. A bad COR means events are not detected where they occur, and this can create myocardial perfusion defects where none exist or, less commonly, fill in perfusion defects where they do exist. In clinical studies, a COR artifact presents with discontinuity and over-riding of adjacent walls. It tends to be most obvious in the horizontal long-axis view, when the septal and lateral walls do not intersect at the apex. All vendors provide a quantitative measure of the COR correction factor and recommend that service be done when the correction factor exceeds some defined limit. When service is performed on any part of the camera that could affect spatial determinations, a new COR should be acquired to account for any electronic shifts. A severe bump on the detector could cause mechanical shifts, and the possibility of an altered COR should be considered and evaluated. Malalignment of the heads of a multihead camera will bring artifacts similar to COR abnormalities.

Pixel Size. Attenuation is defined as the fraction of photons lost per unit of distance, but images are measured in pixels. A conversion factor between pixels and centimeters is essential to calculate the attenuation for each pixel. For this reason and for quantitation of measured distances, pixel size needs to be measured. Pixel size usually does not vary much with time. The usual measurement procedure is to acquire at least 3 point sources in an L shape. The precise distances between the points must be measured in centimeters and entered into the computer, and the computer will correlate the metric distance with the distance between the points in pixels. Pixel dimensions in both X and Y directions should be similar. When pixel size starts to drift, it indicates that the count location circuits inside the camera head or the analog-to-digital converter discrimination circuits are drifting, and a service engineer should be called.

Other Factors. Attention should be given to patient positioning. The patient's arms should be placed out of the field of view. This is aided by a device that supports the arm comfortably above the head, relieving pressure in the axilla (*357*). The collimator should be as close to the patient's chest as possible for optimum resolution. The orbit configuration can itself influence image findings (see Self-Study Program III, *Nuclear Medicine: Cardiology, Topic 1: Physical and Technical Aspects of Nuclear Cardiology*). In some patients with arthritic conditions or other indications, SPECT can be acquired successfully with the arms at the patient's side (*358*). Alternatively, planar imaging may be performed. Occasionally, claustrophobia is encountered with SPECT acquisition, generally with the use of multihead cameras. This should be approached first with demonstrated concern and

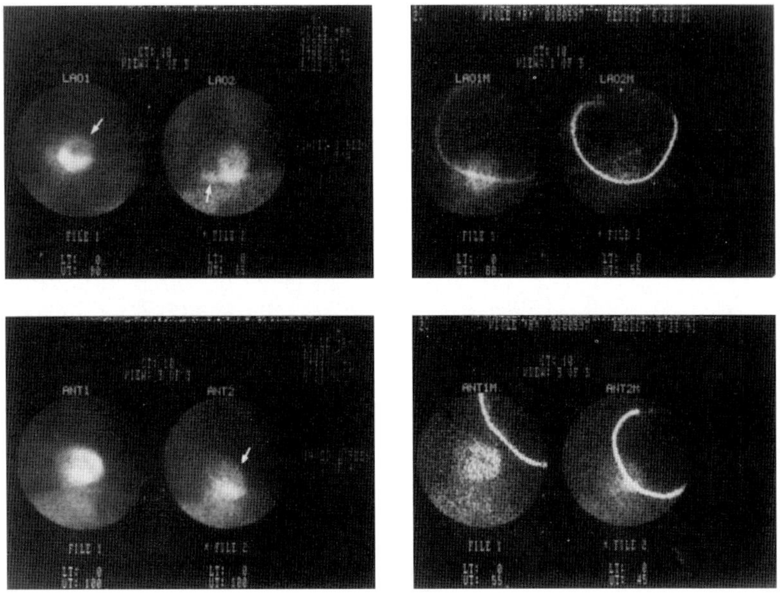

Figure 65 Variable breast position. In the left panels are planar ^{201}Tl images in a woman with large and mobile breasts, with exercise (left anterior oblique 1 [LAO1], anterior 1 [ANT1], left) and at delayed imaging (LAO2, ANT 2, right). Breast markers for each acquisition are shown on the right. On the exercise LAO1 image, a definite attenuation artifact is present (arrow). In the rest LAO2 image, the breast contour is lower and is visualized as a linear area (arrow), with increased activity caused by small angle scatter. The stress anterior view (bottom, ANT 1) is normal, because the breast did not cover the heart and differential attenuation was absent. However, at delayed imaging the contour of the breast crossed the heart in the LAO projection again, causing an attenuation artifact (arrow), now more intense than with exercise. Is this "reverse redistribution"? This is an example of the potential variability of breast position, its related attenuation artifact and possible influence on image interpretation. (Reprinted with permission from Wackers FJTh. Artifacts in planar and SPECT myocardial perfusion imaging. *Am J Cardiol Imaging* 1992;6:42–58.)

understanding in an attempt to gain patient compliance. This often can be overcome with a single-head SPECT gantry, but, rarely, planar images will be necessary. Mild sedation may be necessary if clinically indicated.

During processing, error in assignment of the long axis may result in the generation of short-axis slices that are not perpendicular to the long axis of the left ventricle. This may lead to greater reduction of inferior wall activity of the short-axis slices, because the short-axis plane crosses the inferior wall in a more basal location, which is subject to more attenuation than the anterior wall. Alternatively, such erroneous axial localization may section the septum more distally, omitting the proximal membranous septum. If this error is more prominent in redistribution images, it could lead to apparent redistribution in the basal septum, likely a common cause of artifactual misinterpretation. Both errors will result in misinterpretation in visual and quantitative analysis.

THE MOST COMMON PLANAR AND SPECT IMAGE ARTIFACTS

General Considerations

The final images displayed can misrepresent the physical and clinical reality of myocardial perfusion in various ways (see Self-Study Program III, *Nuclear Medicine: Cardiology, Topic 1: Physical and Technical Aspects of Nuclear Cardiology*). Many of these apply only to SPECT studies and occur when 1 of the principles of SPECT is violated. Most common among SPECT-related artifacts are those that arise from the specific assumption that the target structure will be unchanging in intensity and location during image acquisition. Thus, any technical factor that alters the representation of a structure or displaces it in the field of view can produce SPECT image artifacts. SPECT reconstruction can hide evidence of an attenuation artifact that influences a projection or set of projections in a major manner or, conversely, can magnify a relatively minor problem for planar imaging, such as patient motion, into a significant clinical concern. Although there are few ways to distort unprocessed planar images without the distortion being readily apparent, extensive SPECT image processing can conceal artifacts of acquisition and fabricate others. Artifacts are intrinsic to all imaging modalities. Nowhere has the effort to prevent, recognize and correct image artifacts been greater or more successful than in myocardial perfusion imaging.

For example, extracardiac activity near the myocardium may obscure defects or, alternatively, may cause defects in the reconstruction process by moving

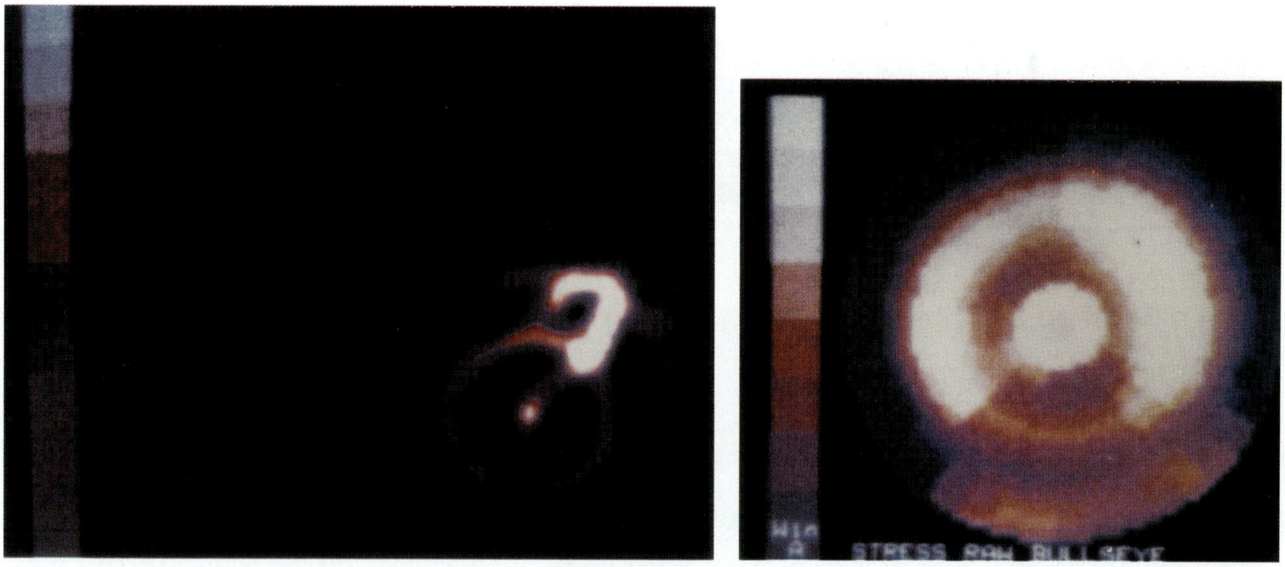

Figure 66 Ring artifact. Ring artifact in a transaxial tomographic slice (left) as a result of a marked flood field nonuniformity. The corresponding polar map (right) also displays the concentric ring artifact. (Reprinted with permission from DePuey EG, Garcia EV. Optimal specificity of thallium-201 SPECT through recognition of imaging artifacts. *J Nucl Med* 1989;30:441–449.)

counts from the myocardium to the hotter areas. This most commonly occurs with hepatic and other subdiaphragmatic activity. Such count reduction is a result of the combination of the SPECT reconstruction algorithm and tissue attenuation. The closer to the heart the extracardiac hot spots, the greater the influence they can have. In spatial terms, a negative penumbra around the backprojection rays (a filter effect designed to enhance contrast and reduce star artifacts) will be emphasized around the hot spot, creating a rim of decreased activity and a dense defect in the inferior wall. Technetium-99m sestamibi is much more likely to present such a problem than is ^{201}Tl, because of the more frequent sestamibi localization near the heart. The reduced and faster biliary excretion of tetrofosmin should reduce the problems related to high levels of paracardiac background.

Successful image interpretation depends on the recognition and avoidance of such artifacts. In the following sections, attenuation and scatter, common to both planar and SPECT methods, are considered along with attempts at their correction. Then the principles of SPECT imaging are considered, and the major SPECT artifacts are catalogued with a review of their cause(s), recognition and, when possible, approaches to correction. Before artifacts are considered, the reader should be aware of variants in the normal image pattern and the relationship of this pattern to the coronary arteries, as well as some pathologic and nonartifactual image findings, the nonperfusion indicators of ischemia.

Variants of Normal SPECT Analysis

Different portions of the left ventricular myocardium may be assigned to the distribution of the LAD, LCX and the posterior descending coronary artery, a branch of the RCA in patients with a right dominant coronary system (*310*). Because of

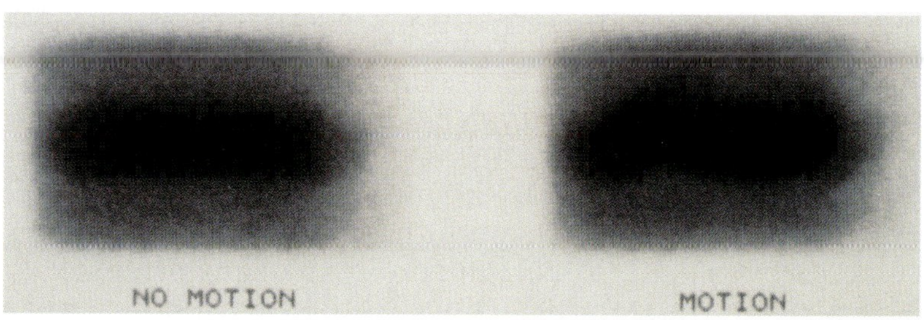

Figure 67 Patient motion: "blurogram." Summed planar projection images without (left) and with (right) patient motion. (Reprinted with permission from DePuey EG. How to detect and avoid myocardial perfusion SPECT artifacts. *J Nucl Med* 1994;35:699–702.)

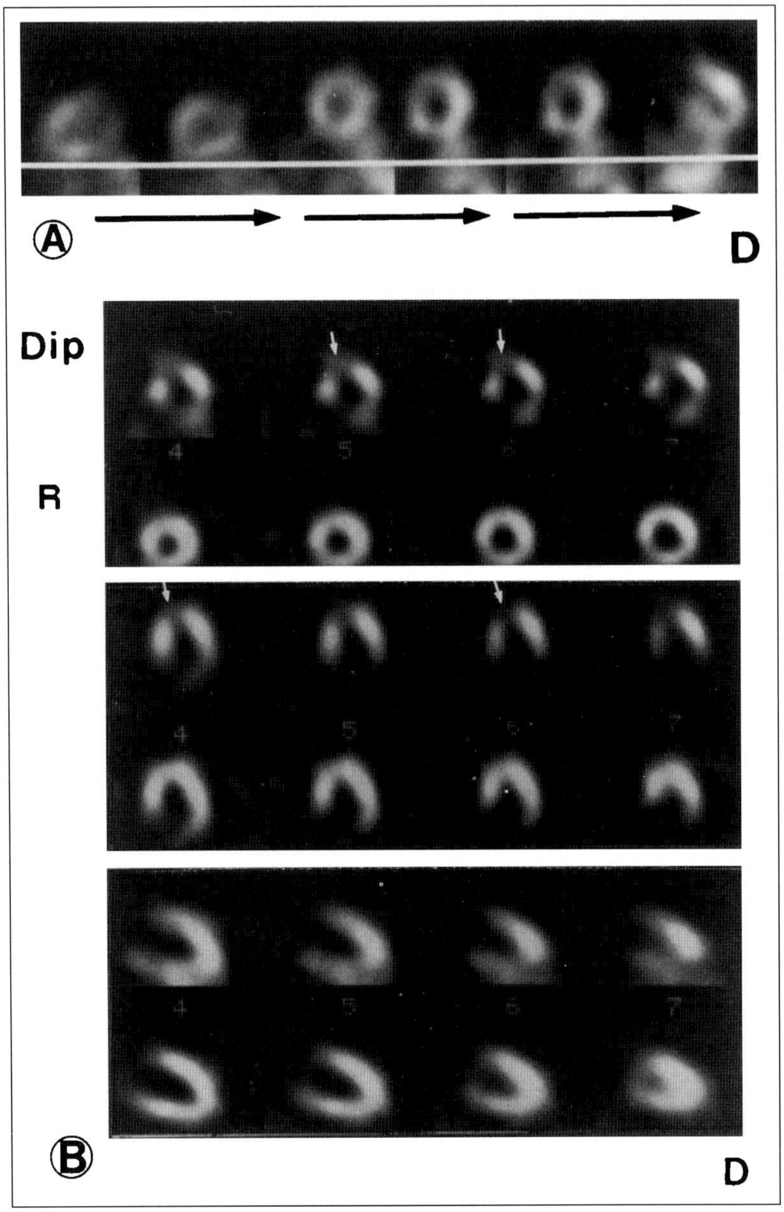

Figure 68 The effects of patient motion. (A) Selected thallium-201 (^{201}Tl) analog images, from the left posterior oblique (left) to the right anterior oblique (right) positions before SPECT reconstruction. During left anterior oblique acquisition, the patient suddenly moved upward on the table. The white bar is a reference for the initial position of the inferior wall. Thallium-201 SPECT images of the same patient are shown in (B). The initial images (after dipyridamole [Dip] infusion) show a defect in the anteroapical and septal regions (arrow). The redistribution (R) images are normal. The "positive" results of this SPECT study are caused entirely by marked body motion during initial image acquisition, not evident at redistribution imaging. Because the stress image, acquired in an anxious, apprehensive patient who never before saw a scintillation camera, is the first to be acquired in the standard ^{201}Tl protocol, motion in this phase is most likely. (Reprinted with permission from Wackers FJTh. Artifacts in planar and SPECT myocardial perfusion imaging. *Am J Cardiol Imaging* 1992;6:42–58.)

variations in the size, branching, collateral supply and dominance of the individual coronary arteries, the precise vascular territory of a given coronary artery will differ among individuals, but general guidelines are helpful in assigning regions of myocardium to individual arteries. The anterior and anteroseptal segments on the short-axis slices are generally supplied by the LAD. The LAD also supplies the anteroseptal segments on the horizontal long-axis slice, the anterior segments on the vertical long-axis slices and the apical segments on the vertical and horizontal long-axis slices. The inferior and inferoseptal segments on the short-axis slices are supplied by the RCA, as are the inferior and inferoapical segments on the vertical long-axis slices. However, the distal inferior segment may fall within the distal LAD region. The LCX usually supplies the lateral and inferolateral segments on the short-axis slices. The anterolateral segments are typically supplied by the diagonal branch of the LAD, although this territory may sometimes derive its blood supply from a ramus intermedius coronary artery or a high-rising obtuse marginal branch of the LCX artery. Certain portions of the left ventricular myocardium have a variable association with a specific coronary distribution and may be called "border zones." These border zones are located at the interface between specific coronary territories and represent regions with a relatively higher likelihood of overlap of the coronary blood supply. These variations of the coronary arterial tree reduce the ability to determine, with a very high specificity, disease in individual coronary arteries. However, when the coronary anatomy is known in an individual patient, optimum assignment of tomographic perfusion defects to individual coronary arteries and their branches can be performed, involving the direct computer overlap of angiographically

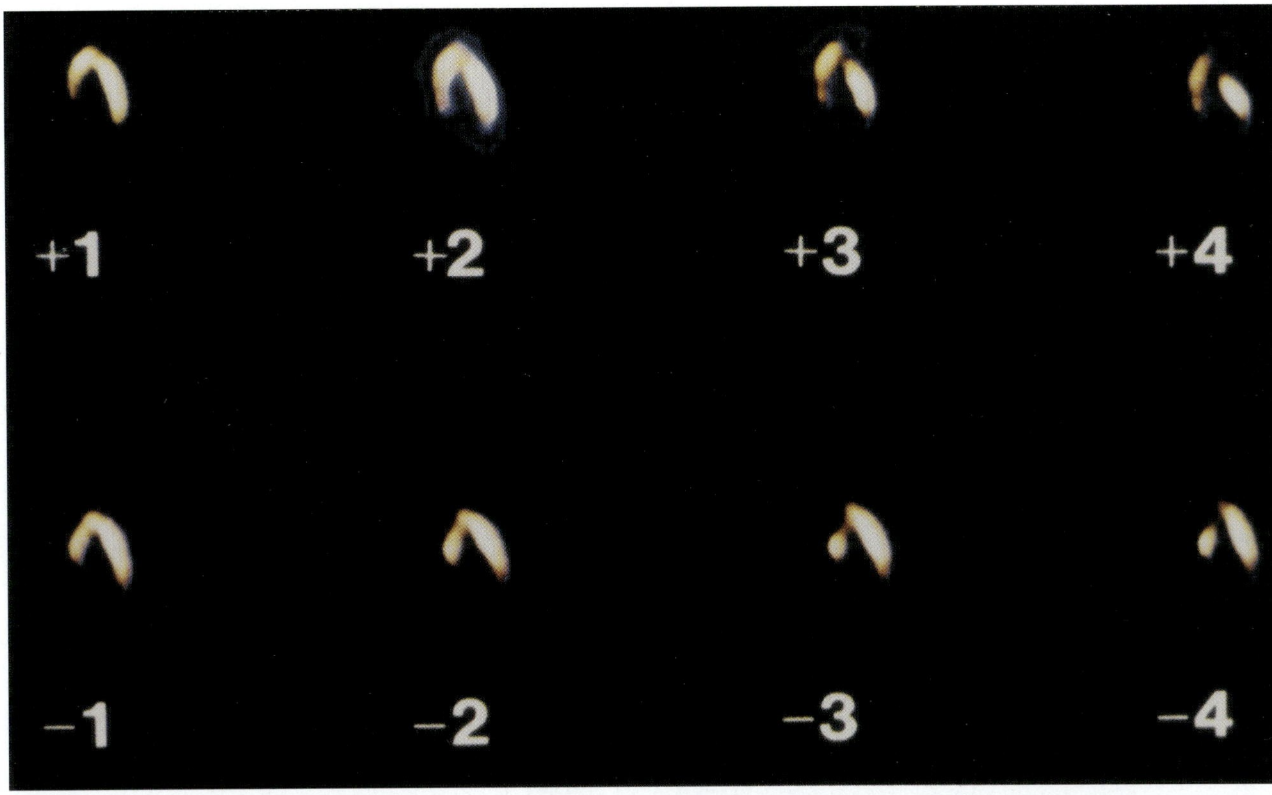

Figure 69 Center of rotation (COR) artifact. Horizontal long-axis slices are shown in a normal individual. The COR was progressively shifted to the right (+1–+4 pixels) or to the left (−1–−4 pixels). With increasing COR artifacts, the septal and lateral walls appear to be misaligned. Rightward COR errors produce linear apicoposterior defects, and leftward errors create linear anteroapical defects. (Reprinted with permission from DePuey EG, Garcia EV. Optimal specificity of thallium-201 SPECT through recognition of imaging artifacts. *J Nucl Med* 1989;30:441–449.)

defined coronary territories on the SPECT perfusion map (*66,91, 95,257, 332,333*).

In each of the 3 vascular territories, receiver operating characteristics (ROC) curve analysis has been used to determine the normal limits of the total percentage of circumferential profile points and polar coordinate map abnormalities that most accurately identify disease in each of the 3 coronary arteries. On early polar maps, the threshold of significant defect size for the LAD, LCX and PDA territories were found to be ≥12%, 12% and 8%, respectively. This will be refined with subsequent versions.

Anatomic Variants. A normal finding on the short-axis slices is a reduction and drop-out of counts in the septal region toward the base of the heart, as a result of the presence of the membranous septum, which does not contain myocardial tissue. Activity in this region is therefore low, resulting in an apparent perfusion defect. These basal septal structures also are apparent on the horizontal long-axis slices, in which the septum appears shorter in length than the posterolateral wall.

Myocardial thinning in the region of the apex of the left ventricle is also a normal finding and may lead to lower counts at the apex, most noticeable in the vertical and horizontal long-axis. Image defects determined by computer analysis must always be sought visually, although when subtle they may be hard to confirm. One study has confirmed the superiority of perfusion image localization

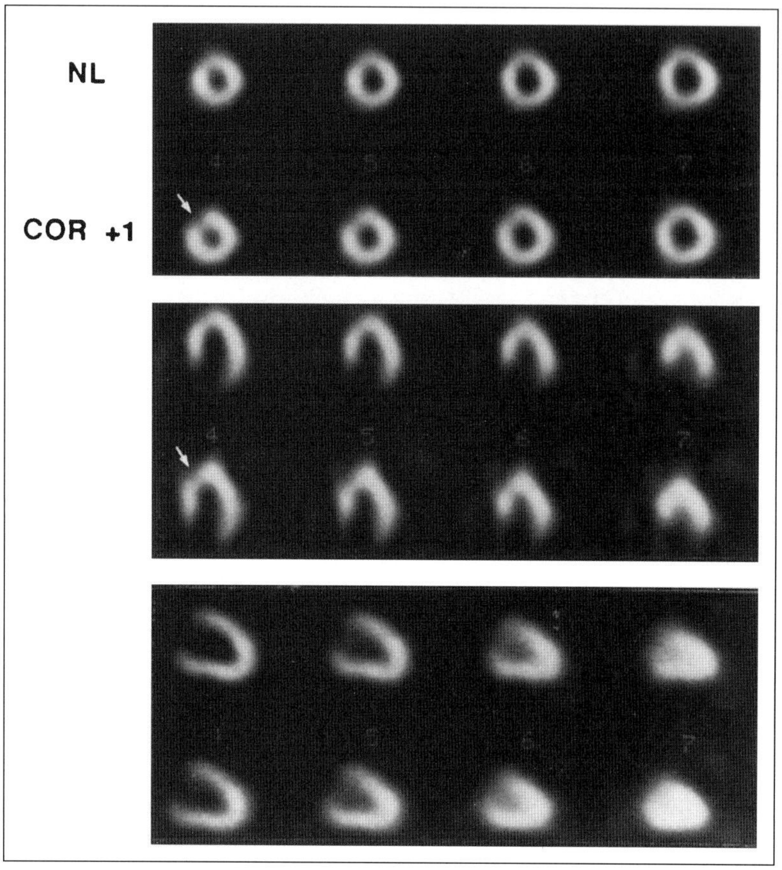

Figure 70 Center of rotation (COR) artifact. SPECT technetium-99m sestamibi images in a normal subject. The original SPECT slices (NL, top) are compared with those acquired after the introduction of a 1-pixel COR offset (COR +1). Small artifactual defects are present on short-axis and horizontal long-axis slices (arrows). (Reprinted with permission from Wackers FJTh. Artifacts in planar and SPECT myocardial perfusion imaging. *Am J Cardiol Imaging* 1992;6:42–58.)

of coronary lesions compared with the stress ECG as well as the localizing value of ST elevation (*359*).

Nonperfusion and Other Indicators of Extensive Coronary Disease and Ischemia

Lung uptake on ^{201}Tl images, cavitary dilation and basal uptake are 3 image indicators of advanced, extensive, or multivessel CAD (Figs. 71,72). Dilation may be associated with induced subendocardial ischemia or underperfusion. Lung uptake is associated with delayed pulmonary transit and increased extraction of the tracer in the setting of extensive coronary disease and severe left ventricular dysfunction or prolonged transit of any origin. Basal uptake demonstrates increased activity where usually there is least, signifying the extent and intensity of distal underperfusion.

"Dense cavitary photopenia" may be seen with planar or SPECT imaging. Because the blood pool has little activity, this finding does not relate to a displacement of blood pool activity, as would happen with a thrombus. Rather, it represents reduced intensity of the region of the apparent left ventricular cavity because of the absence of activity in the overlying, transparent, planar wall. Alternatively, the imperfectly tomographic SPECT image, with the cavity generally "contaminated" by counts in the moving, perfused, overlying wall, may demonstrate photopenia because of a lack of activity or motion in the overlying wall. If induced by stress, photopenia suggests a tight, high-risk lesion. It extends partially and irregularly over the cavity, indicating its relationship as a property of the overlying wall. However, when fixed, as is often the case, it indicates scar and the proper environment for thrombus formation (*360*) (Fig. 73).

Here, a cavity/myocardial intensity or count ratio is taken as a marker for left ventricular dysfunction on rest ^{99m}Tc sestamibi studies. This is a natural extrapolation, relating abnormalities of rest perfusion to rest dysfunction. However, relative underperfusion may be more evident at stress and has similar implications about stress-induced underperfusion and dysfunction in the presence of normal rest function (*361*). These image findings are discussed further in Self-Study Program III, *Nuclear Medicine: Cardiology, Topic 6: Myocardial Perfusion Scintigraphy—Clinical Aspects.*

Attenuation

Planar images can be distorted during acquisition by simple attenuation artifacts when a larger fraction of the emitted photons are absorbed from 1 region of the heart than from another. The obvious causes are easy to remedy: an absorber in a shirt pocket or a necklace or some other object between the heart and the detector. These items cause a distinctly defined area that should be recognized readily.

Breast tissue in women (or men) or a dense, thick chest wall can cause more subtle defects. Such apparent defects will only be visible in projections in which the attenuating stucture, the breast, for example, is between the heart and the detector. A common accompaniment of breast attenuation is a semicircular area of decreased activity, extending into the cardiac background. This may be outlined by a line of enhanced intensity related to scatter off the breast from photons in transit. All myocardial images should be acquired with breast tissue displaced from the heart or homogeneously applied to it.

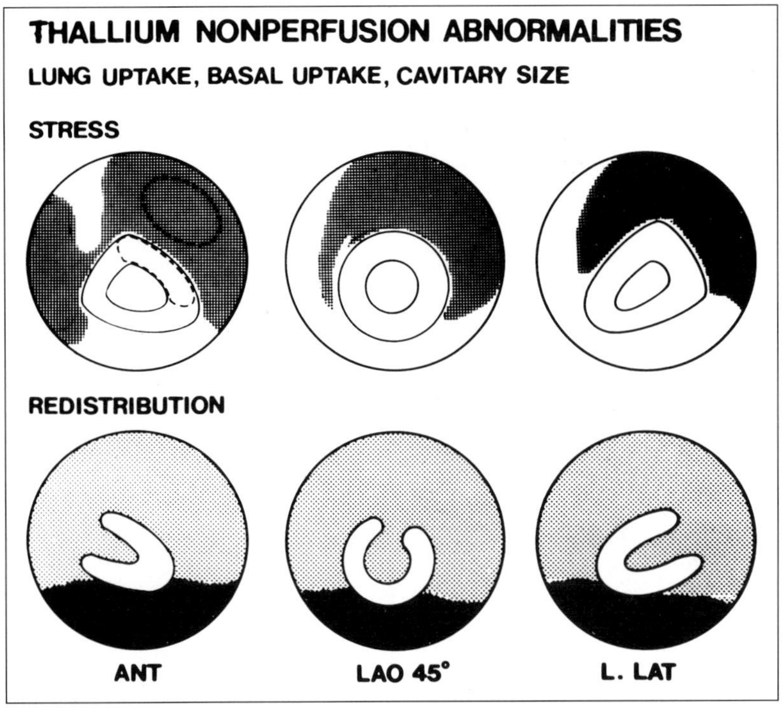

Figure 71 Nonperfusion indicators of high-risk coronary artery disease. Shown diagrammatically are the 3 perfusion scintigraphic indicators associated with high coronary risk which interact with, but are unrelated to, the distribution of perfusion. These are the nonperfusion indicators of high coronary risk and, in addition to lung uptake, include cavitary dilation and basal uptake (evidence of severe, generalized, distal underperfusion.) Lung uptake is not often seen with delayed ^{99m}Tc imaging. Delayed imaging also may reduce the value of true cavitary dilation ANT = anterior; LAO = left anterior oblique; L. Lat = left lateral. (Reprinted with permission from Canhasi B, Dae MW, Botvinick EH, et al. Interaction of supplementary indicators of ischemia and stress electrocardiography in the diagnosis of multivessel coronary disease. *J Am Coll Cardiol* 1985;6:581–589.)

In both planar and SPECT acquisition, breast tissue attenuation is the most commonly occurring artifact in females (*323,348,349,362*). Breast tissue generally attenuates activity of the anterolateral, anteroseptal and upper posterolateral walls and may also attenuate activity of the lateral wall in the LAO projection. In other planar projections, however, attenuation will be reduced or absent, as will related defects. SPECT artifacts from this source most commonly manifest as areas of decreased activity in the anterior, anteroseptal and anterolateral segments but could affect the lateral wall, as well. These defects usually do not change from the initial poststress to the redistribution image, provided the breast position is the same in the 2 acquisitions. However, shifting of the breast position or background activity that varies from the initial to the redistribution study may cause attenuation patterns that simulate reversibility, partial reversibility or reverse redistribution, a treacherous situation that must be guarded against.

For this reason the breast should generally be left in its normal position, stabilized with a bra, or strapped in the same position during each acquisition. A clue to the presence of breast tissue attenuation may be obtained from planar images obtained before the SPECT study or by examining the individual projection images obtained during SPECT acquisition. On the anterior and LAO planar images, the contour of the breast may be superimposed on the cardiac image, causing attenuation of the anterior wall of the heart and the extracardiac tissues. The negative image of the breast also may be seen coming into view on the rotating projection images as the 45° LAO projection approaches. This negative image disappears as the cardiac images are rotated more laterally.

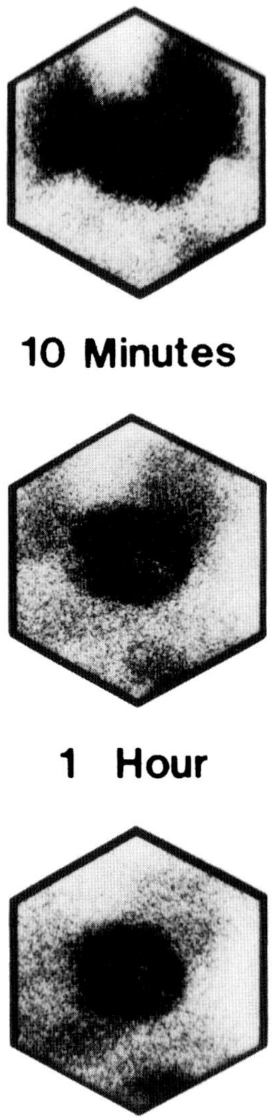

Figure 72 Lung uptake. (A) The familiar butterfly pattern of dense "lung uptake." The finding relates to the nonspecific slow transit of thallium-201 through the lungs, with resultant increased extraction. When associated with coronary disease, it generally indicates increased pulmonary capillary pressure, advanced coronary disease and high related coronary risk. (Reprinted with permission from Gibson RS, Watson DD, Carabello BA, et al. Clinical implications of increased lung uptake of Tl-201 during exercise scintigraphy 2 weeks after myocardial infarction. *Am J Cardiol* 1982;49:1586–1593.)

Although these techniques identify the presence of breast attenuation, they do not identify the origin of reduced radioactivity in breast attenuation. Modestly reduced radioactivity in the anterior myocardial wall, sparing the apex and septum, also strongly supports the impression of an attenuation-related defect rather than an anterior descending perfusion defect (Fig. 74). However, LAD disease in the presence of a patent bypass graft or, less commonly, with extensive collaterals and serial lesions could produce a similar pattern. Preserved function noted in gated sestamibi images, reflective of function at the time of image acquisition, in an area with an apparent modest perfusion defect, objectively supports an attenuation cause for fixed defects (*299,363*). Evidence of normal systolic function during stress would suggest attenuation as the cause of even an apparently reversible defect. Also, evidence of differential attenuation on the sequential, dual-isotope protocol supports the presence of attenuation (*290*). Repeat imaging with the breast retracted or compressed and more homogeneously distributed in the prone position should reduce or eliminate breast-related attenuation artifact in planar or SPECT images (Fig. 75). This reacquisition is more securely applied with ^{99m}Tc sestamibi or tetrofosmin, relatively stable agents once localized, and is aided by the speeded acquisition with multihead cameras and complemented by the rapid processing of modern computers.

When effects of artifact are evident in the projection image database and are not clearly separable from the myocardium, they usually will be evident on SPECT reconstruction, because the same defects are encoded and plotted in 3 dimensions during SPECT processing. Although such defects have been said not to triangulate on SPECT study, even attenuation artifacts will appear to triangulate after SPECT reconstruction but will often present with patterns of image abnormality, atypical for CAD. All such data, whatever their source, will be plotted as intensity levels and will be presented in a consistent form and triangulated from the same 3-dimensional database to the SPECT slices. Only defects or image abnormalities related to display or reproduction artifacts may appear not to triangulate on SPECT presentation.

More commonly seen in short or obese patients (but not exclusively), the diaphragm may attenuate the inferior wall in the anterior planar view and in inferior and inferoseptal basal regions of SPECT slices. To reduce or eliminate attenuation of the inferior left ventricular regions by the diaphragm and subdiaphragmatic structures, the anterior steep LAO or left lateral planar image should be obtained with the patient in the right lateral decubitus position (*259,304,311, 349,364,365*), and SPECT acquisition in the prone rather than the supine position has been effective (*304*). However, because of their common occurrence, these findings often are included in normal databases. In addition, prone positioning may be employed when the patient has difficulty maintaining the supine position and also permits separation of subdiaphragmatic radioactivity, commonly present with sestamibi study (Fig. 76). Imaging in the prone position also may reduce frequency of patient motion and "upward creep" artifacts (*303,304*). Although prone acquisition often produces a small region of reduced anterior activity as a result of attenuation by the imaging table intervening between camera and target, the finding is usually well differentiated from defects related to major breast attenuation or true perfusion defects. An increase in relative hepatic uptake of uncertain cause has been reported in association with severe right coronary lesions (*364*).

The right ventricle and its blood pool, especially when enlarged, may also attenuate the inferior left ventricular wall in the anterior view. This may explain the normal depression of inferior wall activity in the anterior planar projection and could suggest a defect when activity is beyond the usual range of normal attenuation (*311, 365,366*). This may be suspected when an enlarged right ventricle is noted in the 45° LAO view and the inferior wall in the steep LAO view is completely normal.

When high levels of hepatic uptake of perfusion tracers are evident, lower-than-expected counts values may be recognized in the adjacent inferior

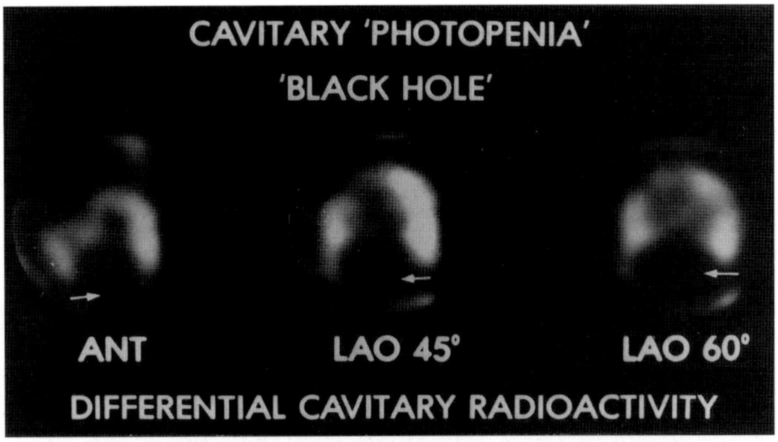

Figure 73 Cavitary photopenia. Shown in anterior (ANT) and 45° and 60° left anterior oblique (LAO) projections are perfusion scintigrams performed on a patient with a large apical aneurysm. Note the area of reduced radioactivity, an apparent "black hole" in the apical wall, appearing to extend into the region of the "cavity." The latter most likely relates to reduced radioactivity in the overlying myocardial wall. (Reprinted with permission from Dae M, Canhasi B, Botvinick E, et al. The etiology and implications of dense cavitary "photopenia" on myocardial perfusion scintigraphy. *Investig Radiol* 1985;20:388–392.)

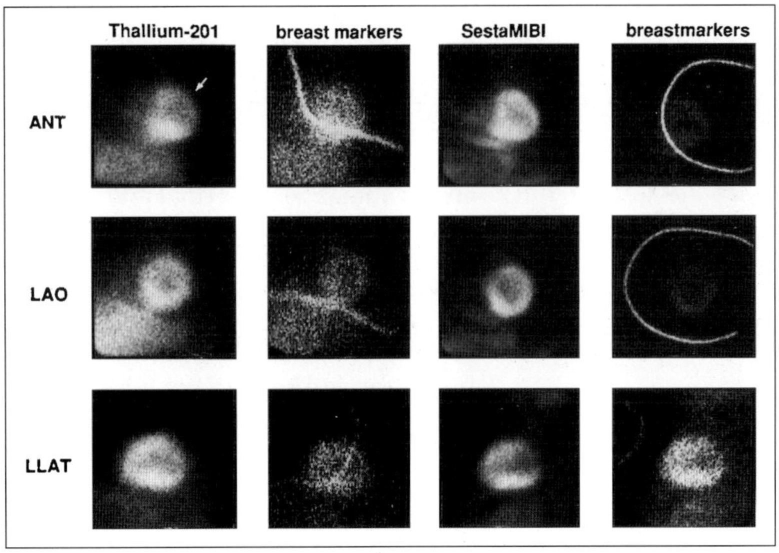

Figure 74 Breast attenuation: thallium-201 (^{201}Tl) and technetium-99m (^{99m}Tc). Thallium-201 and ^{99m}Tc sestamibi planar images in a woman with large, pendulous breasts. Breast markers indicate the breast contour. The anterior (ANT) view shows a typical attenuation artifact (arrow) in the anterolateral wall, created by attenuation by the overlying breast tissue. The breast marker corresponds to the boundary of the defect. This often can be seen in clinical studies with a highlighted linear intensification from scattered radiation, which marks boundaries of the source of scattered activity, the breast or a skin fold. In the left anterior oblique (LAO) view, the breast contour is below the heart. Because the heart is entirely covered by breast tissue, attenuation and cardiac activity is relatively homogeneous and no attenuation artifact occurred. The marker on the left lateral (LLAT) view indicates a skin fold across the heart. However, no obvious attenuation artifact is evident. Technetium-99m sestamibi images in the same patient are essentially normal. Breast markers show the superimposition of the breast on the myocardium in the ANT view to be similar to that seen with ^{201}Tl. However, any related attenuation defect in this view or the LLAT is modest, because of the higher energy of ^{99m}Tc. (Reprinted with permission from Wackers FJTh. Artifacts in planar and SPECT myocardial perfusion imaging. *Am J Cardiol Imaging* 1992;6:42–58.)

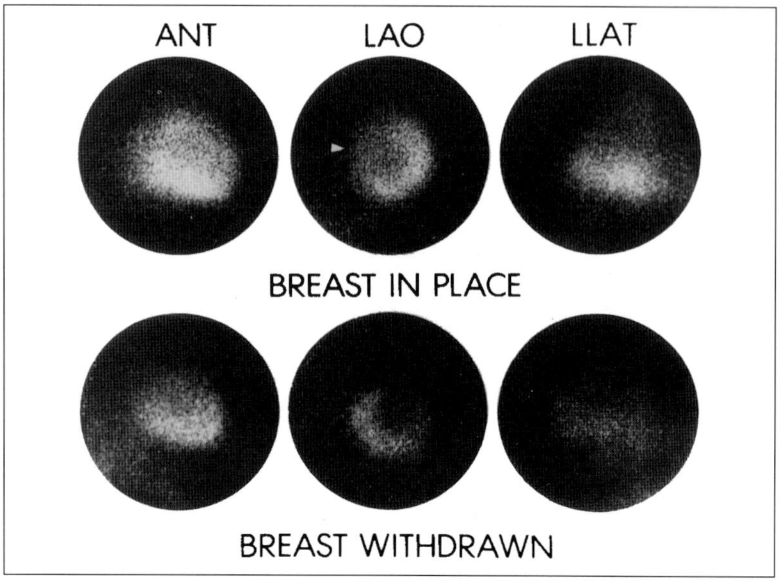

Figure 75 Breast attenuation. Planar images (above) show an apparent defect in the region of the septum in the left anterior oblique (LAO) projection. The defect moves to the lateral wall with altered breast position. Constancy of anatomic positioning is a critical aspect of successful perfusion imaging. SPECT, gating and other methods help reduce errors resulting from soft tissue attenuation. Technical advances in attenuation correction eventually will eliminate it. ANT = anterior projection; LLAT = left lateral projection. (Reprinted with permission from Botvinick E, Dae M, O'Connell JW, Ortendahl D, Hattner RS. The scintigraphic evaluation of the cardiovascular system. In: Parmley WW, Chatterjee K, eds. *Cardiology.* Philadelphia, PA: JB Lippincott; 1991:1–121.)

myocardial wall. This phenomenon was studied in simulations and found to be the result of photon attenuation effects during reconstruction, distorting liver reconstruction and influencing inferior wall activity. It can be eliminated by attenuation correction (*367*).

Although the higher-energy ^{99m}Tc is less readily attenuated than the lower-energy ^{201}Tl, it is still highly attenuated and retains ~85% of the attenuation level of ^{201}Tl. The reader must be on guard for attenuation artifacts with ^{99m}Tc agents as well as when using ^{201}Tl. Similarly, SPECT reconstruction reduces the intensity of attenuation artifacts. The combined ^{201}Tl rest/^{99m}Tc sestamibi or tetrofosmin stress protocol presents the possibility of recognizing attenuation artifact and possibly correcting for it by noting the differential effect of the regional attenuation of the 2 radionuclides (*290*). The better resolution of the ^{99m}Tc-based images, on the other hand, may make more evident the normal variations of radionuclide distribution, such as the apical slit. Caution is advised in labeling all defects more evident on the higher-energy image as abnormal and perfusion related.

SPECT reconstruction reduces attenuation artifact seen in planar images. Attenuation may yet be appreciated as the cause of a defect, by evaluation of the defect appearance in the rotational display of planar projection images and by the anatomic configuration of defects. Alternatively, image gating may aid identification of attenuation artifact. Recently, methods for attenuation correction have been introduced.

Attenuation Correction. Perfusion may be quantitated absolutely if presented with attenuation and scatter correction. This is now possible only with PET. Relative quantitation of perfusion may compare counts in an area with those in another region at the same time or to counts in the same region at another time. The distribution of counts or perfusion is often normalized to the most intense pixel and compared with a database of tracer distribution in a group with a low-likelihood of CAD. However, such databases have a broad range of normal values in patients who may not resemble the habitus of the patient being considered. The databases also are dependent on the specific protocol applied. Attempts to correct for attenuation and scatter have a dual objective: to increase the diagnostic accuracy of the method and permit absolute quantitation of regional perfusion.

Methods for attenuation and scatter correction are varied and currently investigational in nature. Results are inconsistent, sometimes demonstrating improved specificity, sometimes worsening specificity by the introduction of artifacts and rarely increasing sensitivity (*13*). Recent technical developments in

SPECT acquisition and processing provide transmission correction of emission data. In the last few years, several groups have developed prototype transmission–emission CT systems. These attempt to optimize the signal-to-noise ratio of transmission data, overcome the cross-talk of transmission and emission photons, produce a simple user-friendly design, and keep radiation exposure low, all for a reasonable cost. They have been implemented on some commercial systems (by ADAC, Siemens, Picker and others) (*368,369*) and are being sold. For a not inconsequentially increased purchase cost, most manfacturers of commercial 2- and 3-head cameras now present the user with the possible application of attenuation correction algorithms. Either a fanbeam or scanning line-source technology is used. Gadolinium-153 (^{153}Gd), 100 keV, with a half-life of 270 days, is most commonly used for acquisition of the transmission image. The limited field of the fanbeam pattern bears the potential of "truncation" artifacts because of the resultant acquisition of incomplete tomographic data sets, especially when applied in large patients (*370*). Researchers have presented methods to reduce this error (*371,372*) (Fig. 77). The subject is reviewed in an article by Bacharach et al. (*373*) and discussed in Self-Study Program III, *Nuclear Medicine: Cardiology, Topic 1: Physical and Technical Aspects of Nuclear Cardiology.* A fixed-line transmission source geometry had the advantages of no moving parts, high-transmission counting statistics and low radiation exposure, but the symmetric fanbeam collimator produced truncation artifacts of the transmission projection data. An asymmetric fanbeam collimator promises to reduce this problem. However, initial transmission systems based on a triple detector system with a 360° orbit were not accepted.

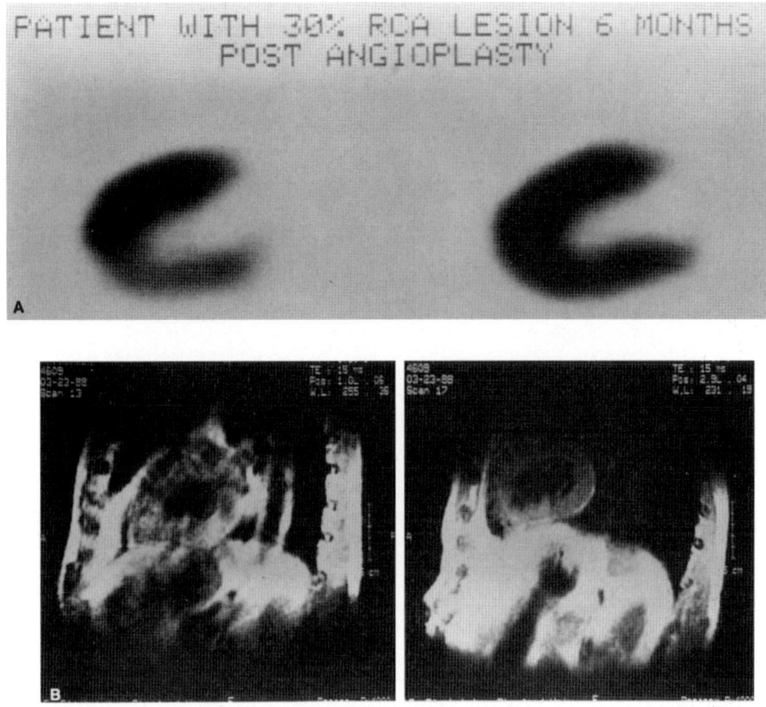

Figure 76 Attenuation demonstrated. (A) Vertical long-axis cuts through the midleft ventricle of a 71-yr-old man with atypical symptoms, a normal electrocardiogram and a coronary arteriogram showing 20%–30% narrowing in the right coronary artery 6 mo after angioplasty of that vessel. The supine study (left), which was done first, shows an inferior defect, whereas the prone study (right) is normal. (B) MR image of this same patient. The images are sagittal cuts through the midleft ventricle, again acquired with the patient supine (left) and prone (right). The supine image shows a "backward flop" of the heart, with partial obscuring of the inferior wall by the diaphragm. In contrast, the prone image shows the heart to lie more anteriorly in the chest, with a good separation between heart and diaphragm, explaining the reduced attenuation in this position. Prone imaging is 1 of several ways to differentiate true perfusion abnormalities from attenuation artifacts. (Reprinted with permission from Segall GM, Davis MJ. Prone versus supine thallium myocardial SPECT: a method to decrease artifactual inferior wall defects. *J Nucl Med* 1989;30:548–555.)

The most widely available and current method of choice is a scanning line source for transmission image generation on a dual-head camera with a 90° configuration and parallel-hole collimation, applied over 180° from the RAO to the LPO. The transmission scan is acquired before or simultaneously with the emission study to estimate the nonuniform distribution of attenuating structures between camera and myocardium. An external radionuclide source is applied to perform transmission imaging and is combined with a "blank" scan to determine the total attenuation distribution in 3 dimensions (*374,375*). The

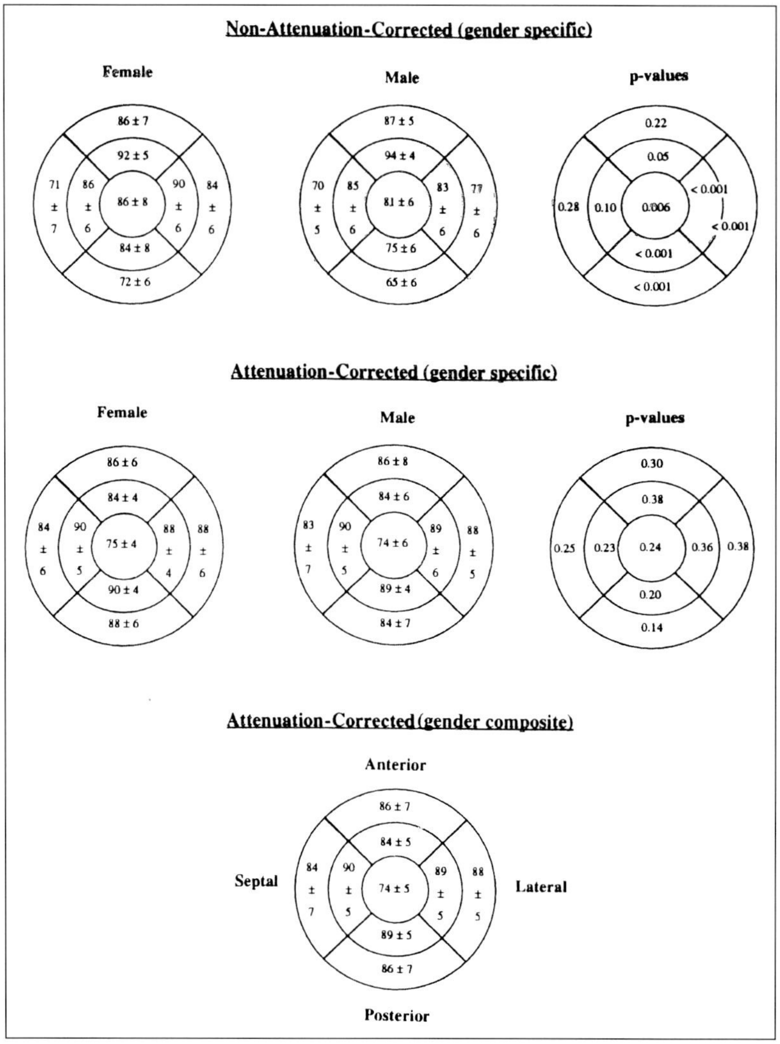

Figure 77 Effects of attenuation correction. The stress technetium-99m sestamibi tracer distribution in the myocardium of patients with a ≤5% pretest likelihood of coronary artery disease. Normal, sex-specific polar map distribution (20 subjects each) are presented for uncorrected (top) and attenuation-corrected (bottom) images. Significant differences (*P* values) between the gender maps are displayed on the right for the uncorrected and attenuation-corrected distributions. (Reprinted with permission from Ficaro EP, Fessler JA, Shreve PD, et al. Simultaneous transmission/emission myocardial perfusion tomography. Diagnostic accuracy of attenuation corrected ^{99m}Tc-sestamibi single-photon emission computed tomography. *Circulation* 1996;93:463–473.)

study-specific attenuation map then can be generated with iterative or backprojection methods. This method minimizes truncation artifacts but requires accurate "coupling" between the moving line source and the "blank scan." However, the source is expensive and gives higher radiation exposure. A multiple-line-source geometry may resolve some of these issues.

Although the presence and effect of attenuation on image findings may be assessed from projection images, objective standardized polar maps, gated function and prone images that often resolve the cause of inferior defects (*304,365*), this is inefficient, suboptimal and based on indirect evidence. Study-specific nonuniform attenuation correction can be a major advantage (*4–12,371,376, 377*), because it may: (1) increase diagnostic sensitivity and specificity; (2) improve accuracy of quantitation and move closer to absolute perfusion quantitation (however, new sex-specific databases will be needed for this goal); (3) contribute to improved patient management; (4) improve estimates of left ventricular size and function with improved defect and myocardial identification; (5) lead to the development of new and more efficient imaging protocols with greater confidence in a stress-only protocol, as in the triage of acute chest pain; and (6) may be especially important for comparing defects in dual-isotope ^{201}Tl rest/^{99m}Tc stress and ^{99m}Tc SPECT protocols, in which physical differences in the radionuclides applied may lead to image differences (*294,295*).

Some studies report an improved accuracy with a variety of attenuation correction methods and radionuclides, usually improving specificity if not sensitivity (*378–390*). These studies demonstrate the ability of the method to correct for attenuation in phantoms, increase image homogeneity in normal studies, achieve occasional improvement in normalcy and rarely in specificity and increase image contrast between normal and abnormal areas in select patient populations. However, multiple errors have also been reported with "overcorrection" of inferior attenuation and normalization of inferior activity, regardless of related regional perfusion. Frequently demonstrated has been resolution of inferior defects in proximity to regional high background, regardless of their pathophysiologic significance. Such methods lead the reader to conclude that if an inferior defect is seen and a normal study desired, then do attenuation correction! Technical factors are also critical. Here, field uniformity of each of the multiple heads must be high and their sensitivities within 15% of each other. Patient motion within and between transmission and emission scans is also a likely source of gross error in the method and has yet to be characterized. The current trend is to perform simultaneous transmission and emission scans with efficiency of time and avoidance of misregistration (*378–380*). A recent multicenter trial (*378*) demonstrated that attenuation correction, when combined with motion- and depth-dependent loss of spatial resolution, provided greater diagnostic accuracy than conventional reconstruction of myocardial SPECT studies in both men and women. A new analytic algorithm for attenuation correction is now being tested by ADAC (Milpitas, CA).

Scattered Photons

Compton scatter is inherent in all planar and SPECT images because of the poor energy resolution of gamma cameras. Emitted photons that bounce or scatter off an atom at a shallow angle will retain enough of their original energy to remain within the energy acceptance window of the gamma camera. However, they will be detected as if they were coming from a point other than their true origin. Scattered photons may be detected at extracardiac or alternate myocardial locations and have the effect of blurring the images. Attenuation correction and collimator design have been the focus of recent efforts to improve SPECT studies, and less attention has been given to the even more difficult task and time-consuming methods of scatter correction (*377*).

Scatter Correction. Scatter also is often the cause of image artifacts. This most often involves an augmentation of inferior counts as a result of scattered radiation derived from an area of intense subdiaphragmatic activity. This may obscure inferior defects and, when most prominent at rest, may make fixed defects appear reversible. Scatter artifacts also may be corrected with application of off-peak image data (*381,382*). Like attenuation, scatter is patient specific, because it is affected by both patient anatomy and tracer distribution. With simultaneous acquisition of transmission and emission images, downscatter into the ^{153}Gd window from myocardial ^{99m}Tc can erroneously suggest a thin body habitus and little attenuation, when the true activity from the ^{153}Gd transmission source, in fact, may be greatly reduced in the presence of a large body habitus and much attenuation (*312,323,350*). The lower-energy, 60-keV photon of ^{241}Am makes scatter less likely in the energy window and may be employed to acquire the transmission study. However, its physical half-life of 243 yr makes it less optimal for this purpose. The transmission image also may be acquired by a scanning line-source method, in which only a fraction of the field of view is sampled sequentially, reducing the effect of scatter. Also, the contribution from noise in the transmission scan increases with decreasing acquisition time and causes errors in the "corrected" emission scan (*383*). This statistical problem increases as the transmission source deteriorates. Attempts to correct for scatter include the dual-window technique, in which downscatter is used to advantage as an energy window is sampled between the energies of the transmission and emission sources. The fraction of the higher-energy emission source found in this intermediate window is applied as an adjustment to correct for downscatter. An effort also has been made to recognize and differentiate the effects of decreased perfusion from attenuation based on the differential regional attenuation of the varying emission energies of ^{201}Tl (*384*).

Scatter radiation from adjacent hepatic or bowel activity may enhance a region in the posterior basal wall with low primary count levels as a result of regional attenuation. Correcting this scatter component for the associated attenuation results in an overcompensation of intensity that may make other areas appear falsely underperfused. To avoid this effect, scatter must be corrected before attenuation can be corrected. Scatter can be corrected with several methods. Commercial systems are limited to the multiple energy window method, in which a separate window tracks lower-energy scattered radiation and the correction is applied before image reconstruction. Although early results show a decreased effect of hepatic activity on inferior wall intensity, improved myocardial-to-background contrast and possibly improved defect contrast, the method also increases noise in the emission images. Only a single modification of a commercially available method has been validated with visual and quantitative analysis (*371*). Although accuracy seems improved with this method when compared with noncorrected data, no multicenter trials have been reported and the method is not yet available commercially.

Attenuation correction is possible but costly and not yet perfected. All current methods of attenuation and scatter correction are imperfect and should not be relied upon alone to differentiate attenuation- from perfusion-based defects except as one of several available analytic tools. Attenuation correction should not be applied clinically as a solution to attenuation effects until the specific methods are thoroughly, objectively and widely tested. Recently, a simplified x-ray computed tomography (CT) system has been combined with a dual-head scintillation camera to provide emission and transmission data in registry for attenuation (and scatter) correction of full-body and cardiac imaging (General Electric, Milwaukee,WI). The equipment is now being marketed. El Fakhri et al. (*391*) have presented an analysis of the respective effects of correction for attenuation, scatter and limited resolution.

SPECT Artifacts

Spect Image Acquisition Artifacts

Attenuation

Cause. This may be the result of breast tissue, adipose of the lateral chest wall, diaphragm, arm, necklaces and objects in pockets. The latter are rarely a problem for SPECT reconstruction. A cardiac pacemaker over the heart is difficult to miss as a source of error in planar or projection images. ECG monitoring leads are small and thin enough that they rarely cause a clinical problem. Less obvious patterns include breast prostheses, intestinal barium and self-attenuation of the inferobasal wall by the overlying ventricle. Attenuation by breast (or chest wall) or diaphragm is a major source of potential interpretive errors. Attenuation is caused by any physical substance between the target organ and the detector. The same myocardial region may demonstrate different intensities, depending on the amount and character of attenuation tissue or other material in different projections. In nuclear medicine, the amount of attenuation is generally related to substance density. Bone attenuates photons more than does lower-density soft tissue. Lungs contain much air with very low attenuation effects. Other factors related to photon energy and electron shell energy that affect attenuation in general are of little importance to imaging ^{99m}Tc and ^{201}Tl. Two common attenuation correction algorithms both assume uniform attenuation in the body (*385,386*). This is especially untrue in the thorax, with 10-fold tissue densities ranging from lung at 0.14 g/cc to bone at 1.50 g/cc. At the energy level of the ^{99m}Tc 140-keV photon, the attenuation coefficient for lungs is 0.10/cm, in which

10% of counts are lost with each centimeter transited; for bone the attenuation coefficient is much greater at 0.22/cm. Although attenuation decreases as photon energy increases, even the high-energy 511-keV photons of positron decay require attenuation correction. The dual-photon nature of PET imaging permits attenuation correction as part of routine image reconstruction.

Recognition. The reader must always examine the raw projection data and correlate apparent perfusion defects with anatomic coronary perfusion patterns. Looking at a cine of the projection images may show a cold area moving across the heart. Anything that moves across the heart in different views is extracardiac. The discrepancy between a markedly abnormal planar view or projection image and the SPECT reconstructed view suggests attenuation, especially when an apparent defect is transiently noted in only a single projection or in limited projections. Perfusion defects should also be compared with the normal sex-specific database illustrated by polar maps or circumferential profiles, paying attention to the distribution and the density of the defect. Nonsegmental defects that do not match coronary perfusion patterns are suspect, although this pattern can result from abnormal coronary anatomy, such as is seen after revascularization or with involvement of only a part of a coronary region, as in branch disease. Cines of gated SPECT studies should show little or no wall motion or thickening in the area of a true, fixed perfusion defect, and prone imaging will reduce the effects of diaphragmatic and breast attenuation (*240,304,365,387*). The best guard against misinterpretation is the suspicion of such an artifact and the application of experience.

As a special case, a dual-nuclide study using rest ^{201}Tl and stress ^{99m}Tc sestamibi has been suggested as a method to detect attenuation. Using a normalized bullseye or polar display to compare the ratio of ^{201}Tl with ^{99m}Tc, areas with relative excess of ^{99m}Tc may correspond to an area of added regional attenuation in the ^{201}Tl study, whereas regions of ^{201}Tl excess suggest true perfusion defects (*342*). However, care must be exercised, as the improved spatial resolution of the ^{99m}Tc image may present details of the normal distribution, such as the apical slit, that are not evident on the ^{201}Tl-based image.

Correction. Once the data are acquired, no consistently reliable correction is yet possible. Correction attempts may provide an aide to recognition but also have been reported to make the results even less reliable. The best approach is to take steps to minimize the effects of attenuation before acquisition. Preventive measures in women involve steps that make attenuation fairly uniform and reproducible over the heart. The right breast rarely will cause an attenuation artifact. Prone imaging will spread breast tissue over a wider area and compress it, resulting in more uniform attenuation. In men, diaphragmatic attenuation can be reduced by prone imaging. However, prone imaging can cause other artifacts related to the imaging table or soft-tissue attenuation over anterior myocardial segments. Images should be processed and reviewed before the patient leaves the laboratory, and acquisition can be repeated in the prone position or with a different breast position.

Some cameras now offer the ability to acquire a 3-dimensional transmission image set to create a true attenuation map of the imaged area for subsequent attenuation correction (*236,388,389*). This could improve specificity, as long as the attenuation map is acquired in exactly the same position as the SPECT study. True attenuation correction results in an increase in spatial resolution, because the origin of detected photons can be mapped more accurately during reconstruction. Its application will require new insights into image processing and a new normal database and image interpretation basis. Attenuation hardware and software packages are available but should be purchased with this awareness. Attenuation correction probably will contribute an imaging advantage, but it will not solve all problems associated with image artifacts.

Center of Rotation Artifact

Cause. Changes in COR may be the result of mechanical shifts in the gantry or electronic drifting in the camera circuitry (*392,393*). The COR must be measured periodically to update the COR correction factor. COR artifact is caused when the measured COR does not match the true COR. This can result from a shift in the true COR after the COR correction was calculated or from applying erroneous or incorrectly acquired COR values. If the source used to calculate COR is moved during acquisition, the reconstruction will shift images to match these incorrect factors. It is possible to apply the wrong COR correction factors to a SPECT reconstruction, and this certainly will cause errors. COR correction factors are specific to each camera. COR may also vary with different collimators or with different photon energy levels. If this is the case, COR correction must be acquired for any combination of factors as well as the specific system used during clinical studies. The malalignment of heads in a multihead camera brings an image artifact similar to that of COR-related artifacts.

Recognition. A severe case of COR error will produce artifactual rings around the true COR in transverse images. If a COR problem is suspected, examination of the transverse images may be helpful. Rings will be difficult to see if the area being imaged has fairly uniform distribution. Technetium-99m–based agents, with their high target-to-background ratio, can produce easily visible rings. Oblique axis views transect the transverse slices so that the rings are also transected. Cross-sections of transverse rings manifest as linear sets of small punctate areas of increased or decreased activity in oblique views, which may not be recognized in the final display. COR errors usually are recognized most easily in long-axis views when opposite septal and lateral walls of the heart do not curve to meet at the apex. Patient movement can cause errors similar to COR error, because in both cases the activity is not detected in the proper place. Movement artifacts, however, tend to be large scale and not show a constant radius.

With multidetector systems, alignment of each detector and all detectors to the others is a new concern. Each detector can be tested by imaging a line source at different positions in relation to each camera head. Interhead alignment should be maintained with the installed alignment correction software. This should be quite stable and needs to be checked only yearly. Accuracy can be checked with the acquisition of a phantom test pattern with each head and then by comparison of this pattern with that acquired with all heads (*394*).

Correction. If the cardiac images suggest a COR error, the first step is to check the COR factors to ensure that the camera and collimator are correct for that study. The next step could be to acquire a new COR to see if it matches the old COR correction. If it does not, apply the new COR factors to the reconstruction. If the camera has been adjusted well by service engineers, reconstruction without COR correction may yield better results than applying a bad COR correction. Some cameras have COR correction built into the raw projection data as it is acquired, and these cannot be corrected after the fact.

Point Spread Function Changes with Distance

Cause. Another commonly encountered artifact is the appearance of a focal area of increased activity or "hot spot," most commonly in the anterior or lateral walls. The physics inherent in gamma cameras causes loss of spatial resolution with increasing distance from the detector. This means that a point close to the detector would be seen as a small dot, and the same point source far away will be seen as a large, indistinct blob covering more pixels. Because the number of counts is constant, the larger blob will have fewer counts detected in any 1 pixel, which is interpreted as lower activity in that area. The anterior wall of the heart is closer to the camera face in most projections, so the counts are more concentrated. The anterior wall can appear hotter than the posterior or lateral walls. With a different orientation, the camera may pass extremely close to the lateral left ventricular wall. This effect is in addition to the extra attenuation of the posterior wall.

Again, a similar artifact may be associated with exaggerated attenuation of the inferoseptum, which results in a "relative hot spot" in the opposite anterolateral wall, or, in some patients, the anterolateral hot spot may be caused by hypertrophy of the anterolateral papillary muscle.

Recognition. This factor, relating proximity to intensity, is built into the normal databases for quantitative analysis, because it is impossible to acquire images without it. If the camera is much closer to the heart in the LAO 30° to LAO 45° projections than during the rest of the acquisition, an artificial hot spot can be created in the anterior or lateral wall. When presented with an artificially "hot" lateral wall, the remainder of the myocardium generally appears within normal limits, with only modest reduction in relative intensity. The alternative to interpretation of the pattern as a normal image is to read all but the lateral wall as abnormal, often incompatible with the clinical presentation. Review of the SPECT slices and projection images often reveals relatively high levels of radioactivity, even in areas other than the lateral wall.

Correction. The only way to avoid this problem is to maintain a constant distance from the target organ to the camera face. This blurs the anterior wall almost as much as the posterior wall and sacrifices the better resolution that is possible in this area. A high-resolution or long-bore collimator loses spatial resolution as a function of distance more slowly than does a general purpose collimator. This better resolution more than compensates for the loss in sensitivity. As cameras are able to follow the body contour more closely, this problem is exacerbated, but usually there is no recognizable effect of variable acquisition distance. Iterative reconstruction techniques can correct for point-spread function blurring to a significant degree. When related to other factors, the cause of the hot spot must be recognized, because it cannot be avoided.

Circular Versus Noncircular Orbit. A noncircular orbit may follow the body contour or conform to a simple ellipse. The type of orbit does not itself produce artifacts. Even a circular orbit rarely centers on the heart, because the heart is not centered in the body and the detector must clear the body over at least 180°. The loss of resolution with distance as described in the section above is always a factor in both types of acquisition. Overall, better resolution is obtained by keeping the detector as close as possible to the patient. A circular orbit is most widely applied. Regardless of the choice of orbit and distance from the body, the movement of the myocardium during imaging causes all walls of the heart to blur.

Cause. Most camera systems offer both types of acquisition orbit.

Recognition. The posterior wall is farthest from the detector, so it will always be less sharply defined than the anterior wall. This is accentuated by the extra attenuation that reduces the counts from the posterior wall. There are no reliable ways to recognize the effect of a noncircular orbit compared with a circular orbit. Defects at the ventricular base, particularly in lateral or posterior (inferior) walls, may be difficult to identify beyond the expected effects of regional attenuation and image degradation. This may contribute to the difficulty in identifying abnormalities previously reported with planar imaging of the LCX (9).

Correction. No current correction is available for the variability introduced by the shape of the orbit applied. It has not been shown to be generally clinically significant. When distance factors are built into reconstruction algorithms, they will have to include the shape of the orbit as an input parameter (*395*).

Nonuniformity. The uniformity of the camera detectors changes over time. Changes in PMT tuning and gains shift the detected location of counts. A PMT failure will create a dramatic nonuniformity, leaving an area empty of counts. Poorly functioning ADCs in the camera head can cause counts to be digitized to the wrong location, resulting in parallel lines of increased and decreased activity across the field of view. Collimator damage can have dramatic effects on sensitivity in the affected area.

Cause. The SPECT uniformity floods are designed to correct for variations in sensitivity over the field of view of the detector. A uniformity artifact will occur when the calculated uniformity correction factors do not match the true uniformity at the time of acquisition. This can result from a shift in the regional sensitivity after the uniformity correction was calculated or from incorrectly acquired uniformity data. If the uniformity correction source is not uniform, the reconstruction will apply these incorrect factors to images. Liquid flood sources must be well mixed to a uniform concentration before use. Solid flood sources are guaranteed by the manufacturer to have only an acceptable amount of variability. It is possible to apply the wrong uniformity correction factors to a SPECT reconstruction, which will cause errors. Severe defects in regional sensitivity must be fixed by addressing the cause, such as replacing a poorly functioning PMT or a badly damaged collimator.

Recognition. Improper uniformity correction can result in ring artifacts in transverse images. These artifacts will be more severe near the center of the field of view than near the outer edge. If the area in question has fairly uniform distribution, these rings may be difficult to see. Nonuniformity artifacts in a ^{99m}Tc-based study with a higher target-to-background ratio than ^{201}Tl may produce rings that are more easily visible. Oblique-axis views transect the transverse slices, so the rings are also transected. Cross-sections of transverse rings manifest as linear sets of increased or decreased punctate activity in oblique views and may not be recognized in the final display.

Correction. If uniformity errors are suspected, the first step is to check (if possible) the uniformity factors to ensure that the camera and collimator are correctly matched for the study. The next step might be to acquire a new uniformity flood to see if the uniformity has changed since the last flood. As a last resort, the study may be reconstructed without flood correction. If the camera head is well tuned, this will introduce only minor nonuniformity errors. On some cameras, uniformity correction is performed during the acquisition, and the raw data already includes this factor, so it is not possible to go back and try different correction factors.

Changes in Radiopharmaceutical Distribution During Acquisition. The distribution of activity can change or appear to change during SPECT acquisition in 3 distinct circumstances: (1) patient movement, (2) internal physiological movement and (3) activity seen in some views but not seen in all views. These have different causes and cures, although the consequent image artifacts may appear similar. Again, the mathematical basis of SPECT reconstruction algorithms assumes that the distribution of activity does not change during the acquisition. Any such change will be reflected in the reconstructed images by an artifact resulting from counts shifted away from the correct location.

Patient movement. Patient movement can be divided into 3 categories: vertical movement in the Y direction, in which the body shifts along the axis of rotation toward the patient's head or feet; horizontal movement in the X direction, in which the body shifts sideways from left to right or vice versa; and twisting or rotational movement, in which the body pivots around any of the 3 axes defining 3 dimensions. Movement of any part of the body may cause artifacts, and patient movement is among the most common causes of SPECT artifacts. Much research has been done on patient motion, both because it is so common and because it can be simulated well using real patient data (*95,357,396–403*).

Cause. Patient motion during SPECT imaging is a frequent cause of image artifacts (*323,351,352*). It is very important that the patient does not move during SPECT acquisition. Explaining the importance of not moving gives the patient incentive to remain still, especially if the explanation includes the information that movement might require starting the study over again (with possible repeat of the exercise test if using ^{201}Tl or teboroxime) or that altered image data may cause misdiagnosis and added expense. This should be emphasized by the patient's physician when initially describing the test to the patient and again by the technologist just before beginning acquisition. If the patient cannot lie still for the necessary time, planar images should be considered. Multihead cameras can reduce acquisition time and the likelihood of patient motion. When motion occurs, it is seen by each imaging head, usually making the motion easier to detect and correct. When motion is seen by only 1 detector, it is not in the Y direction, making correction difficult or impossible. Ensuring patient comfort reduces the likelihood that movement will occur. A good arm support to hold the left arm over the head is helpful. The arm should be supported at both the wrist and elbow with no patient effort. Some patients feel more comfortable with something to grip as well or with both arms over their heads. Patients who place hands under their head usually find this too uncomfortable to maintain during the entire study and move during the acquisition. Talking can encourage head movement and alter breathing patterns, which can affect cardiac position within the chest.

Another form of cardiac motion, upward creep (see SPECT software), has been shown to occur in the absence of visible patient motion (*303*) (Figs. 78,79). This results from an apparent gradual upward motion of the heart in the chest with gradual postexercise reduction of respiratory rate, because of a relocation of the mean cardiac position with resumption of the baseline resting state. This phenomenon is uncommon when the patient is imaged at or near to the resting state. It is rarely seen in association with pharmacologic stress by primary coronary dilators such as dipyridamole, after low-level dynamic exercise stress or when imaged long after vigorous dynamic exercise, as with ^{99m}Tc sestamibi. Delayed thallium images, sestamibi and tetrofosmin are all imaged long enough after exercise that

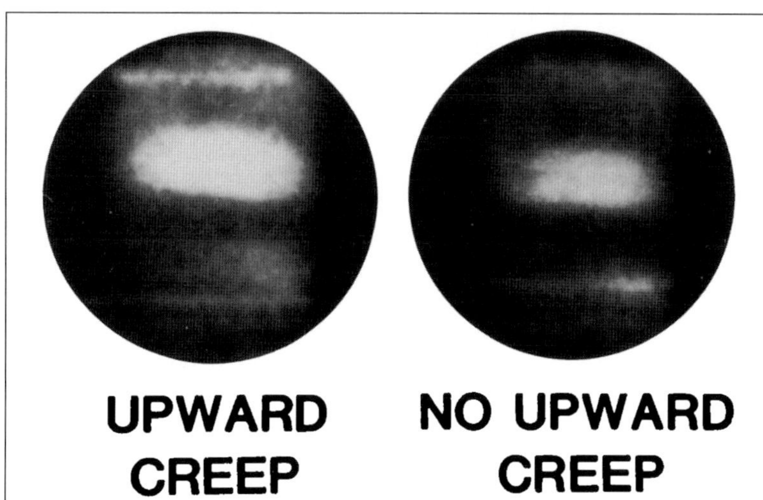

Figure 78 Upward creep: summated images. Summated images or "blurrograms" of a patient, showing upward creep on the immediate poststress acquisition (left), and showing no upward creep on repeat imaging immediately after the poststress acquisition (right). The heart is in the middle of the field of view, and the horizontal lines on the top and bottom of the image are the 2 summated point sources. The right-hand edge of the heart represents the initial frame, and the left-hand edge represents the last image acquired in this projection set. (Reprinted with permission from Friedman J, Van Train K, Maddahi J, et al. "Upward creep" of the heart: a frequent source of false positive reversible defects during thallium-201 stress-redistribution SPECT. *J Nucl Med* 1989;30:1718–1722.)

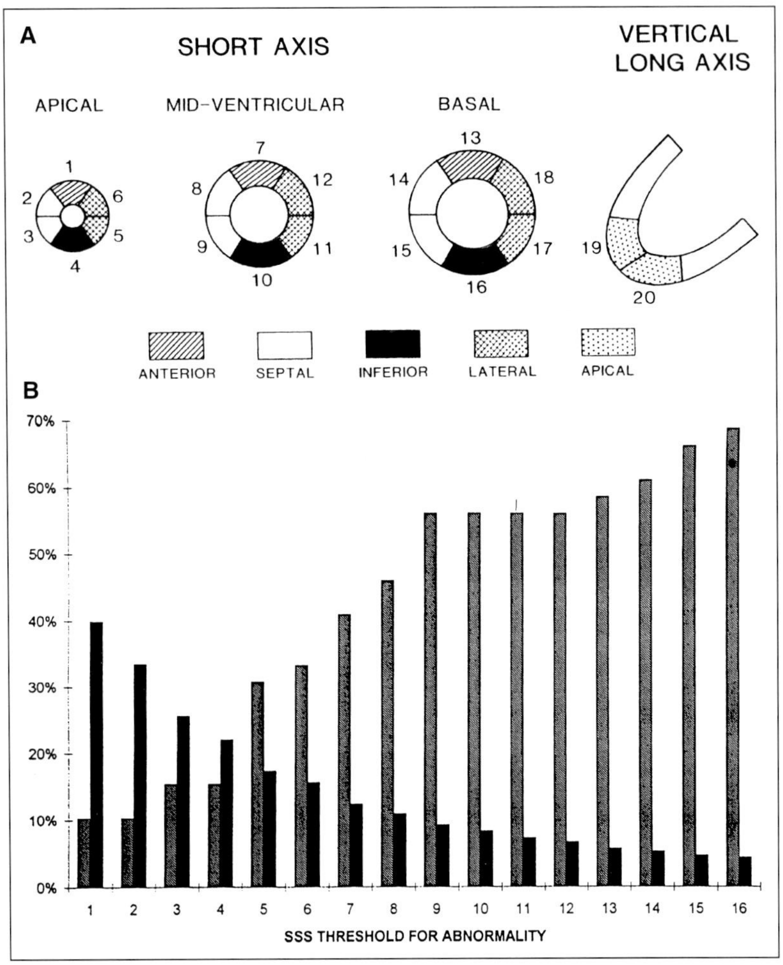

Figure 79 Twenty-segment score. (A) Twenty segments commonly scored to determine defect extent and related prognostic significance. (B) The relationship between the threshold of the summed stress score (SSS) applied in image interpretation and the percentage of hard events occurring in patients with normal scans and so not detected by perfusion imaging (gray bars) and also the percentage of the study population with abnormal scans (black bars). As the threshold applied increases, more events are missed and the population with abnormal scans falls. It is such data that has resulted in the SSS of 3, representing the threshold for abnormality. Not shown here is the direct incremental relationship between defect size and event rate. (Figure 79A is reprinted with permission from Friedman J, Van Train K, Maddahi J, et al. "Upward creep" of the heart: a frequent source of false positive reversible defects during thallium-201 stress-redistribution SPECT. *J Nucl Med* 1989;30:1718–1722. Figure 79B is reprinted with permission from Hachamovitch R, Berman DS, Kiat H, et al. Exercise myocardial perfusion SPECT in patients without known coronary artery disease: incremental prognostic value and impact on subsequent patient management. *Circulation* 1996;93:905–914.)

the patient has returned to a resting state. The ^{201}Tl stress-first protocol brings the patient under the camera early after exercise and may encourage this effect.

Upward creep is a potential source of artifactual image defects when acquisition begins soon after injection and related exercise. In this condition, the heart position within the chest drifts slowly upward during the first 10–15 min after exercise, probably as a result of changing heart and respiratory rates, even in the absence of any patient motion. On the summed projection images, upward creep is recognized by the upward slope of the summed cardiac activity in relation to the horizontal or the line inscribed by the point sources discussed previously. This phenomenon is predominantly seen in patients who achieve a relatively high level of exercise and in whom tomographic acquisition is started very quickly after exercise, most commonly with ^{201}Tl imaging. It is observed exclusively on the initial post-stress images and is not seen at the time of the redistribution study. One possible explanation for this phenomenon is that the increased tidal volume associated with high levels of exercise persists for some time after the termination of exercise. Alternatively, hyperventilation in an anxious patient placed under the camera for the first time, here postexercise, may present the same effect. Thus, the diaphragm and the heart occupy lower positions in the chest early following exercise, gradually reverting to their normal higher positions during the first 10–15 min postexercise. Because the artifact is not seen at the time of redistribution imaging, an artifactual reversible defect is created, localized to the inferoseptal and inferior regions.

Taping a marker dot or 2 to the patient's skin at a level above or below the heart will make it easier to detect and correct patient movement, by providing a well-defined spot away from other body activity. However, movement of the dot may not always correspond with cardiac motion when breathing patterns shift the heart within the chest. Current systems project a horizontal line on the rotating projection image set to aid recognition of vertical motion. Cooper et al. (*357,404*) reported on the effectiveness of different quantitative methods of motion detection.

In the absence of patient motion, when all projection images are added to obtain a single image (referred to as a summed image or "blurrogram"), the 2 point sources inscribe 2 straight lines, 1 above and 1 below the cardiac activity. Vertical patient motion may be recognized on the summed image by identifying a shift in this pattern. One simple way to recognize movement is to play the projection images as a cine. A cine of raw projections makes vertical movement (toward head or foot in the Y direction) easy to see. Horizontal movement, perpendicular to the rotation axis (in the X direction), may be seen if it occurs while the movement is parallel to the camera face but is impossible to see if the movement is directly toward or away from the camera. Any camera with 2 detectors at right angles will always see horizontal movement. Twisting will be detected by the component of movements in the X or Y direction.

It is recommended that, in addition to examining the summed images, the 32 projections be routinely displayed on the computer in a closed-loop cine display format to further assess the presence of patient motion and other artifacts during image acquisition. When current dynamic projection image displays present a horizontal line to help identify vertical motion, the myocardium should move on the line. When seen to bounce on the line, rise above or cross it, vertical motion is clear. This format permits only recognition of patient motion in the vertical axis, whereas motion in other planes can be quite distinctive and productive of SPECT image artifacts (*352*) (Figs. 80–84). A small proportion of patients may not be able to remain still during the 22 min required for single-head SPECT acquisition. Acquisition time is variably abbreviated with multihead cameras (*282*).

Motion correction algorithms simply reprocess the data with vertically aligned projection images. They may show some improvement and so aid interpretation. However, vertical is often combined with rotary motion, which cannot be corrected. A second acquisition may be needed. Alternatively, limited sedation may be considered in these patients, or planar imaging may be more appropriate.

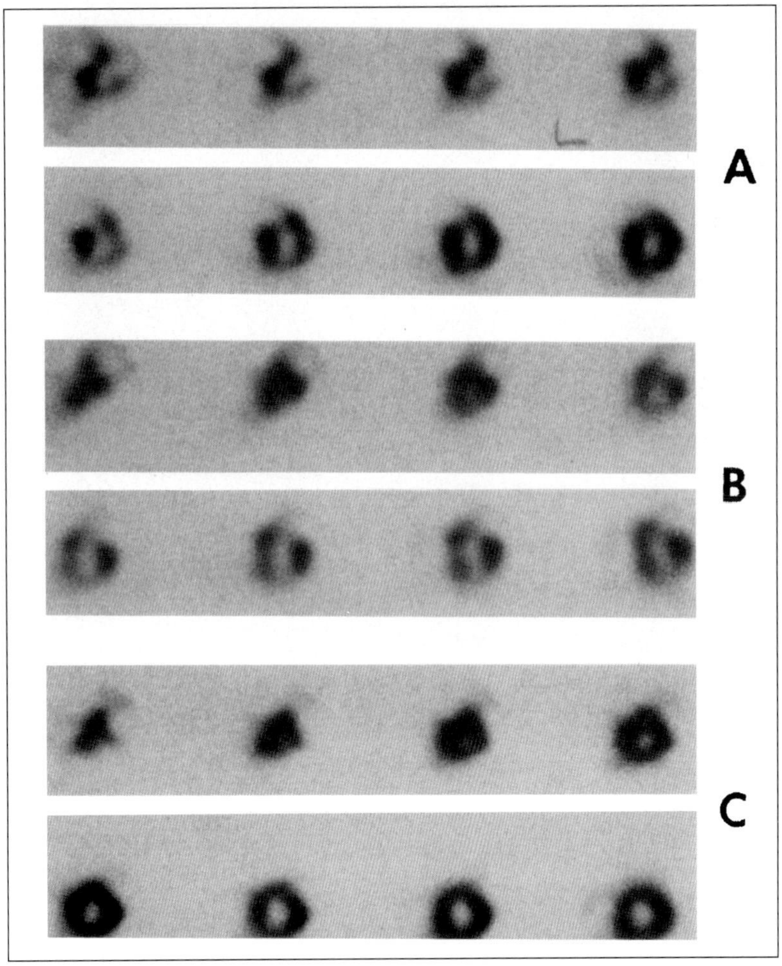

Figure 80 Effects of motion timing: images. Resultant contiguous short-axis slices from apex (upper left) to base (lower right) after upward displacement of 2 pixels in 8 frames of a 32-frame SPECT acquisition. (A) Short-axis slices when frames 7–14 were affected. (B) Slices when frames 18–25 were affected. (C) Normal undisturbed image set. Note the difference in defect size and location. (Reprinted with permission from Botvinick EH, Zhu YY, O'Connell JW, Dae MW. A quantitative assessment of patient motion and its effect on myocardial perfusion SPECT images. *J Nucl Med* 1993;34:303–312.)

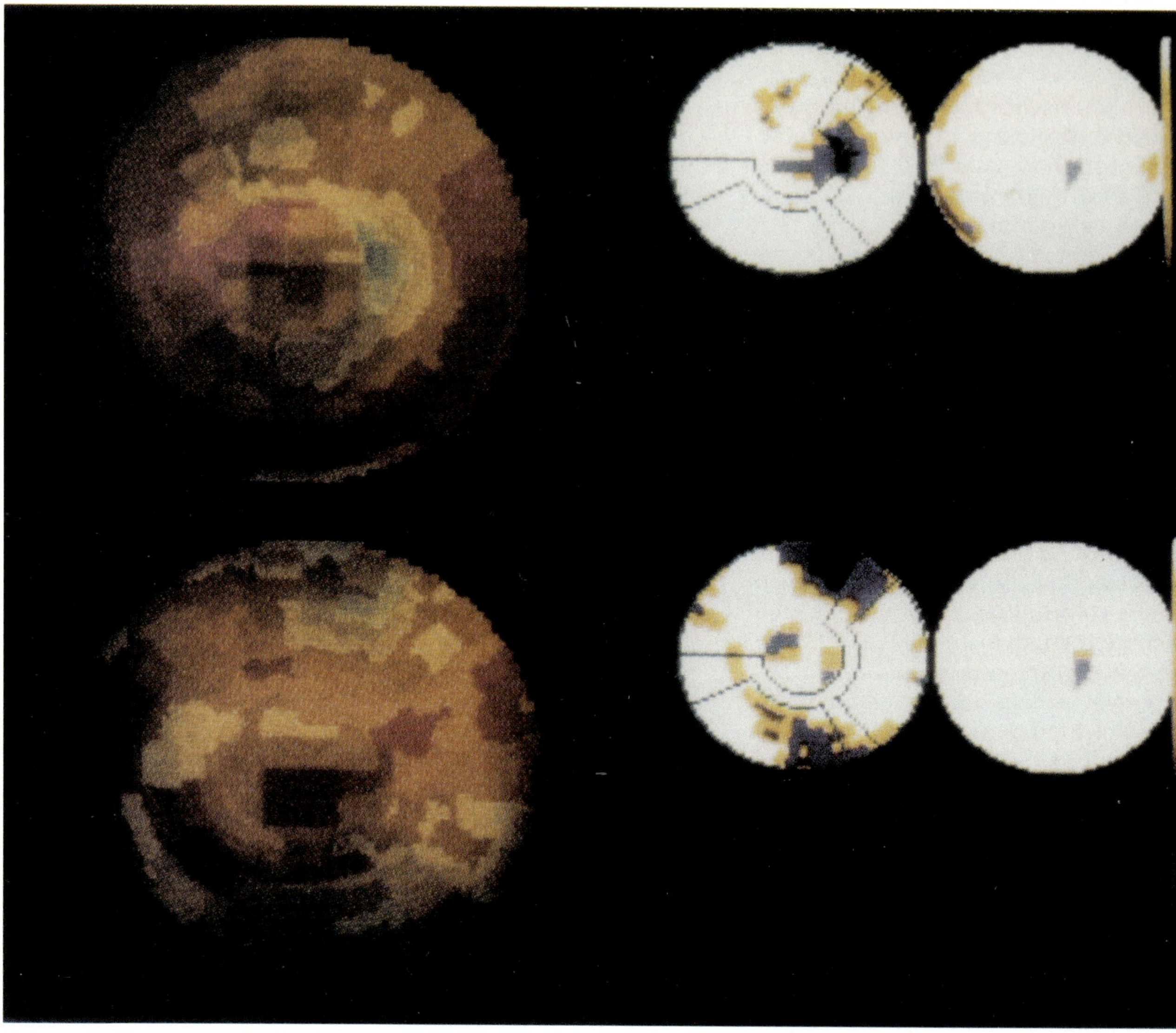

Figure 81 Effects of motion timing: polar coordinate display. Resultant polar displays with the effect of "motion" in frames 7–14 (above) and the effect resulting from alterations in frames 18–25 (below) in a 32-frame SPECT acquisition. Differences in defect size and location are apparent. The color polar displays at left represent the relative difference in count distribution between altered stress and delayed SPECT image sets. Here red or dark gray represents peak activity. The paired maps at right indicate regional abnormalities in altered poststress and delayed images, compared with a normal population. (Reprinted with permission from Botvinick EH, Zhu YY, O'Connell JW, Dae MW. A quantitative assessment of patient motion and its effect on myocardial perfusion SPECT images. *J Nucl Med* 1993;34:303–312.)

Alternatively, a sinogram (for horizontal motion), or a linogram (for vertical motion) may be generated (see Self-Study Program III, *Nuclear Medicine: Cardiology, Topic 1: Physical and Technical Aspects of Nuclear Cardiology*). This procedure collapses each projection frame vertically (sinogram) into a single row of pixels or horizontally (linogram) into a single column of pixels. These rows or columns are stacked vertically or horizontally to form a 2-dimensional image. Image areas of hot or cold activity should form smooth, seamless, sometimes curving lines across the image as the distribution appears in slightly different positions in succeeding projections. A single point in the center of the field of view would show a straight line. Irregularities in the curve indicate changes in the distribution of activity during the acquisition.

The absence of gross perfusion defects seen in SPECT slices but not in planar images also suggests their origin in motion artifact. Such motion artifacts may be produced with relatively modest movement over a few frames. Usually, the artifact increases with extent and duration of motion and shows variable regional abnormality, depending on the frame affected (*352*). A typical SPECT defect pattern, characterized by opposing defects in a noncoronary distribution, is often the result of vertical patient motion. This usually is accompanied by linear uptake extending from the myocardium, again at opposite poles of a SPECT slice. This has been characterized as the "hurricane sign" by Sorrell et al. (*405*). The acquisition of projection images in a fractionated manner was suggested as a method to extract and process data not corrupted by motion that affected the data only during limited phases of the acquisition (*406*). Motion artifact is best prevented and must always be recognized and, when possible, corrected (*331,350,404,407*). State-of-the-art systems have implemented an effective automated vertical and lateral motion-correction algorithm as part of routine image processing (ADAC).

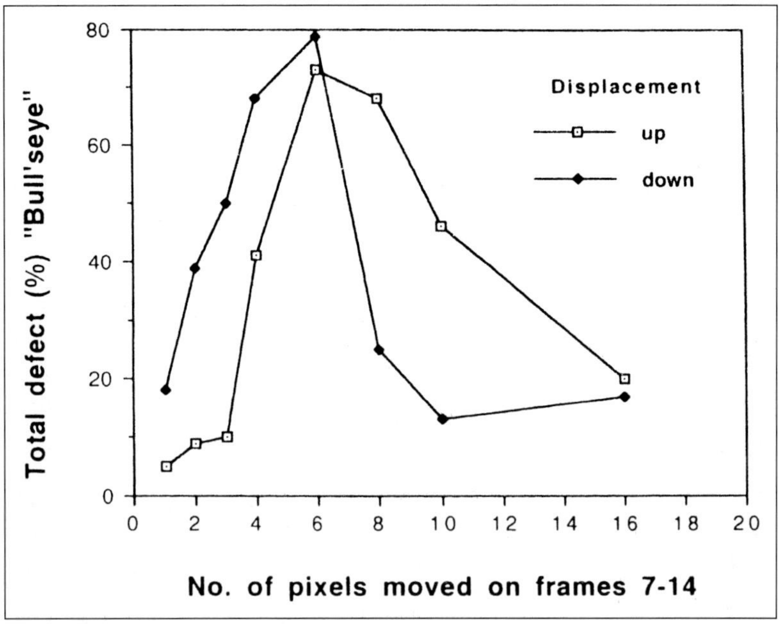

Figure 82 Extent of displacement. The relationship between the extent of displacement (abscissa) and resultant defect size (ordinate) is quantitated on a polar display, for upward and downward displacement in the same projection images (frames 7–14). Note the similar patterns and defect size and the reduction in defect size with increased "motion." (Reprinted with permission from Botvinick EH, Zhu YY, O'Connell JW, Dae MW. A quantitative assessment of patient motion and its effect on myocardial perfusion SPECT images. *J Nucl Med* 1993;34:303–312.)

Correction. The raw data must be corrected before reconstruction. Some types of movement can be corrected, and some can not. If the movement is vertical, several methods of correction are possible. If the movement is horizontal, correction may be possible theoretically, but there is no accepted method to correct it. Twisting motion cannot be corrected. If only 1 frame shows movement, such as from a cough, that blurs the image, that frame can be replaced with an average of the 2 adjacent frames, with little loss of information. Alternatively, such transient motion may be ignored with little impact on the SPECT image data (*352*).

One method of vertical correction is to look at each image and shift them up or down until all images are in line. This is best done using reference lines at the upper and lower boundaries of the cardiac area. Increments of less than 1/2 pixel, variation of a single frame or minor variations over several frames may not be significant (*352*). Although such correction may not entirely eliminate artifactual defects resulting from motion, when motion correction reduces defects it suggests their origin in patient motion. Another method uses mathematical cross-correlation between adjacent slices in the linogram or sinogram. Because each projection is within a few degrees of the adjacent projections, the detected distribution should change little. When each projection view is collapsed to a vertical line or horizontal line, adjacent images can be shifted (using a least-squares correlation fit) to minimize the differences between adjacent lines. This is performed automatically but should always be followed with a visual check of

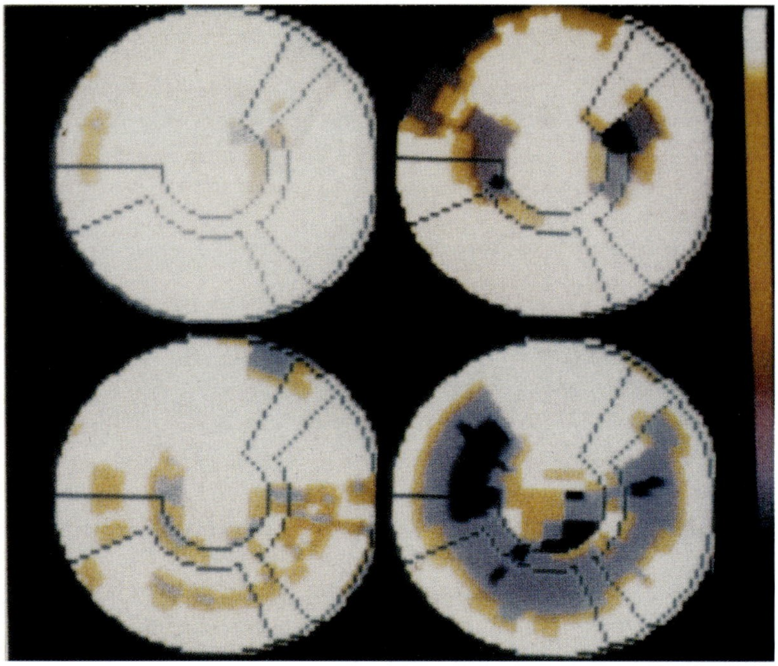

Figure 83 Combined effects of vertical and horizontal displacement: polar maps. Polar displays of resultant SPECT images generated from a computer simulation of horizontal rotational motion of 5-frame magnitude, beginning with frame 16 of 32 acquired, in the direction of orbital rotation (upper left) and counter to the direction of orbital rotation (upper right). A significant defect shown in violet, blue or black, here in the left anterior descending distribution, was only evident with motion opposite to the direction of orbital rotation. Shown below are polar coordinate displays of resultant SPECT images generated from a computer simulation of 3-pixel vertical upward motion in frames 13–20 in the same patient (lower left) and with added horizontal rotational motion of 5-frame magnitude beginning with frame 16, counter to the direction of orbital rotation (lower right). Note the dramatic increase in defect size when vertical and horizontal motion artifacts were combined. (Reprinted with permission from Botvinick EH, Zhu YY, O'Connell JW, Dae MW. A quantitative assessment of patient motion and its effect on myocardial perfusion SPECT images. *J Nucl Med* 1993;34:303–312.)

the results. Concentrated activity moving through the intestine during the acquisition can mislead the sinogram or linogram correction process.

Yet another method takes advantage of the ability to perform multiple sequential SPECT acquisitions and later sum selected cycles. Corresponding projections from each acquisition cycle are compared, and, if 1 projection does not match the others because of patient motion, it can be discarded. Other motion detection methods may be used in addition to and in combination with this method.

The vertical motion of upward creep is well known as an after-effect of a high level of exercise in immediate ^{201}Tl images. It can be treated just as would be any other form of vertical patient motion. Alternatively, an extracardiac radionuclide accumulation of clinical significance may be interpreted erroneously to be an artifact of motion. Commercial algorithms are now available (ADAC) to correct for both vertical and horizontal motion by analysis of the transverse 3-dimensional data set. This method is quick, automated and seemingly accurate. Rotary motion remains problematic, and, of course, no correction algorithm is perfect. Motion is best avoided.

Physiological changes in distribution. This is considered separately from patient movement, because, unlike patient motion, it cannot be controlled. One reason that the agent teboroxime may be difficult to use stems from the fact that its natural biodistribution changes so rapidly that the study must be acquired in the short period of time after cardiac uptake but before there is significant washout of the tracer. The timing and duration of ^{201}Tl imaging is more forgiving, because it redistributes much more slowly. During stress thallium acquisition, the tracer slowly washes out of the lungs and myocardium but not at a rate fast enough to affect clinical images. Redistribution during rest or delayed thallium is so slow as to be undetectable in a single acquisition. The stability of sestamibi and tetrofosmin allows great flexibility in imaging time and duration. Sestamibi may show intense activity in the liver, gall bladder and jejunum near the heart, and it moves rapidly enough through the biliary system and small intestine that its distribution can change during acquisition. As long as the radiopharmaceutical movement remains anatomically below the level of the heart, it will have no effect on myocardial reconstruction. Two ways to avoid this problem are to wait until interfering areas have cleared most of their activity or to image before its accumulation.

Cause. All nuclear medicine radiopharmaceuticals change their distribution over time, at different rates at different times. If distribution changes significantly during acquisition, it can create artifacts.

Recognition. Recognition is best from the raw projection data, which usually will show any type of motion during the acquisition. Emptying of the biliary tree into the small bowel and its subsequent movement can be seen in the cine of projection images. If a significant concentration passes near the heart, this may cause problems, and special care should be used when examining the reconstructed images. High concentrations of activity in the liver that are excreted during the acquisition will affect the final images, because the dome of the liver is seen in some of the same transaxial planes as the heart. Small changes in hepatic concentration have little effect on the final images.

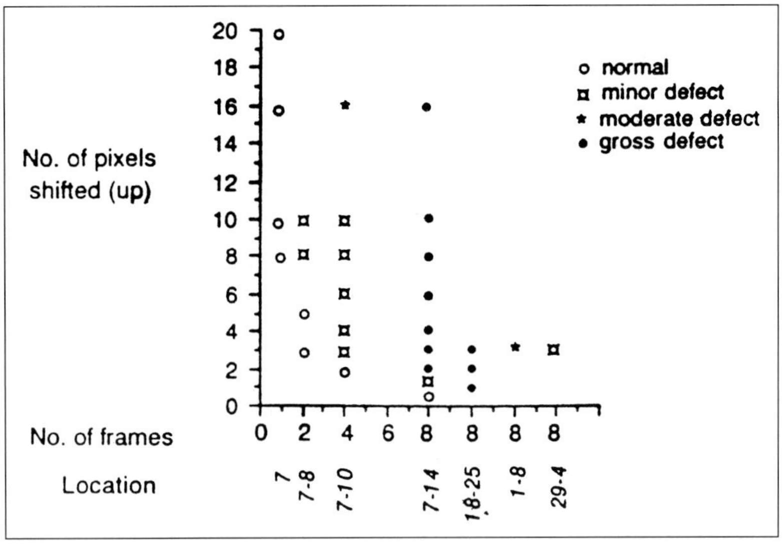

Figure 84 Defect size. The relationship between the visual extent and intensity of the defect generated and the extent (number of pixels), duration (number of frames) and timing (specific frames) of upward image displacement. Defect size and intensity increased with increased extent and duration of motion. Even gross motion limited to a single projection frame had little effect on the final image. (Reprinted with permission from Botvinick EH, Zhu YY, O'Connell JW, Dae MW. A quantitative assessment of patient motion and its effect on myocardial perfusion SPECT images. *J Nucl Med* 1993;34:303–312.)

When activity is seen at the level of the heart in some projections but not in others, the usual result appears to move counts out of the myocardium into the area of changing activity. For example, a hot liver dome may show equal concentration to the myocardium in early views (RAO to anterior) but have little activity in later views (lateral to LPO). The lateral view counts must be reprojected across the volume, perpendicular to the detector in proportion to the distribution seen in the anterior view. This means that some of the counts originating from the myocardium will be allocated to the liver area, even though the liver activity has washed out and not contributed to the lateral counts. Because the planes most likely to be affected by such physiological changes include the inferior wall of the left ventricle, underperfusion in this area may be the result of physiological changes in radiopharmaceutical distribution, and this possibility should be investigated.

Correction. No true correction method is available after the data are acquired, except for repeating the acquisition. If the changing activity is at the level of the heart, it will affect the reconstructed distribution in the myocardium in some way. If the artifact is not in a plane of clinical interest, it can be ignored. With sestamibi, physiological changes can be avoided with good timing of image acquisition. A drink of fatty liquid will induce gall bladder contraction and movement through the small intestine to help clear the area. Occasionally, the gall bladder will be cleared only to increase the background interference as a result of high-intensity activity in the small bowel. This problem may be avoided by imaging early, at a time when extracardiac hepatobiliary activity is restricted to the gall bladder or by delaying imaging until after activity in the small intestine has moved past the area of the heart. One of the beneficial features of sestamibi and tetrofosmin is that images can be repeated later if physiological motion is detected.

Activity in and out of the field of view. When activity is within some projections but not in others, this conflicts with the assumption in SPECT reconstruction algorithms that all activity is seen in all views. Missing activity in some views results in uncorrectable truncation or clipping artifacts. If most of the activity is within the field of view all the time, the errors will be small. This applies to all radioactivity, not just that in the cardiac area of interest. The reconstruction planes near the top and bottom of circular heads will always generate artifacts, because part of the body that is seen in lateral views is not seen in anterior or posterior views. Rectangular detectors with fields of view narrower than the body will also demonstrate this problem. In addition, truncated images will adversely affect attenuation correction, because they fail to include all body volumes that contribute to attenuation.

Cause. Some cameras present this problem because their field of view is less than body width. Another cause is an infiltrated dose in the right arm. When the right arm is at the patient's side, it easily can be out of the field of view in some projections. Usually so little activity is in the arm that it has no effect on the study. If there is significant activity in the right arm visualized in only some projections, there will be reconstruction errors.

Recognition. Ray artifacts always indicate activity seen in 1 place in some views but not seen there in other views. These artifacts can be the result of patient body movement, physiological movement within the body or activity within the field of view in only some projections. When viewed as a cine, the raw projection data usually will show the motion during the acquisition, including hot spots moving in and out of the field of view. The ray artifacts are generated during transverse slice reconstruction and are visible only in transaxial slices. Because oblique slices intersect the transverse slices, the rays may be visible as a line of hot spots in final images.

Correction. There is no correction method. Data can be filtered in such a way as to reduce the effects at the cost of overall distortion. One way to deal with this problem is to smooth the data at the edge of the field of view in every projection to minimize the effect of a hot spot when it enters or leaves the field of view. Another method is to manually outline such hot spots when visible and set the counts in those areas to a background level. Neither of these methods will fix the problem; they will only hide the evidence. If the hot spot is at the level of the heart, it will affect the calculated distribution in the myocardium in some way. If the artifact is not in a plane of clinical interest, it can be ignored.

Artifacts Related to Thallium-201/Technetium-99m Differences

Differential attenuation of thallium-201 and technetium-99m. These differences are related to the use of a dual-isotope protocol. This problem occurs only when a ^{99m}Tc tracer is used for the stress part of the study and ^{201}Tl is used for rest imaging.

Cause. Technetium-99m has higher energy photons than ^{201}Tl and suffers less from attenuation. Even when the 167-keV photons from ^{201}Tl are included, most of the detected thallium photons are in the 70–80 keV range. The normal cardiac-to-skin-surface distance is about 8 cm, and, in water, there is about 10% less attenuation for ^{99m}Tc than for ^{201}Tl (both peaks) photons. Because some of the path from myocardium to skin passes through air, the attenuation difference will be slightly greater than 10%. This still may be sufficient to present visible differences, because attenuation defects will be more prominent in thallium images. The size of the patient should be considered during interpretation, because thallium attenuation will vary more in different projections than will ^{99m}Tc attenuation.

Recognition. A perfusion defect in a ^{201}Tl rest study that is not present in the ^{99m}Tc stress study suggests an attenuation artifact in the rest ^{201}Tl study or resting ischemia that is not reproduced at stress (unlikely). This finding suggests reverse redistribution, a phenomenon of diverse causes that usually are not clinically important. A valid difference assumes exact reproducibility in all aspects of positioning and image acquisition.

Correction. This problem cannot be corrected in the reconstructed images unless true attenuation correction is performed. When recognized, it can be taken into account during study interpretation.

Point-Spread Function for Each Nuclide. This problem occurs only when ^{99m}Tc perfusion images are compared with ^{201}Tl perfusion images. The point-spread function (PSF) maps of ^{201}Tl and ^{99m}Tc are similar near the peak, but near the PSF base the ^{201}Tl map is much wider than the ^{99m}Tc map. Several factors may make the sestamibi or tetrofosmin cavity appear larger and the walls thinner. One of these is the difference in PSF, as the poorer spatial resolution of greater scatter of thallium blurs and thickens the myocardial walls to present a smaller left ventricular cavity. The lower count density of thallium requires a smoother filter, which will thicken the myocardial walls. Other factors may be that the cavity is truly dilated or the myocardial distribution may be different for the 2 radiopharmaceuticals. The perceived cavity size in a teboroxime image is more probably the result of physiologic dilation of the ventricle than it is in ^{99m}Tc sestamibi images. Because teboroxime must be imaged immediately after stress, as with a stress thallium study, the ventricle may well be dilated. This dilation can be exaggerated by the effect of the PSF differences. The better spatial resolution of ^{99m}Tc images may show greater details of normal image heterogeneity, such as the apical slit. These generally can be recognized and taken into account when interpreting the images, so they appear to be of little clinical importance, and the accuracy of the dual-isotope method is sustained (*286*).

Cause. The wider point spread of ^{201}Tl causes more of the counts in the ^{201}Tl image to be spread over a larger area of the image. With true ^{201}Tl photon events scattered throughout the field of view, this effectively increases the background everywhere. It also produces an image that has less-well-defined edges, because the edges are spread over more pixels than in ^{99m}Tc images. Because the myocardial walls are less well resolved, they will appear thicker in the ^{201}Tl image and the apparent cavity will appear smaller. This should produce an apparent difference in transcavity diameter of $<30\%$ (*408*).

Recognition. A difference in cardiac cavity size may be partly the result of the physical characteristics of ^{99m}Tc and ^{201}Tl. A stress sestamibi or tetrofosmin image is actually acquired at a time delayed from stress while the patient is at rest, so the cavity size should generally be the same for sestamibi and rest ^{201}Tl images. A slightly larger sestamibi cavity is likely to be primarily the result of the better resolution and a sharper reconstruction filter applied with sestamibi. When the sestamibi cavity diameter is much larger than the ^{201}Tl cavity, in the range of 40% or more, no physical cause is known, and this is almost certainly a pathologic phenomenon. This value is quantitated routinely on current systems.

Correction. Because this problem is inherent in the physics of SPECT, it cannot be corrected. Some efforts have been taken to minimize the effect of the PSF (deblurring) and to transform the ^{99m}Tc point spread to that of ^{201}Tl, to recognize the cause of this apparent dilation in this physical effect. Deblurring works well in images with edges that are already fairly well defined and have high counts density, such as bone or brain images. It does not work in areas with much background noise, because it creates clumps of higher-count areas in which there is no real structure. Applying a ^{99m}Tc-to-^{201}Tl transformation to ^{99m}Tc images will widen the myocardial wall and blur the edges, making it appear ~1 pixel wider. Small differences in cavity size can be assigned to this cause, but large differences cannot.

Tilted Camera Head

Cause. Collimator holes must be perpendicular to the axis of rotation. Except for slant-hole collimators, this means the detector face must be parallel to the axis of rotation. All commercial reconstruction packages make this assumption. The technologist setting up the study should verify the detector position by eye. Most computers will automatically detect camera tilt, and, when a tilt goes undetected by the computer, a service call is necessary. Of course, those cameras with heads locked at right angles perpendicular to the orbit cannot tilt, so this should not be a problem.

Recognition. This can be very difficult to recognize. Unexplainable reconstruction impossibilities may have this as a root cause.

Correction. This cannot be corrected. It is possible to write reconstruction code to take camera head angle into account, but the problems of limited-angle tomography have become evident, as they did in relation to 7-pinhole and rotating slant-hole tomography. Such software is not now commercially available. The study must be repeated to correct this problem.

Acquisitions on Cameras with Varying Specifications and Capabilities. This is not so much an artifact as a factor to recognize. Current camera–computer systems present comparable specifications and performance capabilities, as, for the most part, do systems from the same generations. However, when performing serial studies over years with varying equipment, image characteristics may vary. In addition, multihead cameras provide higher data density, improved resolution and more rapid acquisition with less chance for motion artifact. These factors must be considered when comparing serial studies performed with different equipment or, for that matter, with different radionuclides and protocols.

Processing and Display Artifacts. These 2 types of artifact can be combined, because they are interdependent. The last stage of processing creates the display. These artifacts share a very important property: they can be corrected fairly easily by reprocessing the study. They include artifacts related to various aspects of the imaging process and/or the equipment used.

Color Table. The application of color and the specific color table applied influences the visual perception of edges and intensity boundaries. It is quite easy to demonstrate a perfusion defect in 1 color table that is quite invisible in another. When used properly, color will call attention to areas that should be examined closely. However, color can also display apparent regional myocardial heterogeneity that is actually within the range of normal. Gaining familiarity with a color table and its effects will reduce the likelihood of errors based on color perception. If a certain percentage drop in counts is considered evidence of a true perfusion defect or evidence of regional viability, a color table can be designed to show changes in color at this level for emphasis.

Cause. The boundary between 2 colors is perceived as an edge and interpreted as a large change in myocardial activity, when it may actually represent a minor difference and fall within the normal limits of distribution heterogeneity. Alternatively, significant changes in counts may be hidden within 1 hue of the color scale.

Recognition. All color tables, except monochrome gray scale, have this potential for deception.

Correction. Look at the images in a monochrome gray scale as well as in color. Analyze any apparent defect objectively with the use of quantitative methods and assess its potential to be caused by artifacts of acquisition or display.

Gray Scale. Because the most intense location in the indicated region of interest is presumed by the nondescriminating software to be myocardium, all pixels included will be scaled to this highest intensity level. When 1 myocardial area appears intense because of overlap by or scatter from an extracardiac source, all other regions may appear abnormal and may even be so identified on polar map analysis! An extensive polar map abnormality, not evident as a cardiac structure in the projection images, may relate to the inclusion of a region of high-level paracardiac background, such as bowel activity after a sestamibi injection. Alternatively, such high-level background included in the analytic region of interest may delete from the polar map a defect evident on the SPECT slices.

The gray scale used to display an image can enhance or hide information, depending on the upper and lower thresholds of the intensity window. Extracardiac activity in sestamibi studies frequently shows higher activity than the myocardium, because the liver excretes concentrated agent. When images are scaled to the most intense pixel in the image set, the intense extracardiac activity reduces the range of intensities allotted to myocardial counts. Although this preserves the relative intraslice intensity, the myocardium in the affected image dims with respect to its rest or stress counterpart, making comparison more difficult and making intensity differences in the myocardium more difficult to see. It is also possible to set the upper threshold below some of the pixel values in the myocardium, with all such pixels above this value showing the same display intensity. No differences can then be seen among these pixels. An extreme case would be to set the upper threshold to saturate the lowest-count pixel in the myocardium, and then all cardiac pixels would appear to be the same high intensity (*409*).

The problem of extracardiac activity may be somewhat relieved with the introduction of ^{99m}Tc-based tetrofosmin, which has reduced biliary excretion (*410*).

Problems of absolute intensities do not affect the relative intensity distributions and should not be evident in polar coordinate maps or relative activity profiles, as long as extracardiac activity is excluded in their generation.

Cause. High extracardiac background suppresses regional myocardial intensity by simple relative-counts scaling to intensities or colors.

Recognition. The hottest pixel, and only the hottest pixel, in the myocardium should have the maximum intensity in the display. The brightest pixel should not be extracardiac.

Correction. This can be avoided by imaging in the presence of low adjacent background but must always be sought, recognized and accounted for in image interpretation. Alternatively, high background activity may simply result in the presentation of all of the normalized myocardium in relatively low-intensity shades or colors. Although such a condition would preserve the relative intensity and perfusion pattern in an accurate polar analysis, it may make for a difficult comparison with the other image set of the stress–rest duo. This may be overcome more easily by either redrawing regions to exclude background or rescaling and normalizing myocardial counts to the highest-intensity pixel, with an appropriate upper-threshold adjustment to make the adjusted image look most like its alternate.

Try to spread the full intensity range between 0 and the hottest cardiac pixel. All display systems have methods to let the user window the images. Although simply lowering the upper threshold may cure the problem, on some systems this reduces the number of intensity levels in the image, reducing the ability to recognize defects.

Normalize by Each SPECT Slice or Over the Entire Image Set. A set of images can be windowed in 2 ways. The image set may include the slices from 1 study or slices from all 3 views for both stress and rest–redistribution studies. Images can be scaled to the hottest pixel in the entire set, or each image can be scaled individually to the hottest pixel in that image. For example, ischemia in the apex can be hidden, if that slice (with universally fewer counts in all regions) is scaled individually so that it appears to have the same uniform high intensity as slices with normal perfusion. This usually does not apply between different views, because the same myocardial region is matched with different regions in other orientations. The abnormal apex would be relatively reduced, even if the scale is set per slice, when compared with the normally perfused, more proximal myocardium in long-axis slices. Regions might appear normally perfused and with high relative intensity in 1 axis and not another, if the set is normalized per axis and the slice involves only underperfused regions. If an area of myocardium appears to have decreased perfusion in 1 view and normal perfusion in another, that area should be considered abnormal. It would be uniformly abnormal in all views if normalized for the image set, rather than each image slice. If all images are scaled to a common maximum, then the same area of myocardium will have the same intensity in all axes. This is preferred.

Cause. Normalizing each image individually will disguise differences in perfusion between apex and base in the short-axis slices and differences between septum and lateral wall or anterior and inferior walls in the corresponding long-axis views. Any uniformly underperfused slice would appear with the same intensity as a normal slice.

Recognition. If every slice has some pixel that appears equally and maximally intense, then each image is probably scaled separately. This may obscure interslice differences. If the brightest pixels in different slices in each axial set have different intensities, or if there is a large difference between myocardial intensity in different axes, images are probably scaled to the full image set. If an intense slice or slices appear in each axial set but fail to triangulate between axes, the images are likely normalized to each axial set.

Correction. All nuclear medicine display software has options to scale a full set of images in all axes to the same value. This should be applied.

Background Subtraction to Enhance/Create Defects. This is more likely to be a problem with planar than SPECT images. A slight decrease in counts in some area of the myocardium may not be visible, but a constant number subtracted from each pixel will increase the relative difference and make a defect more evident. For example, a 10% difference in relative counts in 1 image is not significant, but subtracting a constant value from all pixels can increase this difference to 50%, which is significant. In SPECT, much of the background is removed as part of the processing, because background is in front of and behind the heart. This background activity is not present in the myocardial slices, so it does not appear in the display. Windowing can mimic background subtraction in the final display and emphasize the depth of perfusion defects.

Cause. Background subtraction removes too many counts from the image.

Recognition. Some background counts should always be visible in both SPECT and planar images. If only the myocardium is visible, then too much background has been removed. SPECT images can be victimized similarly by windowing the images, but background subtraction as such is not part of SPECT processing.

Correction. Return to the original image and use a smaller background subtraction value. If it is a SPECT reconstruction, reduce the lower threshold of the display window.

Image Misalignment Between Studies. Myocardial perfusion interpretation is largely based on the appreciation of differences between stress and rest or redistribution images. For this comparison to be valid, the same regions of myocardium in the 2 image sets must be compared. The usual format for final display is a row of stress images above a row of rest–redistribution images, representing the same myocardium in the 2 different states. Once the slices for each view are created, each row must be shifted in relation to its comparison row to align the corresponding slices. Misalignment may result in the erroneous impression of defects when the slices are of different size or with apparent cavitary dilation. Misalignment of slices at the septal base is among the leading causes of false positive image readings. Relying on apical slice alignment may create apparent basal redistribution when slices are not quite aligned at the base. A slice in the area of the membranous septum will appear as an incomplete circle, like a backward C. If compared with a complete circle adjacent to the membranous area, there will appear to be redistribution in that area.

Alignment usually is more difficult (and more meaningful) in the short-axis orientation. Frequently the best way to align the rest and stress short-axis slices for comparison is to minimize both sets to see all of the myocardium and align all slices starting with the left ventricular base. Alignment from the apex may be problematic because of the presence of perfusion defects, partial volume effects or cavitary dilation. If the apex is well defined, alignment can start there by aligning the first short-axis slice in each study that shows the left ventricular cavity. In most hearts, both the base and apex should line up, regardless of which end is used as the anchor point. If this does not appear to be the case, check the alignment carefully. If the stress images show a dilated ventricle, it may be worthwhile doing the alignment and comparison twice, once from the base to compare basal slices and once from the apex to compare apical slices.

Cause. Not checking the alignment carefully.

Recognition. Most important is that the base of the septum be aligned in both studies. The first slices showing the apex should line up approximately in both rows of short-axis slices. An apical defect in the stress study that fills in during redistribution can easily hide the stress-related apex. Extracardiac activity below the apex may obscure the beginning of the apex. The edges of the ventricular cavity should line up approximately in all slices, unless cavitary dilation is present. The short-axis basal slices can be more difficult to judge, because of the presence of the membranous septum and the more distant and seemingly thinner myocardium in the base compared with the rest of the heart. If the papillary muscle is visible, it should line up in both studies. In the horizontal and vertical long-axis slices, similar slice alignment is necessary but is usually much easier. There are fewer slices, and centering the largest cavity in both rows usually creates a satisfactory alignment. The cavity should disappear at about the same lateral or anterior slice in both studies. A variant of this problem is the erroneous display of the same study represented both as rest and stress. This would change a reversible to a fixed defect or even to a normal study, depending on which image set was displayed.

Correction. Every display program has a simple way to move a row of slices. Align each pair of image rows. Sometimes changes in cardiac size with stress intervention make a perfect match impossible, and this must be considered in interpretation.

Inconsistent Wall Definition for Polar Map Creation. The apex, or center of the polar map, is frequently derived from long-axis slices, because an apical short-axis slice might not contain the cavity and a circumferential profile is difficult to generate without a distinct hole in the center of the ring. The very apical short-axis slices are solid myocardium without a cavity. The apical endocardial wall is marked in a long-axis view to define the line in the polar map between data from the short-axis slices and the apex data from the long axis. A more accurate method uses a 3-dimensional image of the apex and samples along planes rotating around the long axis of the left ventricle instead of planes parallel to the long axis. To generate apical regions, the comparison normal database should use the same method that is used in clinical studies.

The apical endocardial line is used along with a line at the base of the heart to define the inner and outer circumferential profiles that create the polar image rings. If the slice selected for the base is too proximal, few counts will be there, and the outer ring of the polar map will be dark and will be read as abnormal compared with the normal database. Faulty basal slice selection is 1 cause of false-positive image readings in polar maps. Automated slice selection is possible, but it works most reliably when the heart is normal.

Cause. The endocardial wall, base or apex is not marked correctly.

Recognition. A dark vertical line is in the center of the polar map, or the inner or outer rings of the map are dark.

Correction. Repeat the polar map processing with correct edges.

Incorrect Inferior Junction Definition for Polar Map Creation. The polar map is derived from data related to circumferential profiles. The 2 subjective steps involved in the generation of circumferential profiles are the assignment of the left ventricular center and the assignment of the junction of the right and left ventricles. Assignment of the center of the left ventricle too close to a given myocardial wall will result in fanning of the profiles and potential artifactual defects. Error in assigning the junction between the left and right ventricles would result in shift and misassignment of different segments of the profile, which would then be compared with noncorresponding portions of the normal database profiles. As a result, artifactual defects may be introduced.

The inferior junction of the right and left ventricles at the interventricular septum is used as a reference point to compare different polar maps. The computer will rotate the polar map so that the orientation is the same in both stress and rest–redistribution studies and also matches the normal database orientation. The better target-to-background ratio and greater count density of ^{99m}Tc-based agents compared with thallium makes this anatomical point easier to see in ^{99m}Tc images. The commercial normal database provides a polar map of usual coronary artery perfusion areas, and, if a different reference point is used, then the concentric rings of the polar map will be rotated clockwise or counterclockwise (*334,344,411,412*). The comparison with normal values and the overlaid map of coronary artery perfusion areas will be incorrect.

Polar maps simply reflect the distribution of regional radioactivity, regardless of its cause. They will reflect artifacts of attenuation, motion, field homogeneity, COR artifact and other defects. Polar maps serve as an objective arbiter of image heterogeneity and a quantitative parameter of defect size. Yet, for this reason, findings on polar maps must be confirmed by a thorough analysis of the SPECT slices, their related projection images and the technical aspects of acquisition and processing or risk a great loss of specificity.

A prominent source of error in image quantitation also results from the inclusion of the most basal short-axis slices. At these very basal levels, myocardial activity usually is seen in the lateral wall, but significant reduction is noted in the inferior and septal regions, because the inferior wall often is attenuated and the basal septum is the membranous septum. This will produce artifactual defects in both visual qualitative or quantitative methods. Inclusion of these regions in quantitive analysis causes artifactual and extremely peripheral inferior and septal defects on the polar map display.

Cause. Selecting the wrong reference point during polar map processing will rotate the polar map and invalidate comparisons between studies and with the database of normal values.

Recognition. If perfusion defects appear to shift position clockwise or counterclockwise between stress and rest polar maps, the most likely cause is an incorrectly rotated polar map. There is no easy way to discern whether a patient polar map orientation matches the normal database. Artifacts must be sought in polar map reconstruction as well as in image slices.

Correction. Repeat the polar map processing and carefully select the septal junction with the right and left ventricles. Avoidance and correction of artifacts will aid in polar mapping as well as slice interpretation.

Incorrect Axis Selection for Short-Axis Slices. The long axis of the heart is not parallel to the axis of the body, so the SPECT transverse slices of the heart do not lend themselves to easy identification or comparison of myocardial regions. The slices must be reoriented, in essence viewing the same data at a different angle. The long axis of the heart is defined by drawing a line in 2 orthogonal planes that bisect the heart. This axis must be the same for both stress and rest–redistribution studies, or different parts of the myocardium will be displayed in the corresponding comparison views. The angles in relation to the transverse planes will not be the same if the patient's heart is not exactly in the same position for both stress and rest imaging. Defining the correct long axis, regardless of physical angles, will correctly orient the heart for all subsequent processing. An error in axial slicing is the classic reason for the production of a reversible basal septal defect (*413*).

This error may be recognized and true basal defects identified by viewing a rotating 3-dimensional image. This presents the complete myocardium without any axis definition or slice alignment necessary. Although some attempts have been made at automatically selecting the long axis, they all make some assumption about the shape of the heart. A prominent defect, such as a major infarct, can produce unpredictable results from automatic axis definition. Changing the axis can translate a defect from 1 slice to another. This is another technical cause for apparent reverse redistribution. Seven-pinhole tomography reconstruction could even move a defect from 1 side of the heart to the opposite side by changing the angle of reconstruction (*413–415*).

Some software lets the user draw the lines for both studies on the screen at the same time or shows the previous axis while the new axis is being drawn. Some software automatically redraws the axis of the initial (rest or stress) study on the subsequent transverse image. Although this is a potential advantage for reproducibility of image reconstruction, it assumes that the angle of the heart has not changed between studies. Axes redrawn from the prior study may be used as an initial starting point and adjusted to the ventricle.

Cause. Incorrect axis selection for short-axis slices is caused by selecting a long axis of the heart that does not match the anatomical axis or does not match the axis definition from the other half of the stress–rest–redistribution study.

Recognition. The short-axis views provide the easiest presentation to diagnose this problem. The shape of a short-axis slice should be nearly circular. An oblong shape is possible but quite rare, and a check of the axis definition is indicated. A defect present in a rest study that is not seen in a stress study is physiologically unlikely, and changing the axis can translate a defect from 1 slice to another. One good way to check axis alignment is to photograph the lines used to define the axis in both studies and compare them. Most software will redisplay the reference slices and axes at any later time. Viewing the short-axis slices as a cine should show the center of the left ventricular cavity in the same screen location for all slices.

Correction. Select the correct axis and reprocess the study.

Incorrect Filter Selection for Reconstruction. *(See Acquisition Artifacts)* The term "filter" may include both the type of filter (Butterworth, Hamming, etc.) and the frequency cutoff. Using 1 type of filter with 1 cutoff can result in images similar to those of a different type of filter with a different cutoff. The best filter produces the best spatial resolution with the least amount of noise in the final image. Too smooth a filter will hide defects, and too sharp a filter will produce irregularities that are noise instead of real physiological underperfusion. The optimum filter is a function of the count density in the area of clinical interest, the myocardium. Several problems are encountered in attempting to use the optimum filter for each study. Determining this filter is time consuming, because it must be done by looking at the results of many different filters. Picking the filter is a subjective judgment with inter- and intraoperator variability. Minor variations in filters will have little effect on the clinical interpretation. Using the same filter for all studies of the same type will give the interpreter consistent levels of noise and resolution and increased confidence that perceived defects are real. Sometimes specific situations, as noted above in obese patients or with reduced data density in 24-hr-delay ^{201}Tl images, may force the selection of a different filter—in these 2 cases, 1 with greater smoothing characteristics. Selecting the wrong filter can also change a polar map from normal to abnormal.

Cause. Selecting the wrong filter from a range of choices, either the wrong type or the wrong cutoff.

Recognition. If the filter is sufficiently different, the image looks much smoother or noisier than expected. The usual cause is incorrect filter selection, although a sufficiently different count density can have the same effect. Once a filter has been established for a study type, a little experience is enough to detect a significantly different filter.

Correction. Check the filter used, and, if necessary, select another filter for the study and reprocess it. If necessary, make a unique choice.

Image Interpretation

When artifacts are clearly recognized and there are no other apparent abnormalities, the image must be read as normal but revealing an artifactual defect. Insecurity in interpretation of an obvious attenuation artifact is a leading cause of false-positive images and the needless performance of angiography in the presence of normal coronary arteries (*416*). Higher-energy ^{99m}Tc photons reduce but do not eliminate such difficulties. Similarly, SPECT images, integrating as they do image data from a wide angle of view, also tend to minimize but do not eliminate such artifactual defects.

FLUORODEOXYGLUCOSE IMAGING WITH CONVENTIONAL CAMERAS

Overview

With the clinical development of PET methods and reimbursement for imaging in evaluation of patients with malignant melanoma, lung and colon cancer, as well as FDG applications, much effort has been placed in the development of

FDG imaging with conventional scintillation cameras. Much progress has been made in FDG imaging with a conventional gamma camera (*417–422*). The simplest way to accomplish this is with a high-energy collimator (511 keV) fitted to a conventional scintillation camera (511-keV SPECT). Here, no use is made of the coincident 511-keV photons. Another method is based on the recognition of the coincidence photons and their registry in 2 opposed conventional camera heads (gamma-camera PET). Here, no collimator is required, but, like standard PET, the coincidence detection is itself localizing and intrinsically tomographic. Collimators block most photons, so 511-keV SPECT is inherently much less sensitive and count rates much lower than those of gamma-camera PET and, of course, true PET. Yet, even current gamma camera design is not able to take advantage of the high count rates of gamma-camera PET, because of the high number of singles (counts in a single head) and random, noncoincidence events. Management of this large number of events of various kinds is a major challenge to the use of gamma-camera PET.

Image resolution is set by the collimator in 511-keV SPECT at about 15–20 mm, whereas that of gamma-camera PET is set by the intrinsic camera resolution at about 5 mm. However, with 511-keV SPECT, simultaneous acquisition of the ^{99m}Tc (140-KeV) perfusion and the flourine-18 (^{18}F) (511-keV) metabolic tracers can be performed, with less severe effects of attenuation compared with gamma-camera (or traditional) PET, in which simultaneous imaging cannot be performed by the coincidence method and attenuation is great and must be corrected. This is because the pair of 511-keV photons must traverse and be attenuated by the entire body, as opposed to the collimated photons in 511-keV SPECT, which are simply those that leave the myocardium and traverse the anterior thorax to the crystal. Coincidence imaging appears to cause increased attenuation, especially of the inferior left ventricular wall, compared with that seen with collimated acquisition (*423*).

In spite of its high energy, ^{18}F FDG imaging is still associated with considerable attenuation that must be addressed and corrected in gamma-camera PET. Owing to the large solid angle of gamma camera imaging, scatter is also important. Attenuation correction may be omitted with 511-keV SPECT, but image quality may suffer and affect interpretation. In spite of the reduced sensitivity of 511-keV SPECT, images are readable, clinically useful and may be acquired in the time frame of standard SPECT perfusion images. Image resolution is better and scatter rejection less of a problem in imaging high-energy 511-keV than lower-energy photons. Extra thick crystals will increase the number of positron interactions and so be advantageous for 511-keV imaging on conventional cameras by both methods.

In order to image the 511-keV photon, camera electronics must be modified and optimized for uniformity of detection of this high-energy photon. A special ultra-high-energy collimator had to be designed for the purpose. However, FDG PET studies performed with a scintillation camera equipped with such a specially-designed ultra-high-energy collimator continue to suffer from a gross lack of intrinsic resolution, with full width at half maximum (FWHM) of 12–16 mm, compared with a dedicated PET camera and intrinsic resolution of 3–5 mm FWHM. Adding coincidence detection to the system increases intrinsic resolution to a range comparable with that of the dedicated PET system. However, in operation, even such a camera-based 511-keV detector system suffers significantly compared with PET, because of the much-reduced sensitivity. With the same conventionally applied FDG doses, the conventional camera-based system equipped with an ultra-high-energy collimator will acquire only 1–3 $\times$ 10^6 cpm, compared with 30–50 $\times$ 10^6 cpm for a dedicated PET system. For this reason, most recent camera-based PET systems have utilized a 5/8-in crystal, thicker than the conventional 3/8-in system. This increases the sensitivity to ^{201}Tl by ~100% and of ^{99m}Tc by an additional 10%, without adversely affecting spatial resolution (*423*). However, this still does not compare with the sensitivity of a dedicated PET device. Coincidence detection increases sensitivity of the camera-based system again 2- to 5-fold, to 3–15 × 10^6 cpm. This limited count rate restricts as well the FDG dose permitted with camera-based devices to ~1/2–2/3 of the 10 mCi usually administered with dedicated PET cameras. This relatively counts-poor nature of the camera-based PET image would be expected to adversely affect resolution of small abnormalities. However, in studies by Sandler et al. (*424*), the clinical information in camera-based FDG PET images compared well with that in images acquired with dedicated PET cameras. When Chen et al. (*425*) compared SPECT and FDG PET images in the same 18 patients, PET demonstrated superior acquisition, sensitivity and image resolution, but SPECT with the ultra-high-energy collimator presented image data with comparable viability information compared with PET. Given the increasing desirability of imaging FDG with a conventional camera and the importance of increased crystal thickness for this purpose, what, beyond some increased cost, is the negative aspect of using the 5/8-in crystal for conventional single-photon studies? Preliminary experience suggests a minimal resolution loss with the greater thickness crystal. However, sensitivity is increased dramatically, particularly when imaging higher-energy photons such as indium-111, gallium-67 and ^{131}I.

To increase the efficiency of the FDG protocol, a dual-isotope, single-acquisition study has been tested and applied (*424*). Here, FDG was administered initially, followed by stress imaging with a ^{99m}Tc-based agent and subsequent simultaneous acquisition in dual-energy windows. Prior evaluation had demonstrated only 6% of counts in the ^{99m}Tc window to be downscattered from the 511-keV source. This made possible the simultaneous acquisition and assessment of stress perfusion and metabolism (viability), the ultimate and most efficient stress–rest study.

In a comparison of methods for FDG imaging with a conventional camera, collimator-based imaging demonstrated reduced specificity for viability determination, whereas the coincidence method compared well with conventional PET imaging (*425,426*).

Burt et al. (*418*) compared the accuracy of FDG SPECT, FDG PET and rest ^{201}Tl imaging methods in 20 patients with left ventricular dysfunction and fixed ^{201}Tl defects at rest. Although FDG metabolic imaging was found to identify 13 additional viable segments among 60 dysfunctional segments with fixed defects on rest ^{201}Tl imaging, SPECT and PET FDG imaging were equally accurate. Bax et al. (*417*) performed another such comparison. When 20 patients with prior infarction and wall-motion abnormalities were studied by FDG metabolic imaging and perfusion with both SPECT and PET methods, the agreement between ^{201}Tl/FDG SPECT and nitrogen-13 ammonia/FDG PET was 76%. Among those 12 patients with LVEF<35%, all SPECT and PET data were identical.

Two studies by the same group evaluated the ability of FDG SPECT to determine the viability and restoration of function with revascularization (*427,428*). Negative predictive value was greater than positive predictive value, and the latter was lower than the values seen with several FDG PET studies. In the few studies that compare FDG SPECT with FDG PET for their ability to predict functional recovery with revascularization, the concordance was high (*429*).

Compared with FDG PET, FDG SPECT is more widely available, less expensive (although still quite costly), permits gating and has a relatively brief acquisition. Gamma-camera PET permits simultaneous acquisition of perfusion and metabolism data but provides reduced counts, reduced resolution and may yield a false mismatch pattern when the lower-energy perfusion tracer is more highly attenuated then the positron-emitting ^{18}F. Two studies demonstrate the value of gated SPECT wall motion and thickening as markers of viability before revascularization and as markers of functional improvement after revascularization (*430,431*).

The cardiac application of FDG PET studies with camera-based systems is likely to gain increasing popularity because of: (1) the evident excellence and superiority of the method in determination of regional myocardial viability; (2) the importance of determination of myocardial viability in dysfunctional segments; (3) the great potential of the dual-isotope ^{201}Tl (^{99m}Tc sestamibi/tetrofosmin)/FDG protocol (Fig. 85); (4) the high cost and technical nature of dedicated PET systems; and (5) the increasing clinical value and application of FDG PET for oncology and brain evaluation.

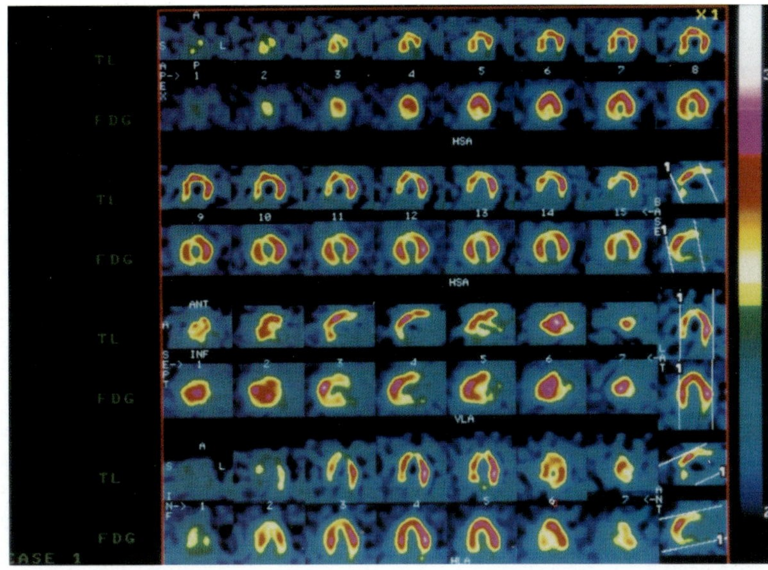

Figure 85 Thallium-201 (^{201}Tl) rest/fluorodeoxyglucose (FDG) protocol. Shown are paired stress ^{201}Tl (upper rows in each panel) and rest PET FDG (lower rows in each panel) in short- (2 upper panels), vertical long- (third panel) and horizontal long-axis (lower panel) slices acquired in a 36-yr-old man with chronic ischemic cardiomyopathy. Clear apical, anterior, septal and inferior defects visible on stress imaging improve greatly on the rest FDG image, the ultimate rest and viability study. Only a limited fixed inferior basal defect appears nonviable. Myocardium at risk and regional viability were optimally evaluated in a single study. (From M. Sandler, Vanderbilt University Medical Center, Nashville, TN; courtesy of El-Scint, Inc., Tel Aviv, Israel.)

THE CURRENT STATE OF THE TECHNOLOGY

In 1997 ~30% of MPS was performed in an office-based setting (*432*), 65% in hospitals and the rest in freestanding imaging centers. The number of office-based studies has increased as part of an effort to reduce costs, to increase method accessibility and serve an increasing number of cardiologists trained in the field. The benefits of telemedicine will be applied more widely, because these laboratories will benefit greatly from the many software possibilities that aid image acquisition, processing and display (*433*). Automation of these tasks will help throughput and quality of studies performed (*13*). The developing potential of expert systems and neural networks could make a great and beneficial impact here. Databases that can document test indication, accuracy and relation to outcomes will be increasingly important as laboratory credentials are established and examined. Such databases also will play a significant role in demonstrating the benefits and insufficiencies of the field. Laboratories should maintain connections both between systems in their lab to ensure uniform study form and quality and with other labs to permit interchange of data and ideas. Interfile exchange and Digital Imaging and Communications in Medicine (DICOM) compatability are important features to permit this information flow. In time, this interchange will permit the cross-correlation of quantitative data from one lab with another and the validation of measures in one lab by another. In this way, the relative advantages of differing radionuclides (*434*), protocols, the potential differing effects of attenuation correction and other processing methods used in the setting of these varying protocols and hardware will be identified. This will aid uniformity and quality of the method, and the isolated practitioner will be isolated no more. Quantitation, once thought potentially expendable (*435*), is at the heart of nuclear cardiology diagnosis, prognosis and viability evaluation and is an added advantage of PET methods. It will gain increasing accuracy and application, and with this the field will gain increased credibility and utility as it moves irrevocably from the subjective impression to the objective, measured likelihood.

ANNOTATED REFERENCES

1. Zaret BL, Strauss HW, Martin WD, et al. Noninvasive regional myocardial perfusion with radioactive potassium. *N Engl J Med* 1973;288:809–812.
   (This early article demonstrates the potential of the field. The radionuclide has poor physical characteristics for imaging, the imaging devices are relatively primitive and the images are irregular, noisy and difficult to read. However, this was a time when the great risk of coronary artery disease was just being identified, the diagnostic insufficiencies of the stress electrocardiogram had recently been determined, the potential benefits of revascularization were just being realized and the risk groups with greatest potential for that benefit were being sought. A noninvasive method to identify patients at risk was sought. In spite of its deficiencies, the image presents radionuclide distribution in parallel with regional perfusion. The promise of the ability to visualize the primary abnormality in coronary disease and to present a noninvasive clarification of the stress electrocardiogram brought a frenzy of deserved interest and activity.)

2. Botvinick EH, Shames DM, Gershengorn K, et al. The clinical advantages of myocardial perfusion scintigraphy with rubidium-81 over stress electrocardiography. *Am J Cardiol* 1977;39:364–373.
   (As opposed to the short half-life of potassium-K, rubidium-81 has a half-life of several hours, permitting its shipment and use early in the day. However, its high energy required special collimation, and images were still suboptimal.)

3. Lebowitz E, Greene MW, Bradley-Moore P, et al. Tl-201 for medical use. *J Nucl Med* 1973;14:421–432.
   (This agent, a potassium analog, presents more optimal, yet imperfect, physical characteristics for imaging.)

4. Maddahi J, Rodrigues E, Berman DS, et al. State of the art myocardial perfusion imaging. Clin Cardiol 1994;12:199–222.
   (This is a thorough review of the technical and clinical aspects of perfusion imaging.)

5. Mullins LJ, Moore RD. The movement of thallium ions in muscle. *J Gen Physiol* 1960;43:759–766.

6. Gehring PJ, Hammond PB. The interrelationship between thallium and potassium in animals. *J Pharm Exp Ther* 1967;155:187–193.

7. Zimmer L, McCall D, D'Addabbo L, et al. Kinetics and characteristics of thallium exchange in cultured cells. *Circulation* 1979;60:138–145.
   (5–7: These articles evaluate the kinetics of thallium-201 on the cellular level. An actively transported intracellular cation, the radionuclide presents unique physical characteristics that have made a lasting niche for the agent among perfusion imaging agents, in spite of its supoptimal physical characteristics.)

8. Heo J, Iskandrian AS. Technetium-labeled myocardial perfusion agents. *Cardiology* 1994;12:187–198.
   (This is an excellent review of the new technetium-based perfusion agents.)

9. Taillefer R, Lambert R, Essiambre R, et al. Comparison between thallium-201, technetium-99m sestamibi, and technetium-99m teboroxime planar myocardial perfusion imaging in detection of coronary artery disease. *J Nucl Med* 1992;33:1091–1098.
   (This article presents a comparison of the diagnostic accuracy of 2 technetium-based perfusion agents with the earlier standard thallium-201.)

10. Iskandrian AE, Kegel JG, Tecce MA, et al. Simultaneous assessment of left ventricular perfusion and function with technetium-99m sestamibi after coronary artery bypass grafting. *Am Heart J* 1993;126:1199–1203.

(First-pass acquisition of technetium-99m sestamibi is applied to determine left ventricular ejection fraction, and both perfusion and function are determined from the same study performed after coronary artery bypass graft surgery. This is but one example of the potential application of the method.)

11. Najm YC, Timmis AD, Maisey MN, et al. The evaluation of ventricular function using gated myocardial imaging with Tc-99m sestamibi. *Eur Heart J* 1989;10:142–148.

(This is one of the early papers that demonstrated the method and value of gated perfusion imaging. Function derived from first-pass acquisition at the time of injection reflects function at peak intervention. Unlike the first-pass method, the gated method reflects function at the time of imaging, not the time of injection.)

12. Cooke CD, Garcia EV. Three-dimensional display of cardiac single photon emission computed tomography. *Am J Cardiogr Imaging* 1993;7:152–221.

(The 3-dimensional display of perfusion imaging is presented as a technical advance in processing and display. However, this method also presents the ability to display a large amount of image data in a condensed and anatomically relevant manner. It has gained popularity as computer memory has expanded and software has developed.)

13. Watson DD, Germano G, DePuey G, et al. Wintergreen panel summaries. Panel on instrumentation and quantification. *J Nucl Cardiol* 1999;6:94–102.

(This is a summary from the Wintergreen Symposium topical panels, an interactive exchange of ideas between leading researchers and practitioners of nuclear cardiology and industry. They review the current state of nuclear cardiology and present goals for future work.)

14. Maddahi J, Van Train KF, Prigent F, et al. Quantitative single-photon emission computerized thallium-201 tomography for detection and localization of coronary artery disease: optimization and prospective validation of a new technique. *J Am Coll Cardiol* 1989;114:1689–1798.

15. DePasquale EE, Nody AC, DePuey E, et al. Quantitative rotational Tl-201 tomography for identifying and localizing coronary disease. *Circulation* 1988;77:316–319.

(14,15: These 2 articles present computer methods for quantitating perfusion image data. Circumferential profiles and polar maps are 2 methods that permit data quantitation. Computer applications and similar processing are major advantages, not disadvantages, of the digital scintigraphic method.)

16. Mahmarian JJ, Verani MS. Myocardial perfusion imaging during pharmacologic stress testing. *Clin Cardiol* 1994;12:223–245.

(This is an excellent and thorough review of pharmacologic stress perfusion imaging methods.)

17. Hearse DJ. Myocardial ischemia: can we agree on a definition for the 21st century [editorial]? *Cardiovasc Res* 1994;28:1737–1744.

(The author considers the differences between the several forms of dysfunctional myocardium, including viable [hibernating, stunned, ischemic] and nonviable [scar].)

18. Parmley WW, Tyberg JV. Determinants of myocardial oxygen demand. *Prog Cardiol* 1976;5:19–36.

(This article presents the factors that affect myocardial oxygen demand, from a mechanical viewpoint.)

19. Sonnenblick EH, Ross J Jr, Covell JW, et al. Velocity of contraction as a determinant of myocardial oxygen consumption. *Am J Physiol* 1965;209:919–927.

(The author presents a single determinant of myocardial oxygen demand and reviews the basic determinants of myocardial oxygen demand on mechanical and cellular levels.)

20. Taylor RR, Cingolani HE, Graham TP, et al. Myocardial oxygen consumption, left ventricular fiber shortening and wall tension. *Cardiovasc Res* 1967;1:219–228.
(Wall stress is considered a major factor contributing to myocardial oxygen demand.)

21. Graham TP Jr, Covell JW, Sonnenblick EH, et al. Control of myocardial oxygen consumption: relative influence of contractile state and tension development. *J Clin Invest* 1968;47:375–385.
(The study presents the relative contributions to myocardial oxygen demands of increased contractility and wall stress.)

22. Weiss HR, Sinha AK. Regional oxygen saturation of small arteries and veins in the canine myocardium. *Circ Res* 1978;42:119–126.
(The authors present evidence for the differential consumption of oxygen across myocardial layers.)

23. Feigl EO. Coronary physiology. *Physiol Rev* 1983;63:1–205.
(This is a review of the coronary circulation, its distribution and its response to increased flow demands.)

24. Klocke FJ. Coronary blood flow in man. *Prog Cardiovasc Dis* 1976:19:117–166.
(This excellent study analyzes the form, magnitude and distribution of the coronary vascular resistance[s].)

25. Austin RE Jr, Smedira NG, Squiers TM, et al. Influence of cardiac contraction and coronary vasomotor tone on regional myocardial blood flow. *Am J of Physiol* 1994; 266:H2542–H2553.
(This article presents the factors that determine regional vasomotor tone, related resistance and the resultant coronary flow.)

26. Hoffman JIE, Baer RW, Hanley FL, et al. Regulation of transmural myocardial blood flow. *J Biomech Eng* 1985;107:2–9.
(Here, insight is gained into the complex mechanical features that regulate regional myocardial blood flow.)

27. Falsetti HL, Carroll RJ, Marcus ML. Temporal heterogeneity of myocardial blood flow in anesthetized dogs. *Circulation* 1975;52:848–853.
(The authors present the evidence for and mechanism of regional temporal variability of coronary blood flow in an animal model.)

28. Canty JM Jr. Coronary pressure-function and steady-state pressure-flow relations during autoregulation in the unanesthetized dog. *Circ Res* 1988;63:821–836.
(The concept and pattern of coronary flow autoregulation is presented.)

29. Bache RJ, Vrobel TR, Arentzen CE, et al. Effect of maximal coronary vasodilation on transmural myocardial perfusion during tachycardia in dogs with left ventricular hypertrophy. *Circ Res* 1981;49:742–750.
(The limits of coronary vasodilation are evaluated in these animal studies.)

30. Parks C, Manohar M, Lundeen G. Regional myocardial blood flow and coronary vascular reserve in unanesthetized ponies during pacing-induced ventricular tachycardia. *J Surg Res* 1983;35:119–131.
(The compensatory mechanisms of the coronary circulation during tachycardia with ventricular dysfunction are examined.)

31. Murray JF, Rapaport E. Coronary blood flow and myocardial metabolism in acute experimental anemia. *Cardiovasc Res* 1972;6:360–367.
(Examined are the compensatory mechanisms of the coronary circulation during anemia and tachycardia.)

32. Fan FC, Chen RYZ, Schuessler GB, Chien S. Effects of hematocrit variations on regional hemodynamics and oxygen transport in the dog. *Am J Physiol* 1980;238:H545–H552.
(This text presents the effects of anemia and polycythemia on coronary flow dynamics and oxygen delivery.)

33. Bellamy RF. Diastolic coronary pressure-flow relations in the dog. *Circ Res* 1978;43: 92–101.
(The author outlines the effects of an altered coronary perfusion pressure on coronary flow reserve.)

34. Kroll K, Feigl EO. Adenosine is unimportant in controlling coronary blood flow in unstressed dog hearts. *Am J Physiol* 1985;249:H1176–H1187.
(The authors demonstrate that autoregulation persists even after intrinsic adenosine is depleted.)

35. Node K, Kitakaze M, Sato H, et al. Increased release of nitric oxide in ischemic hearts after exercise in patients with effort angina. *J Am Coll Cardiol* 1998;32:63–68.
(Nitric oxide release during supine bicycle exercise in 17 patients with proximal left anterior descending coronary artery stenosis is compared with that in 17 individuals with normal coronary arteries. Although neither variable changes with exercise in the control group, nitric oxide release increases across the coronary bed in proportion to the level of lactate production.)

36. Buckberg GD, Fixler DE, Archie JP, et al. Variable effects of heart rate on phasic and regional left ventricular muscle blood flow in anaesthetized dogs. *Cardiovasc Res* 1975;9:1–11.
(This work documents the effects of heart rate on regional coronary blood flow.)

37. Sasayama S, Ross J, Franklin D Jr, et al. Adaptations of the left ventricle to chronic pressure overload. *Circ Res* 1976;38:172–178.
(The adjustments of the myocardium and its blood supply to left ventricular hypertrophy are demonstrated.)

38. Manohar M, Thurmon JC, Tranquilli WJ, et al. Regional myocardial blood flow and coronary vascular reserve in unanesthetized young calves with severe concentric right ventricular hypertrophy. *Circ Res* 1981;148:785–796.
(This study evaluates the effects of left ventricular hypertrophy on coronary on coronary flow reserve.)

39. Hoffman JIE. Regulation of myocardial blood flow and oxygen delivery during hypoxia. In: Arieff AI, ed. *Hypoxia, Metabolic Acidosis, and the Circulation.* Oxford, UK: Oxford University Press; 1992:21–32.
(The authors review the effects of hypoxia, resultant hypoxemia and acidosis on coronary blood flow and coronary flow reserve.)

40. Gould KL, Kirkeeide RL, Buchi M. Coronary flow reserve as a physiologic measure of stenosis. *J Am Coll Cardiol* 1990;15:459–474.
(The authors present the coronary flow reserve as a pathophysiologic measure of coronary stenosis.)

41. Pijls NHJ, Van Son AM, Kirkeeide RL, et al. Experimental basis of determining maximum coronary, myocardial, and collateral blood flow by pressure measurements for assessing functional status severity before and after percutaneous transluminal coronary angioplasty. *Circulation* 1993;87:1354–1367.
(Measures of coronary flow reserve and regional coronary flow were derived before and after coronary angioplasty.)

42. De Bruyne B, Paulus WJ, Pijls NHJ, et al. Rationale and application of coronary transstenotic pressure gradient measurements. *Cathet Cardiovasc Diagn* 1994;33:250–261.
(A differentiation was made between absolute and relative coronary flow reserve.)

43. deKemp RA, Ruddy TD, Hewitt T, et al. Detection of serial changes in absolute myocardial perfusion with ^{82}Rb PET. *J Nucl Med* 2000;41:1426–1435.

(This dog study demonstrates that the method is able to detect absolute differences in serial measurements of myocardial perfusion with dobutamine and atrial pacing.)

44. Christie A. *The Pale Horse.* New York, NY: Pocket Books Inc.;1952.

(Rat poison with thallium as its main ingredient is the murder weapon in this Agatha Christie mystery. In 1977, a friend and fellow cardiologist gave the editor of this self-study topic a newspaper article from a British newspaper. It told of a child who was hospitalized with a bizarre illness. The diagnosis of toxic ingestion of rat poison was made by a nurse who was familiar with the case and who had also read the Christie story. How, the colleague asked, could nuclear medicine physicians recommend the widespread administration of this poison? The answer lies in the tracer nature of clinical radionuclides, in which, unlike pharmaceuticals, the small amount administered does not participate in bodily processes or reactions.)

45. McCall D. Cation exchange and glycoside binding in cultured rat heart cells. *Am J Physiol* 1979;236:C87–C95.

(Thallium-201 [^{201}Tl] transmembrane transport is an energy-requiring process involving the Na+/K+ pump and adenosine triphosphatase. However, this article confirms that the rate of transport for ^{201}Tl is about twice that for K+ [and the rate for teboroxime is even faster].)

46. Strauss HW, Harrison BS, Pitt B, et al. Noninvasive determination of the distribution of regional cardiac output. *J Nucl Med* 1977;18:1167–1174.

(This article analyzes the uptake of thallium-201 [^{201}Tl] in animals after intravenous administration in the parenchyma of the body organs, measured in a well counter post mortem. Because the agent localizes in parenchyma according to its relative perfusion, it presents an excellent method for determining the fractional cardiac output to each organ. Regardless of the intervention or heart rate, myocardial perfusion represents roughly 4%–5% of the cardiac output. Although absolute flow may change, so too does output to other organs, keeping the fractional myocardial perfusion relatively constant. Because oxygen extraction is maximum at baseline and because the fractional myocardial perfusion is relatively constant, myocardial oxygen supply with stress is linked to the cardiac output. This article demonstrates the relationship between ^{201}Tl distribution and the regional fraction of cardiac output. Similarly, technetium-99m sestamibi distribution parallels regional perfusion and fractional cardiac output.)

47. Weich HF, Strauss HW, Pitt B. The extraction of Tl-201 by the myocardium. *Circulation* 1977;56:188–196.

(This article establishes the extraction fraction of thallium-201 by the myocardium.)

48. Nielsen AP, Morris KG, Murdock R, et al. Linear relationship between the distribution of Tl-201 and blood flow in ischemic and non-ischemic myocardium during exercise. *Circulation* 1980;61:797–801.

(This article establishes the linearity of the thallium-201–blood flow relationship under a variety of interventions. However, at high flow rates, a "roll off" in extraction fraction underestimates the regional flow, whereas at low flow rates, an inordinately high extraction is associated with a longer transit time.)

49. Pohost GM, Zir LM, Moor RH, et al. Differentiation of transiently ischemic from infarcted myocardium by serial imaging after a single dose of Tl-201. *Circulation* 1977;55:294–302.

(This article was the first to demonstrate the phenomenon of redistribution and its practical clinical application to the determination of reversible myocardial ischemia.)

50. Gould KL. Noninvasive assessment of coronary stenoses by myocardial perfusion imaging during pharmacologic coronary vasodilatation. *Am J Cardiol* 1978;41: 267–273.

51. Strauss HW, Pitt B. Noninvasive detection of subcritical coronary arterial narrowings with a coronary vasodilator and myocardial perfusion imaging. *Am J Cardiol* 1977;39:403–409.

(50,51: These were the first articles to demonstrate the presence of even apparently nonsignificant coronary lesions by perfusion imaging, here in association with pharmacologic stress.)

52. Meerdink DJ, Leppo JA. Comparison of hypoxia and oubain effects on the first-pass myocardial uptake kinetics of Tc-99m hexakis 2-methoxyisobutyl isonitrile and thallium-201. *J Nucl Med* 1989;30:1500–1506.

(This study evaluates the effects of hypoxia and membrane-active drugs on radiotracer kinetics. These can affect the myocardial extraction of perfusion imaging agents but not to the degree of altered regional perfusion. However, after their localization, these agents are fixed and not influenced by drugs, hypoxia or even altered perfusion. Of course, with time, thallium-201 and, much less so, technetium-99m sestamibi will alter distribution in accordance with prevailing perfusion and other factors relating to membrane transport and diffusion.)

53. Leppo JA, MacNeil PB, Moring AF, et al. Separate effects of ischemia, hypoxia and contractility on thallium-201 kinetics in rabbit myocardium. *J Nucl Med* 1989;30: 312–319.

(This article also reviews the influence of nonperfusion-related factors on thallium uptake, washout and distribution to myocardial cells. Although contractility does not itself influence thallium kinetics, it does influence apparent radionuclide distribution and image characteristics, such as cavitary dilation and photopenia, which are most prominent on SPECT.)

54. Berger BC, Watson DD, Sipes JN, et al. Redistribution of thallium at rest in patients with coronary artery disease. *J Nucl Med* 1979;19:680–687.

55. Pohost GM, O'Keefe DD, Gewirtz H, et al. Thallium redistribution in the presence of severe fixed coronary stenosis. *J Nucl Med* 1979;19:687–684.

56. Pohost GM, Okada RD, O'Keefe DD, et al. Thallium redistribution in dogs with severe coronary artery stenosis of fixed caliber. *Circ Res* 1981;48:439–446.

(54–56: These 3 articles demonstrate the phenomenon of thallium-201 redistribution, at rest [*54*] and after stress [*55,56*]. The initial distribution of the radionuclide parallels perfusion, whereas the delayed distribution parallels K+ space or viable cell mass. The 2 are generally identical and will demonstrate a difference only over time and after reinjection, if the initial localization and regional perfusion differed from the distribution of viable cells, as is true in the setting of "hibernation.")

57. Beller GA, Pohost GM. Mechanism for Tl-201 redistribution after transient myocardial ischemia. *Circulation* 1977;56:141–148.

(This article analyzes serial regional perfusion in normal and ischemic zones after stress-induced ischemia. Ischemic areas do not augment as much as normally perfused regions, but demonstrate slower washout or even accumulation of the radionuclide ["wash-in"] in severely underperfused and ischemic regions. Infarcted regions display similarly reduced radioactivity but with a flat or, less commonly, a maintained washout, presenting a persistently reduced level of radioactivity compared with that of the normal region. With these dynamics, some hours after initial localization, the levels of regional radioactivity in ischemic and normal regions are the same, whereas regional radioactivity in infarcted regions continues to be suppressed.)

58. L'Abbate A, Biagin A, Michelassic C, et al. Myocardial kinetics of thallium and potassium in man. *Circulation* 1979;60:776–783.

(This article describes the similar transcellular transport and intracellular localization of thallium-201 and K+.)

59. Beller GA, Watson DD, Pohost GM. Kinetics of thallium distribution and redistribution: clinical applications in sequential myocardial imaging. In: Strauss HB, Pitt B, eds. *Cardiovascular Nuclear Medicine.* 2nd ed. St. Louis, MO: CV Mosby; 1979:225–242.

(This chapter reviews the mechanism of thallium-201 redistribution as described in the text.)

60. Watson DD, Beller GA, Berger BC. A mechanism for thallium redistribution. *Am J Cardiol* 1979;43:357–364.

(Thallium-201 redistribution is explained, described and documented in terms of the differing uptake and washout rates of normal, ischemic and infarcted tissue.)

61. Garcia E, Maddahi J, Berman D, et al. Space-time quantitation of Tl-201 myocardial scintigraphy. *J Nucl Med* 1981;22:309–317.

(Regional uptake and washout of the radiopharmaceutical are analyzed and quantitated in "normals," and patient studies are compared objectively with the findings. This results in an anatomic map of regional perfusion abnormalities.)

62. Massie BW, Wisnewski J, Kramer B, et al. Comparison of myocardial Tl-201 clearance after maximal and submaximal exercise: implications for the diagnosis of coronary disease [communication]. *J Nucl Med* 1982;23:381–383.

63. Maddahi J, Don Michael TA, Gurewitz J, et al. Significance of slow myocardial washout of Tl-201 at submaximal exercise heart rate. *J Nucl Med* 1986;27:953–961.

64. Kaul S, Chesler DA, Pohost GM, et al. Influence of peak exercise heart rate on normal Tl-201 myocardial clearance. *J Nucl Med* 1986;27:26–30.

65. Iskandrian AS, Heo J, Kong B, et al. Effect of exercise level on the ability of thallium-201 tomographic imaging in detecting coronary artery disease: analysis of 461 patients. *J Am Coll Cardiol* 1984;14:1477–1484.

(62–65: Each of these studies considers the variations in regional thallium-201 myocardial washout rate and its implications to coronary artery disease diagnosis. Certainly, washout appears to be faster in association with dynamic exercise and lower in relation to reduced achieved heart rates. Although low regional washout rates suggest ischemia, globally reduced washout may relate to a reduced level of exercise instead of induced global ischemia. Washout is calculated from the change in background subtracted myocardial counts in a selected myocardial region. Because of this method for calculation of regional washout, the washout value is highly affected by the background level, with higher washout levels noted in relation to lower background levels, which relate in turn to higher workloads and longer exercise times. For this reason, in addition to those conditions that intrinsically determine regional washout, washout calculations are insecure and probably overestimate disease associated with low achieved workloads and pharmacologic stress.)

66. Maddahi J, Van train K, Don Michael TA, et al. Normal initial myocardial distribution and washout of Tl-201 at rest versus exercise. *Clin Nucl Med* 1985;10:11–18.

(For the reasons stated in the notes for reference 65, washout values after a rest injection would not unexpectedly be low.)

67. Gewirtz H, Maksad AK, Most AS, et al. The effect of transient ischemia with reperfusion on thallium clearance from the myocardium. *Circulation* 1979;61:1091–1097.

68. Okada RD, Pohost GM. Effect of decreased blood flow and ischemia on myocardial thallium clearance. *J Am Coll Cardiol* 1984;3:744–750.

(67,68: These articles consider the effects of interventions on the rate of clearance of thallium-201 [^{201}Tl] from the myocardium. Reduced flow or actual ischemia, induced after ^{201}Tl has already been localized, has little effect on the distribution of the agent. However, it does affect its clearance and redistribution to levels related to the prevailing conditions, thus lowering clearance and apparent washout and blunting redistribution.)

69. Sklar J, Kirch D, Johnson T, et al. Slow late myocardial clearance of thallium: a characteristic phenomenon in coronary artery disease. *Circulation* 1982;65:1504–1510.

(Slow myocardial clearance is a finding that often indicates induced regional ischemia. However, factors related to the form and vigor of related stress strongly influence the findings.)

70. Budinger TF, Knittel BL. Cardiac thallium redistribution and model [abstract]. *J Nucl Med* 1987;28:588.

71. Budinger TF, Pohost GM, Bichoff P. Tl-201 integral blood concentration over 2 hr explains persistent defects in patients with no evidence of MI by ECG [abstract]. *Circulation* 1987;76(suppl IV):64.

(70,71: These studies report low blood levels of thallium-201 2 hr after injection and helped to explain the lack of redistribution.)

72. Angello DA, Wilson RA, Palme RT. Effect of eating on Tl-201 myocardial redistribution after myocardial ischemia. *Am J Cardiol* 1987;60:528–533.

(Eating near the time of a thallium-201 injection lowers blood levels and reduces the possibility for redistribution.)

73. Gutman J, Berman DS, Freeman M, et al. Time to completed redistribution of Tl-201 in exercise myocardial scintigraphy: relationship to the degree of coronary artery stenosis. *Am Heart J* 1983;106:989–995.

(This article demonstrates the spectrum of time to thallium-201 redistribution. A relationship was established between the severity of the coronary stenosis and the time to redistribution. However, there are other factors that govern the time to and potential for redistribution in the presence of viable myocardium.)

74. Yang LD, Berman DS, Maddahi J, et al. The frequency of late reversibility in SPECT thallium-201 stress redistribution studies. *J Am Coll Cardiol* 1988;12:1456–1463.

(This article demonstrates the not infrequent need for late delayed 24-hr imaging. The need for this late study varies with the population evaluated and demonstrates further redistribution in approximately 10%–30% of patients presenting with fixed or partially reversible defects at 4 hr. Of course, these images would be most valuable in the presence of fixed defects when imaged earlier, because partially reversible defects do, by their nature, give some evidence of ischemia and viability. Much of the literature confuses fixed with partially reversible defects, although these are not necessarily reflective of similar clinical subgroups.)

75. Perrone-Filardi P, Pace L, Prastaro M, et al. Assessment of myocardial viability in patients with chronic coronary disease: rest–4 hour–24 hour Tl-201 tomography versus dobutamine echocardiography. *Circulation* 1996;94:2712–2719.

(In this study, an almost linear relationship is found between the degree of myocardial thallium uptake and the likelihood that the related segment will improve functionally after revascularization. With the general consideration that relative myocardial uptake of >50% suggests viability and functional improvement after revascularization, those segments with uptake between 50% and 60% are associated with an incidence of functional improvement after revascularization of only 56%, whereas 83% of segments improve among those that demonstrated regional thallium uptake >80%!)

76. Weiss AT, Maddahi J, Lew AS, et al. Reverse redistribution of Tl-201: a sign of non-transmural myocardial infarction with patency of the infarct-related coronary artery. *J Am Coll Cardiol* 1986;7:61–67.

(See annotation after reference 78.)

77. Pace L, Cuocolo A, Marzullo P, et al. Reverse redistribution in resting thallium-201 myocardial scintigraphy in chronic coronary artery disease: an index of myocardial viability. *J Nucl Med* 1995;36:1968–1973.

(Two patterns of segments with reverse redistribution are defined and their clinical implications noted. Stress perfusion defects related to resting asynergy and which appear to worsen at redistribution are less likely to improve function after revascularization [40%] than segments that demonstrate reverse redistribution but are entirely normal at stress [100%].)

78. Faraggi M, Karila-Cohen D, Brochet E, et al. Relationship between resting ^{201}Tl reverse redistribution, microvascular perfusion, and functional recovery in acute myocardial infarction. *J Nucl Med* 2000:41:393–399.

(In a study of 33 patients, reverse distribution is found to be marked early after myocardial infarction, with complete patency of the involved vessel, and is associated with restoration of microvascular reperfusion and with myocardial salvage and viability.)

79. Ohte N, Hashimoto T, Banno T, et al. Clinical significance of reverse redistribution on 24-hour delayed imaging of exercise thallium-201 myocardial SPECT: comparison with myocardial fluorine-18-FDG-PET imaging and left ventricular wall motion. *J Nucl Med* 1995;36:86–92.

(Reverse redistribution is found in 15 of 80 regions studied in 16 patients with prior myocardial infarction and 24-hr redistribution thallium-201 images. In these regions, both FDG uptake and wall motion are present but reduced, suggesting partial but incomplete myocardial loss.)

80. Pace L, Perrone-Filardi P, Mainenti PP, et al. Effects of myocardial revascularization on regional thallium-201 uptake and systolic function in regions with reverse redistribution on tomographic thallium-201 imaging at rest in patients with chronic coronary artery disease. *J Nucl Cardiol* 1998;5:153–160.

(The authors evaluate reverse redistribution in 47 patients before coronary artery bypass graft. They find a variable relationship to left ventricular function and a good relationship to viability. This evidence is consistent with the possibility that the finding relates more to technical factors than to any perfusion-related condition.)

81. Soufer R, Dey HM, Lawson AJ, et al. Relationship between reverse redistribution on planar thallium scintigraphy and regional myocardial viability: a correlative PET study. *J Nucl Med* 1995;36:180–187.

(Thirty-two patients with reverse redistribution undergo fluorodeoxyglucose PET evaluation in 50 segments on planar thallium-201 images. Among 36 [72%] segments with reverse redistribution and patterns of PET viability analyzed, 19 are PET normal, whereas 17 reveal PET criteria for ischemia. On follow-up, 31% of patients with reverse redistribution have events, half of these with "severe reverse redistribution." Segments with reverse redistribution are generally viable, but evidence associating them with risk is tenuous, especially considering that most such segments do not relate to coronary disease.)

82. Lear JL, Raff U, Jain R. Reverse and pseudoredistribution of thallium-201 in healed myocardial infarction and normal and negative thallium-201 washout in ischemia due to background oversubtraction. *Am J Cardiol* 1988;62:543–550.

(76–82: Reverse redistribution indicates a perfusion pattern in which defects appear to improve with stress compared with those at rest or redistribution. Generally affecting a limited myocardial region, it suggests an induced perfusion abnormality in the remaining myocardium, which fails to gain relative radioactivity even as well as the abnormal region. Although it may be associated with nontransmural infarction [*76*], particularly after revascularization, many such images are associated with normal coronary anatomy and likely are the result of associated technical factors or variable regional washout [*77–82*].)

83. Araujo W, DePuey EG, Kamram M, et al. Artifactual reverse distribution pattern in myocardial perfusion SPECT with technetium-99m sestamibi. *J Nucl Cardiol* 2000; 7:633–638.

(The phenomenon of reverse redistribution is examined in SPECT studies performed in 202 patients with low pretest coronary disease likelihood and in phantom experiments. The finding is most common among large patients, in whom breast and diaphragmatic attenuation are evident. Phantom experiments demonstrate that such attenuation would have a greater effect among low count density SPECT studies, as in the rest portion of protocols performed with any single tracer or in the thallium-201 or rest limb of the dual-isotope sequential process.)

84. Gewirtz H, Grotte GJ, Strauss HW, et al. The influence of left ventricular volume and wall motion on myocardial images. *Circulation* 1979;59:1172–1177.

85. Sinusas AJ, Shi QX, Vitols PJ, et al. Impact of regional ventricular function, geometry and dobutamine stress on quantitative ^{99m}Tc-sestamibi defect size. *Circulation* 1993;88:2224–2234.

(84,85: The findings on perfusion imaging are influenced by the related ventricular geometry and regional function, probably as a result of a partial volume effect. The partial volume effect results in a partial filling of a computer pixel or voxel. The unit will then be gray scale or color coded according to the mean pixel intensity, a lower intensity than the peak value within the imaging unit.)

86. Lenaers A, Block P, Theil EV, et al. Segmental analysis of Tl-201 stress myocardial scintigraphy. *J Nucl Med* 1977;18:509–516.

(This early effort relates the distribution of perfusion defects to the related coronary anatomy on an empiric basis.)

87. Massie BM, Botvinick EH, Brundage BH. Correlation of Tl-201 scintigrams with coronary anatomy: factors affecting region by region sensitivity. *Am J Cardiol* 1979;44:616–623.

(This careful analysis of planar perfusion images seeks to relate image findings with the distribution of the coronary anatomy. It also presents, at an early date, the various factors that determine regional sensitivity for coronary disease.)

88. Dash H, Massie BM, Botvinick EH, et al. The noninvasive identification of left main and three-vessel coronary artery disease by myocardial stress perfusion scintigraphy and treadmill exercise electrocardiography. *Circulation* 1979;60:276–284.

(This early article demonstrates the image recognition of multivessel disease in somewhat <50% of such patients with a similar sensitivity for markedly positive stress tests. Together, a markedly positive scintigram or stress electrocardiogram identifies ~66% of these patients. Although the results of stress testing should not be ignored and should be used in association with the scintigraphic findings, the application of SPECT imaging has demonstrated the ability of the method toclarify the clinical significance of even the markedly positive stress test [see reference 94].)

89. McKillop HJ, Murray RG, Turner JG, et al. Can the extent of coronary artery disease be predicted from Tl-201 myocardial images? *J Nucl Med* 1979;20:715–723.

90. Rigo P, Bailey IK, Griffith LSC, et al. Value and limitations of segmental analysis of stress thallium myocardial imaging for localization of coronary artery disease. *Circulation* 1980;61:973–981.

91. Maddahi J, Garcia EV, Berman DS, et al. Improved noninvasive assessment of coronary artery disease by quantitative analysis of regional stress myocardial distribution and washout of Tl-201. *Circulation* 1981;64:924–932.

(86–91: Again diagnosis and prognosis of coronary disease and the ability to identify the presence of multivessel coronary disease are benefited by consideration of the quantitation of regional activity and comparison to a normal data base, by the assessment of thallium-201 washout and by relation to the associated stress test results. However, intrinsic factors limit the ability of the method to identify all stenotic lesions involved in all cases. This has been improved by SPECT, new quantitative methods, and probably by the application of technetium-99m sestamibi-based perfusion agents.)

92. Maddahi J, Abdulla A, Garcia E, et al. Noninvasive identification of left main and triple-vessel coronary artery disease: improved accuracy using quantitative analysis

of regional myocardial stress, redistribution and washout of Tl-201. *J Am Coll Cardiol* 1986;7:53–61.

93. Mahmarian JJ, Boyce TM, Goldberg RK, et al. Quantitative exercise thallium-201 single photon emission computed tomography for the enhanced diagnosis of ischemic heart disease. *J Am Coll Cardiol* 1990;15:318–326.

94. Pollock SG, Abbott RD, Boucher CA, et al. A model to predict multivessel coronary disease from the exercise thallium-201 stress test. *Am J Med* 1991;90:345–352.

95. Garcia EV, Van Train K, Maddahi J, et al. Quantification of rotational Tl-201 myocardial tomography. *J Nucl Med* 1985;26:17–26.

96. Abdulla A, Maddahi J, Garcia E, et al. Slow regional clearance of myocardial Tl-201 in the absence of perfusion defects: contribution to detection of individual coronary stenoses and the mechanism for its occurence. *Circulation* 1985;71:72–80.

(The relative nature of perfusion scintigraphy suggests the possibility of normal images in the presence of widespread or "global" ischemia. In this study, generalized washout abnormalities occur rarely in the setting of extensive coronary disease in the presence of otherwise normal planar images. In fact, the excellent prognosis of normal perfusion images and the disuse of washout analysis in association with SPECT images suggest that the presence of widespread and "balanced" ischemia is a rare phenomenon, not generally to be asserted as a cause for image–anatomy discrepancies.)

(86–96: These studies consider the ability and inability to identify the full extent of myocardium at ischemic risk. Of course, the relative nature of the method, the variability of individual coronary anatomy, the vagaries and possible insufficiencies of the related stress test, the subjective nature of the angiographic gold standard and the difference between angiographic anatomy and scintigraphic pathophysiology do much to explain the apparent lack of scintigraphic perfection. Yet, the method is rarely normal in the setting of multivessel disease and frequently identifies all vessels involved. Its sensitivity has been aided by quantitative regional counts and washout analysis, comparison to a normal patient population and SPECT imaging with greater contrast resolution and anatomic differentiation. Yet, even with SPECT imaging, the results of the associated stress test must be considered to further stratify the diagnostic and prognostic power of the related scintigram.)

97. Bateman TM, Maddahi J, Gray RJ, et al. Diffuse slow washout of myocardial thallium-201: a new scintigraphic indicator of extensive coronary artery disease. *J Am Coll Cardiol* 1984;4:55–63.

(The presentation of a completely normal planar perfusion image in the presence of severe 3-vessel coronary disease is unusual. Washout analysis has been presented as a method to recognize homogeneously reduced perfusion and possibly to augment recognition of abnormal regions, even in the presence of perfusion defects. These authors demonstrated that among 1265 consecutive patients with quantitatively analyzed planar stress-redistribution thallium-201 [^{201}Tl] scintigrams, 13 [1%] have patterns of diffuse, slow ^{201}Tl washout in the absence of a regional perfusion defect. Diffuse slow washout is defined as the presence of washout abnormalities in the distribution of all 3 major coronary arteries but not uniformly in all. Of these 13 patients, 9 [69%] are found to have left main or triple-vessel coronary disease. Diffuse slow washout is a rare indicator of extensive ischemia and related coronary disease in the absence of planar image defects. This incidence appears smaller yet with SPECT acquisition and is associated with a very low negative predictive value. In fact, washout analysis is not usually performed in association with SPECT imaging because of the increased sensitivity of SPECT and the even greater infrequency of such findings. Therefore, washout analysis is not recommended with ^{201}Tl SPECT. If one wishes to perform washout analysis, images acquired before reinjection must be analyzed. Reinjection makes washout analysis impossible. In addition, the low event rate associated with a normal or "probably normal" perfusion image suggests that the pattern does not generally conceal high-risk disease. Nonetheless, a simple planar image can be acquired before stress imaging and prior to reinjection before delayed SPECT imaging. These can be analyzed for washout in the setting of a strongly suggestive history or stress test result, providing yet another piece of supportive data.)

98. Canhasi B, Dae MW, Botvinick EH, et al. Interaction of supplementary indicators of ischemia and stress electrocardiography in the diagnosis of multivessel coronary disease. *J Am Coll Cardiol* 1985;6:581–589.

(This article presents the concept of "nonperfusion indicators" of ischemia. The presence of lung uptake, cavitary dilation or basal uptake increases the likelihood of extensive coronary disease and may indicate more extensive disease than that shown by simple analysis of perfusion defects.)

99. Brown KA, Boucher CA, Okada RD, et al. Prognostic value of exercise thallium-201 imaging in patients presenting for evaluation of chest pain. *J Am Coll Cardiol* 1983;1:994–1001.

(The body of data presented here suggests that a normal scan is related to a benign prognosis in the setting of coronary and even multivessel disease. Pollock et al. [*94*] perform a multivariate analysis in 383 consecutive patients who underwent coronary angiography and perfusion scintigraphy. Age, ST depression and the number of perfusion defects are interacting, independent predictors of multivessel disease. The number of defects on perfusion scintigraphy [or their absence] is better related to prognosis than is the angiographic anatomy [see references 100–103]. A similar relationship is observed when exercise blood pool imaging is demonstrated to differentiate between high- and low-risk subgroups of anatomically similar triple-vessel disease.)

100. Krishnan R, Lu J, Dae MW, Botvinick EH. Does myocardial perfusion scintigraphy demonstrate clinical utility in patients with markedly positive exercise tests? An assessment of the method in a high risk subset. *Am Heart J* 1994;127: 804–815.

(When patients with early deep ST depression are analyzed for the potential benefit of stress perfusion scintigraphy, 2 patient groups are identified. The initial and smaller group have such test results in the presence of known coronary artery disease, sometimes with prior infarction or recurrent symptoms after revascularization. They go directly to angiography without imaging. A larger group has no history of coronary disease and has atypical or absent symptoms, sometimes years after apparently successful revascularization. Here, a spectrum of scintigraphic findings guide patient management and correlate well with related anatomy and patient outcome.)

101. Zir LM, Miller SW, Dinsmore RE, et al. Interobserver variability in coronary angiography. *Circulation* 1975;53:627–633.

(Four experienced coronary angiographers, 2 radiologists and 2 cardiologists, independently assess location and degree of coronary artery stenoses and the degree of left ventricular wall motion abnormality. The degree of interobserver variability is great and should be considered when clinical decisions are based on visual impressions of coronary stenosis. Not only does the anatomic information lack full pathophysiologic content, but its visual interpretation is unreliable.)

102. Beauman GJ, Vogel RA. Accuracy of individual and panel visual interpretations of coronary arteriograms. *J Am Coll Cardiol* 1990;16:108–116.

(An excellent article documenting the variability of visual interpretation of coronary angiograms.)

(101,102: These articles analyze the reproducibility of coronary angiographic interpretations in the hands of trained experts of varying experience. The wide range of variability is surprising, with sufficient disagreement that vessels believed to be disease free and without lesions by some are noted to be totally occluded by others. This variability of interpretation is not the result of vascular misidentification, as each reading relates to identical vessels. In addition, the most experienced experts enjoy no greater degree of agreement than do the novices. It is on the basis of such evidence that we base major management decisions.)

103. Gould KL. Noninvasive assessment of coronary stenoses by myocardial imaging during pharmacologic coronary vasodilation: IV. Limits of detection of stenosis with idealized experimental cross sectional myocardial imaging. *Am J Cardiol* 1978; 41:761–768.
(Additional analysis presents the interaction of coronary vasodilation and imaging technique. The article defines the limits of the method as it was then performed, in terms of coronary pathophysiology rather than anatomy.)

104. Vogel RA. The radiographic assessment of coronary blood flow parameters. *Circulation* 1985;72:460–465.
(Coronary flow reserve, measured noninvasively in patients with digital angiographic methods, correlates extremely well with the findings on stress perfusion and stress blood pool scintigraphy but relatively poorly with those of coronary angiography.)

105. Fuster V, Badimon L, Badimon JJ, Chesebro JH. The pathogenesis of coronary artery disease and the acute coronary syndromes. *N Engl J Med* 1992;326:242–250,310–318.
(Prognosis is probably associated with the number and severity of coronary lesions, the ischemic burden [measured by conventional stress imaging] and by some factors related to lesion stability and the tendency to occlude. These factors are probably related to clotting parameters, endothelial characteristics and a multitude of other factors of which we are becoming aware. The number and severity of lesions are characterized by stress testing and imaging. Factors related to lesion stability remain elusive.)

106. Davies MJ, Thomas AC. Plaque fissuring: the cause of acute myocardial infarction, sudden ischemic death, and crescendo angina. *Br Heart J* 1985;53:363–371.

107. Wilson RF, Holiday MD, White CW. Quantitative angiographic morphology of coronary stenoses leading to myocardial infarction or unstable angina. *Circulation* 1986;73:286–294.

108. Stratmann HG, Tamesis BR, Younis LT, et al. Prognostic value of dipyridamole technetium-99m sestamibi myocardial imaging in patients with stable chest pain who are unable to exercise. *Am J Cardiol* 1994;73:647–652.
(Dipyridamole perfusion scintigraphy demonstrates strong prognostic value, even in more than 300 patients with stable angina who are not exposed to the stress of surgery. This is interesting and somewhat unexpected, as the stress of the pharmacologic agent is not related to, but is probably in excess of, that experienced daily in normal activities. Risk, then, is better related to the ischemic burden and the extent of myocardium at ischemic risk than to the extent of ischemia [or equivalent] induced with daily activities.)
(105–108: It is surprising that strong evidence indicates that subsequent infarction is not necessarily associated with a severe stenosis. Yet most pathophysiologic tests for coronary disease, including perfusion scintigraphy, present documented prognostic value related to their ability to identify the most severe of pathophysiologically significant stenoses. It may not be the individual stenosis that is prognostically significant but its value as a marker for the full extent of disease, "the total ischemic burden.")

109. Gal R, Port SC. Arm vein uptake of Tl-201 during exercise: incidence and clinical significance. *J Nucl Med* 1986;27:1353–1361.
(As with infiltration of the thallium-201 dose, arm vein uptake reduces the washout rate. It is a relatively common event that has little practical adverse clinical effect.)

110. Berman DS, ed. A symposium: technetium-99m myocardial perfusion imaging agents and their relation to thallium-201. *Am J Cardiol* 1990;66:1E–96E.
(This symposium focuses entirely on technetium-99m myocardial perfusion imaging agents.)

111. Berman DS. Introduction. A symposium: technetium-99m myocardial perfusion imaging agents and their relation to thallium-201. *Am J Cardiol* 1990;66: 1E–4E. (This symposium introduction reviews the major aspects to be considered and presented an overview of issues.)

112. Jones AG, Davison A, Abrams MJ, et al. Biological studies of a new class of technetium complexes: the hexakis (alkylisonitrile) technetium (I) cations. *Int J Nucl Med Biol* 1984;11:225–234.

113. McKusick K, Holman BL, Jones AG, et al. Comparison of three Tc-99m isonitriles for detection of coronary artery disease in humans. *J Nucl Med* 1986;27:878–885.

114. Holman BL, Sporn V, Jones AG, et al. Myocardial imaging with technetium-99m CPI: initial experience in the human. *J Nucl Med* 1987;28:13–18.

115. Pichard M, Dupras G, Taillefer R, et al. Compared biodistribution of 201-thallium,-Tc-99m tertiary-butyl-isonitrile (TBI) and Tc-99m-methoxy-isobutyl-isonitrile (sestamibi). *J Nucl Med* 1987;28:654–662.

116. Stierner H, Buell U, Kleinhans E, et al. Myocardial kinetics of Tc-99m hexakis-(2-methoxy-isobutyl-isonitrile) (HMIBI) in patients with coronary heart disease: a comparative study versus Tl-201 with SPECT. *Nucl Med Commun* 1988;9:15–23.

117. Beanlands RSB, Dawood F, Wen WH, et al. Are the kinetics of technetium-99m methoxyisobutyl isonitrile affected by cell metabolism and viability? *Circulation* 1990;82:1802–1814.

118. Beller GA, Glover DK, Edwards NC, et al. Tc-sestamibi uptake and retention during myocardial ischemia and reperfusion. *Circulation* 1983;87:2033–2042.

119. Carvalho PA, Chiu ML, Kronauge JF, et al. Subcellular distribution and analysis of technetium-99m-MIBI in isolated perfused rat hearts. *J Nucl Med* 1992;33: 1516–1521.

120. Piwnica-Worms D, Kronauge JF, Chiu ML. Uptake and retention of hexakis (2-methoxyisobutyl isonitrile) technetium (I) in cultured chick myocardial cells: mitochondrial and plasma membrane potential dependence. *Circulation* 1990; 82: 1826–1838.

121. Glover DK, Okada RD. Myocardial technetium-99m sestamibi kinetics after reperfusion in a canine model. *Am Heart J* 1993;125:657–666.

122. Marshall RC, Leidholdt EM Jr, Zhang DY, et al. Technetium-99m hexakis 2-methoxy-2-isobutyl isonitrile and thallium-201 extraction, washout and retention at varying coronary flow rates in rabbit heart. *Circulation* 1990;82:998–1007.

123. Maublant JC, Gachon P, Moins N. Hexakis (2-methoxy isobutylisonitrile) technetium-99m and thallium-201 chloride: uptake and release in cultured myocardial cells. *J Nucl Med* 1988;29:48–54.

124. Wackers FJTh, Berman DS, Maddahi J, et al. Technetium-99m hexakis 2-methoxyisobutyl isonitrile: human biodistribution, dosimetry, safety and preliminary comparison to thallium-201 for myocardial perfusion imaging. *J Nucl Med* 1989;30:301–311.

125. Holman BL, Campbell CA, Lister-James J, et al. Effect of reperfusion and hyperemia on the biodistribution of the myocardial imaging agent Tc-99m TBI. *J Nucl Med* 1986;27:1172–1177.

126. Holman BL, Jones AG, Lister-James J, et al. A new Tc-99m-labeled myocardial imaging agent, hexakis (t-butylisonitrile)-technetium (I) (Tc-99m TBI): initial experience in the human. *J Nucl Med* 1984;25:1350–1355.

127. Sia STB, Holman BL, McKusick K, et al. The utilization of Tc-99m TBI as a myocardial perfusion agent in exercise studies: comparison with Tl-201 thallous chloride and examination of its biodistribution in humans. *Eur J Nucl Med* 1986;12: 333–336.

128. Okada R, Glover D, Gaffney T, et al. Myocardial kinetics of Tc-99m-hexakis-2-methoxy-2-methylpropylisonitrile. *Circulation* 1988;77:491–498.

129. Li QS, Solot G, Frank TL, et al. Myocardial redistribution of technetium-99m-methoxyisobutyl isonitrile (sestamibi). *J Nucl Med* 1990;31:1069–1076.

130. Taillefer R, Dupras G, Sporn V, et al. Myocardial perfusion imaging with a new radiotracer technetium-99m hexamibi (methoxy isobutyl isonitrile) comparison with thallium-201 imaging. *Clin Nucl Med* 1989;14:89–96.

131. Kiat H, Maddahi J, Roy L, et al. Comparison of Tc-99m methoxy isobutyl isonitrile with Tl-201 imaging by planar and SPECT techniques for assessment of coronary disease. *Am Heart J* 1989;117:1–11.

132. Taillefer R, Lambert R, Dupras G, et al. Clinical comparison between thallium-201 and Tc-99m-methoxy isobutyl isonitrile (hexamibi) myocardial perfusion imaging for detection of coronary artery disease. *Eur J Nucl Med* 1989;15:280–286.

133. Kronauge JF, Chiu ML, Cone JS, et al. Comparison of neutral and cationic myocardial perfusion agents: characteristics of accumulation in cultured cells. *Nucl Med Biol* 1992;19:141–148.

134. Dahlberg ST, Leppo JA. Physiologic properties of myocardial perfusion tracers. *Clin Cardiol* 1994;12:169–186.

135. Leppo J, Meerdink DA. Comparison of the myocardial uptake of technetium-labeled isonitrile analogue and thallium. *Circ Res* 1989;65:632–639.

136. Marshall RC Leidhodt EM, Barnett CA. Single-pass myocardial extraction and retention of a Tc-99m isonitrile vs Tl-201 [abstract]. *Circulation* 1987;76:IV218.

(112–136: The isonitriles, considered in these articles both as a chemical class and individually, distribute according to regional perfusion. Their varied kinetic behavior and biologic handling present great differences in clinical applicability. In these articles they are often compaired at the cellular and tissue levels with thallium-201 [^{201}Tl]. In addition, several articles consider the differences between ^{201}Tl localization and kinetics and that of the isonitriles and the implications of these differences for the determination of tissue viability.

136: The extraction, washout and retention of technetium-99m [^{99m}Tc] sestamibi and ^{201}Tl are studied in 20 isolated, isovolumic, retrograde, blood-perfused rabbit hearts. Mean ^{99m}Tc sestamibi peak instantaneous extraction is lower and more flow-rate affected than ^{201}Tl peak instantaneous extraction. The rate of ^{201}Tl washout is significantly faster than that of ^{99m}Tc sestamibi and more dependent on the initial perfusion rate. Reflecting its higher extraction, ^{201}Tl retention immediately after injection is 55%–79% higher than that of ^{99m}Tc sestamibi, and the relative change in ^{201}Tl is more highly associated with peak flow than is ^{99m}Tc sestamibi. However, because of washout, the superiority of ^{201}Tl as a tracer of perfusion is lost after 10 min.)

137. Baillet G, Mena IG, Kuperus JH, et al. Simultaneous Tc-99m sestamibi angiography and myocardial perfusion imaging. *J Nucl Med* 1989;30:38–46.

138. Borges-Neto S, Coleman RE, Jones RH. Perfusion and function at rest and treadmill exercise using technetium-99m sestamibi: comparison of 1- and 2-day protocols in normal volunteers. *J Nucl Med* 1990;31:1128–1135.

(137,138: This review and article present the theory and practice of combined first-pass function analysis with stress perfusion analysis using a single technetium-99m–based radionuclide and a multicrystal camera. In theory, the functional data could serve to complement the perfusion data, aiding diagnosis and refining prognosis. Much work needs to be done evaluating this relationship. Cost is a potential problem with this method, in which different cameras are to be applied for functional and perfusion imaging.)

139. Williams KA, Taillon LA, Draho JM, et al. First-pass radionuclide angiographic studies of left ventricular function with technetium-99m teboroxime, technetium-99m sestamibi and technetium-99m DTPA. *J Nucl Med* 1993;34:394–402.

(This study analyzes the application of a variety of technetium-99m–based perfusion tracers to first-pass radioangiography. These tracers are generally and widely applicable, with the possible exception of teboroxime. With teboroxime, prolonged pulmonary transit may retard the rapid delivery of the tracer to the left heart and interfere with the generation of accurate first-pass data.)

140. Williams, KA, Taillon LA. Left ventricular function in patients with coronary artery disease assessed by gated tomographic myocardial perfusion images: comparison with assessment by contrast ventriculography and first-pass radionuclide angiography. *J Am Coll Cardiol* 1996;27:173–181.

(Left ventricular ejection fractions, determined from gated rest SPECT sestamibi perfusion scans by a semiautomatic method, compare well with those calculated from first-pass evaluation in 38 patients [$r = 0.87$] and with left ventriculography in 54 patients [$r = 0.93$]. There is high inter- and intraobserver agreement. The "image inversion" method applied assigns "counts" values to "cavitary" intensities that could be affected by factors other than ventricular volume. The method is unique and needs testing.)

141. Nichols K, DePuey EG, Rozanski A, et al. Image enhancement of severely hypoperfused myocardium for computation of tomographic ejection fraction. *J Nucl Med* 1997;38:1411–1417.

(This early study derives the left ventricular ejection fraction [LVEF] from gated perfusion image data using an automated reproducible computer program. An image enhancement algorithm then succeeds in providing accurate, reproducible, gated SPECT LVEF in the most dramatic cases of severe hypoperfusion related to the most dense image defects.)

142. Nichols K, Depuey EG, Krasnow N, et al. Reliability of enhanced gated SPECT in assessing wall motion of severely hypoperfused myocardium: echocardiographic validation. *J Nucl Cardiol* 1998;4:387–394.

(Regional image enhancement succeeds in the correct identification of endocardial borders and the resultant accurate calculation of left ventricular ejection fraction in 40 patients with severe hypoperfusion on stress myocardial perfusion scintigraphy.)

143. Wackers FJTh, Becker AE, Samson G, et al. Location and size of acute transmural myocardial infarction estimated from thallium-201 scintiscans: a clinicopathological study. *Circulation* 1977;56:72–78.

(This article demonstrates an excellent relationship between pathologic and thallium-201 scintigraphic infarct size. Similar relationships have been drawn for technetium-99m sestamibi.)

144. Khan JK, McGhie I, Akers MS, et al. Quantitative rotational tomography with thallium-201 and technetium-99m 2-methoxy-isobutyl-isonitrile: a direct comparison in normal individuals and patients with coronary artery disease. *Circulation* 1989;79:1282–1293.

(This study demonstrates an excellent relationship between image radionuclide distribution and defect size, measured with thallium-201 and technetium-99m sestamibi imaging.)

145. Dae MW, Valesquez-Rocha S, Botvinick EH, O'Connell JW. Comparison of thallium and technetium-99m sestamibi in isoproterenol-induced subendocardial ischemia in rat myocardium [abstract]. *J Am Coll Cardiol* 1992;19:337A.

(Sophisticated autoradiographic studies compare the distribution of thallium-201 and technetium-99m sestamibi in identical myocardium subjected to the same ischemic or pharmacologic intervention, with a 50 μm resolution. Only with prolonged epinephrine infusion is there a difference, with sestamibi underestimation of infarct size. However, all other cases demonstrate identical radionuclide distribution. Is this difference clinically significant?)

146. Wolfe CL, O'Connell WJ, Sievers RE, et al. Assessment of perfused left ventricular mass in normal, ischemic and reperfused myocardium by means of single photon emission computed tomography of technetium-99m isonitrile. *Am Heart J* 1993; 126:1275–1283.

(This technetium-99m sestamibi SPECT animal study demonstrates a good relationship between pathologic and scintigraphic infarct size and little evidence of sestamibi redistribution.)

147. Villanueva-Meyer J, Mena I, Diggles L, Narahara KA. Assessment of myocardial perfusion defect size after early and delayed SPECT imaging with technetium-99m-hexakis-2-methoxyisobutyl isonitrile after stress. *J Nucl Med* 1993;34: 187–192.

(Defect size in 20 coronary patients studied 1 and 4 hr after stress technetium-99m sestamibi imaging do not differ and support the lack of clinically significant redistribution in sestamibi stress images.)

148. Gibbons RJ, Verani MS, Behrenbeck T, et al. Feasibility of tomographic Tc-99m-hexakis-2-methoxy-2-methylpropyl-isonitrile imaging for the assessment of myocardial area at risk and the effect of acute treatment in myocardial infarction. *Circulation* 1989;80:1277–1286.

(Comparing prethrombolytic with post-thrombolytic "infarct size" acquired at least 18 hr after thombolytic therapy, technetium-99m sestamibi myocardial perfusion scintigraphy was used also to determine the extent of myocardium salvaged by thrombolysis compared with that salvaged with conservative treatment.)

149. Christian TF, Schwartz RS, Gibbons RJ. Determinants of infarct size in reperfusion therapy for acute myocardial infarction. *Circulation* 1992;86:81–90.

(The extent of collaterals can be determined by assessment of the risk region with radionuclide administration during occlusion. This method may be applied clinically and so provide information regarding the final infarct size.)

150. Freeman I, Grunwald AM, Hoory S, et al. Effect of occlusion and myocardial viability on myocardial activity of technetium-99m-sestamibi. *J Nucl Med* 1991;32: 292–298.

(Cellular sestamibi uptake is viability dependent. Depolarization of myocyte or mitochondrial membranes, as occurs with coronary occlusion as presented in this article, inhibits cellular uptake and retention of the agent.)

151. Piwnica-Worms D, Chiu ML, Kronauge JF. Divergent kinetics of Tl-201 and Tc-99m sestamibi in cultured chick ventricular myocytes during ATP depletion. *Circulation* 1992;85:1531–1541.

(Unlike thallium-201, technetium-99m sestamibi is not inhibited by other imposed conditions that mimic the metabolic deficiencies of ischemia.)

152. Sinusas AJ, Watson DD, Cannon JMJ, et al. Effect of ischemia and postischemic dysfunction on myocardial uptake of technetium-99m-labeled methoxyisobutyl isonitrile and thallium-201. *J Am Coll Cardiol* 1989;14:1785–1793.

153. Sinusas AJ, Bergin JD, Edwards NC, et al. Redistribution of ^{99m}Tc sestamibi and ^{201}Tl in the presence of a severe coronary artery stenosis. *Circulation* 1994;89:2332–2341.

(152,153: Technetium-99m sestamibi localizes in viable myocardium characterized by a model of "stunning" [*152*] and "hibernation" [*153*]. This supports its ability to monitor and reflect myocardial viability. However, unlike thallium-201, its redistribution is nominal.)

154. Glover DK, Okada RD. Myocardial kinetics of Tc-MIBI in canine myocardium after dipyridamole. *Circulation* 1990;81:628–637.

(See annotation for reference 159.)

155. Medrano R, Lowry R, Young J, et al. Assessment of myocardial viability with ^{99m}Tc sestamibi in patients undergoing cardiac transplantation: a scintigraphic/pathologic study. *Circulation* 1996;94:1010–1017.

(The relative uptake of technetium-99m sestamibi well parallels the distribution of viable myocardium and scar in this series of explanted human hearts studied post-transplantation.)

156. Mast ST, Borges-Neto S. Invited commentary: myocardial hibernation and stunning; still much to learn. *J Nucl Med* 2000;41:1235–11236.

(This is an excellent editorial commentary that reviews the state of current knowledge of "stunned" and "hibernating" myocardium.)

157. Maes A, Borgers M, Flameng W, et al. Assessment of myocardial viability in chronic coronary artery disease using technetium-99m sestamibi SPECT: correlation with histologic and positron emission tomographic studies and functional follow-up. *J Am Coll Cardiol* 1997;29:62–68.

(Technetium-99m [^{99m}Tc] sestamibi uptake is significantly higher in viable areas, as confirmed by PET, and in areas with improved contractility 3 mo after bypass graft surgery. A linear relationship is seen between percentage fibrosis and ^{99m}Tc sestamibi uptake, with an optimal threshold of 50% for prediction of functional recovery, with positive and negative predictive values of 82% and 78%, respectively. This article suggests that ^{99m}Tc sestamibi uptake is comparable with that of thallium-201 for viability evaluation and that regional uptake is the same with the 2 agents.)

158. Dakik HA, Howell JF, Lawrie GM, et al. Assessment of myocardial viability with ^{99m}Tc sestamibi tomography before coronary artery bypass surgery. *Circulation* 1997;96:2892–2898.

(The authors demonstrate the relationship between uptake of technetium-99m [^{99m}Tc] sestamibi and viability in dysfunctional segments. They perform rest ^{99m}Tc sestamibi imaging within 2 days of coronary artery bypass graft [CABG] in 21 patients with left anterior descending coronary artery disease and related wall motion abnormalities. Biopsied segments with improved function after CABG have significantly higher ^{99m}Tc activity [81% $\pm$ 5% versus 49% $\pm$ 16%] and less fibrosis [7% $\pm$ 4% versus 31% $\pm$ 21%]. Technetium-99m activity correlates well with the presence and extent of viable myocardium and predicted functional improvement after revascularization.)

159. Sinusas AJ, Trautman KA, Bergin JD, et al. Quantification of area at risk during coronary occlusion and degree of myocardial salvage after reperfusion with technetium-99m methoxyisobutyl isonitrile and thallium-201. *Circulation* 1990;82:1424–1437.

(These authors demonstrate that after 3 hr of coronary occlusion, technetium-99m [^{99m}Tc] sestamibi defect size correlates well [r = 0.94] with the autoradiographic risk area in dogs. However, when injected after 90 min of reperfusion, uptake correlates with the final infarct size. In both this study and that of Verani et al. [272] the defect area after reperfusion does not correspond to the region of vessel perfusion but to the region of perfusion of viable myocytes. This and other evidence suggest that sestamibi distribution reflects both viable myocardium and regional perfusion and correlates with the area at ischemic risk after occlusion, identifying the area salvaged after reperfusion. Technetium-99m sestamibi appears to act as a microsphere only in the sense that it does not redistribute but is relatively fixed in the cell. However, unlike microspheres, in many studies it appears to localize only in viable tissue.)

(154,159: These are 2 of several studies performed in animals and report an excellent association between ^{99m}Tc sestamibi distribution and regional perfusion

[*154*]. Regional sestamibi was noted to be depressed only in the presence of cellular necrosis [*159*].)

160. Gimple LW, Beller GA. Myocardial viability; assessment by cardiac scintigraphy. *Clin Cardiol* 1994:12:161–170.

(This excellent review presents evidence suggesting a lack of correlation between technetium-99m sestamibi localization and regional myocardial viability and discusses the larger body of literature demonstrating the ability of the agent to monitor viability. The subject remains a topic of ongoing research.)

161. Dilsizian V, Arrighi JA, Diodati JG, et al. Myocardial viability in patients with chronic coronary artery disease: comparison of Tc-99m sestamibi with thallium reinjection and fluorodeoxyglucose. *Circulation* 1999;89:678–687.

(In this study, the distribution of sestamibi parallels well those of thallium-201 and fluorodeoxyglucose.)

162. Acampa W, Petretta M, Florimonte L, et al. Sestamibi SPECT in the detection of myocardial viability in patients with chronic ischemic left ventricular dysfunction: comparison between visual and quantitative analysis. *J Nucl Cardiol* 2000;7:401–413.

(This study analyzes rest sestamibi SPECT and echocardiography in 65 patients with a recent prior myocardial infarction and left ventricular [LV] dysfunction. All undergo revascularization and subsequent echocardiography. Here, visual and quantitative analysis of rest sestamibi images have similar accuracy in predicting the recovery of LV function after coronary revascularization.)

163. Meerdink DJ, Leppo JA. Experimental studies of the physiologic properties of technetium-99m agents: myocardial transport of perfusion imaging agents. In Berman D, ed. A symposium: technetium-99m myocardial perfusion imaging agents and their relation to thallium-201. *Am J Cardiol* 1990;66:9E–15E.

164. Narra RK, Nunn AD, Kuczynski BL, et al. A neutral technetium-99m complex for myocardial imaging. *J Nucl Med* 1989;30:1830–1837.

(163,164: These reviews consider the properties of the second group of technetium-99m–labeled myocardial perfusion agents, boronic acid adducts of technetium oximes [BATO]. The most promising BATO compound is teboroxime. However, it has the property of rapid myocardial washout, which requires rapid imaging after injection. This characteristic requires special acquisition protocols and laboratory restrictions that make it unpopular for clinical work. In addition, its localization is unrelated to tissue viability, another undesirable trait. However, its rapid localization in myocardium presents a most reliable noninvasive method to assess vascular patency after thrombolysis. It has been withdrawn from the market.)

165. Leppo JA, Meerdink DJ. Comparative myocardial extraction of two technetium-labeled BATO derivatives (SQ30217, SQ32014) and thallium. *J Nucl Med* 1990;31:67–74.

(This study evaluates the myocardial transport of 2 technetium-labeled boronic acid adducts of technetium oxime compounds and thallium-201 [^{201}Tl] during varying levels of coronary flow in an isolated blood-perfused rabbit heart model. Over a wide range of coronary flow rates [.3–2.4], mean teboroxime extraction is 25% higher than that of ^{201}Tl. The mean capillary flux for teboroxime is also 46% higher than that of ^{201}Tl. Unfortunately, other unfavorable properties make the agent unsatisfactory for clinical application.)

166. Maublant JC, Moins N, Gachon P, et al. Uptake of technetium-99m teboroxime in cultured myocardial cells: comparison with thallium-201 and technetium-99m sestamibi. *J Nucl Med* 1993;34:255–259.

(In an experimental cell culture model, these workers show that technetium-99m [^{99m}Tc] teboroxime has faster uptake and greater myocardial cell accumulation than both thallium-201 [^{201}Tl] and ^{99m}Tc sestamibi. They also show that, in general, teboroxime is the least and ^{201}Tl the most sensitive to metabolic inhibition at the cellular level.

Teboroxime uptake is decreased at low temperatures but not by cell lysis. Both ^{201}Tl and ^{99m}Tc sestamibi uptake are reduced with cyanide, a blocker of mitochondrial uptake, and iodoacetate, an inhibitor of the glycolytic pathway. Oubain reduces ^{201}Tl uptake only at high doses. Of these 3 perfusion agents, teboroxime shows the greatest resistance to metabolic impairment.)

167. Stewart RE, Hutchins GD, Brown D, et al. Myocardial retention and clearance of the flow tracer Tc-99m SQ30217 in canine heart. *J Nucl Med* 1989;30:860–861.

(Stewart et al. show relatively high extraction of teboroxime after intracoronary injection in open-chest dogs. Myocardial washout of teboroxime also appears to be flow related and quite rapid.)

168. Johnson G III, Glover DK, Hebert CB, et al. Myocardial clearance kinetics of technetium-99m-teboroxime following dipyridamole: differentiation of stenosis severity in canine myocardium. *J Nucl Med* 1995;36:111–118.

169. Gewirtz H. Myocardial clearance kinetics of technetium-99m-teboroxime following dipyridamole injection [editorial]. *J Nucl Med* 1995;36:119–120.

(168,169: Using an open-chest canine preparation, Johnson et al. [168] report the ability to differentiate among stenoses severities by a measure of the clearance kinetics of this rapidly vanishing radionuclide. Implanted radiation detectors in dogs make measurements not possible in the patient. Administered after dipyridamole and applied to a stationary target, measures of washout are possible in the period immediately after administration. Exciting, too, is the possibility of extracting from such measurements an absolute value of the clearance rate, which could identify disease in a nonrelativistic manner. This is yet another aspect of the potential of teboroxime application that was not evaluated before its withdrawal from use. It deserves reconsideration [*169*].)

170. Johnson LL, Seldin DW. Clinical experience with technetium-99m teboroxime, a neutral, lipophilic myocardial perfusion imaging agent. In Berman D, ed. A symposium: technetium-99m myocardial perfusion imaging agents and their relation to thallium-201. *Am J Cardiol* 1990;66:63E–67E.

(This is a thorough review article of the physical and biologic properties and clinical traits of teboroxime and its chemical class.)

171. Narra RK, Feld T, Wedeking P, et al. SQ30217, a technetium-99m labeled myocardial imaging agent which shows no interspecies difference in uptake. *Nuklearmedizin* 1989;23:(suppl);489–491.

172. Stewart RE, Heyl B, O'Rourke RA, et al. Demonstration of differential post-stenotic myocardial technetium-99m teboroxime clearance kinetics after experimental ischemic and hyperemic stress. *J Nucl Med* 1991;32:2000–2008.

(171,172: Myocardial clearance of teboroxime is rapid, with biexponential half times of 2 [68%] and 78 min [32%] [*171*], and differential, flow-dependent washout is also rapid and proportional to regional flow [*172*].

173. Seldin DW, Johnson LL, Blood DK, et al. Myocardial perfusion imaging with technetium-99m SQ30217: comparison with thallium-201 and coronary anatomy. *J Nucl Med* 1989;30:312–319.

(The authors consider the properties of teboroxime and adapted a suitable imaging protocol. The agent's properties necessitate the completion of imaging within 10–15 min after injection.)

174. Heller LI, Villegas BJ, Weiner BH, et al. Sequential teboroxime imaging during and after balloon occlusion of a coronary artery. *J Am Coll Cardiol* 1993;21:1319–1327.

(Planar teboroxime scans are acquired during balloon occlusion and after reperfusion in 15 patients undergoing angioplasty. The scan is 100% accurate in distinguishing left anterior descending from left circumflex or right coronary occlusions. Rapid planar teboroxime images can identify the occluded vessel and document vessel patency.)

175. Faber TL. Multiheaded rotating gamma cameras in cardiac single-photon emission computed tomography. *J Nucl Cardiol* 1994;1:117–119.
(In order to perform SPECT imaging with teboroxime, it is necessary to begin imaging 2 min after injection and to finish imaging in about 13 min. Multihead cameras expedite this rapid acquisition.)

176. Cannon PJ, Dell RB, Dwyer EM. Measurement of regional myocardial perfusion in man with 133-xenon and a scintillation camera. *J Clin Invest* 1972;51:964–977.
(The same methods applied to the calculation of quantitative regional myocardial perfusion with the xenon washout method may potentially be applied to teboroxime.)

177. Botvinick EH. The proper tool for the job [editorial]. *J Am Coll Cardiol* 1993;21: 1328–1331.

178. Heller LI, Villegas BJ, Weiner BH, et al. Sequential teboroxime imaging during and after balloon occlusion of a coronary artery. *J Am Coll Cardiol* 1993;21:1319–1327.
(177,178: This editorial [*177*] is written in reference to an article [*178*] that described the ability of teboroxime to identify coronary patency after thrombolysis. The advantages and disadvantages for clinical application are considered.)

179. Beller GA, Sinusas AJ. Experimental studies of the physiologic properties of technetium-99m isonitriles. In: Berman D, ed: A symposium: technetium-99m myocardial perfusion imaging agents and their relation to thallium-201. *Am J Cardiol* 1990;66:5E–8E.

180. Weinstein H, Dahlberg ST, McSherry BA, et al. Rapid redistribution of teboroxime. *Am J Cardiol* 1993;71:848–852.
(179,180: The lack of relation to myocardial viability and the technical difficulties presented by its kinetic behavior make SPECT imaging with teboroxime problematic [*180*] and a poor comparison with technetium-99m sestamibi [*179*].)

181. Gerson MC, Lukes J, Deutsch E, et al. Comparison of imaging properties of technetium-99m Q12 and technetium-99m Q3 in humans. *J Nucl Cardiol* 1995;2:224–230.
(The "Q" complexes are a group of mixed ligand tracers with physical traits and imaging characteristics more favorable than current technetium-99m [^{99m}Tc] and thallium-201 tracers. They differ structurally from the diphosphine tetrofosmin complexes in that the Q complexes contain monophosphine as well as Schiff base ligands and show little evidence of washout. They have been chemically manipulated to reduce hepatic excretion. Q-12 has been formulated as a "furifosmin" kit, but no kit has been formulated for Q-3. In 10 patients with chest pain and angiographically evaluated coronary anatomy, ^{99m}Tc Q-12 and ^{99m}Tc Q-3 images provide similar coronary detection in the range of 90%–100%. Unlike ^{99m}Tc sestamibi, imaging is begun only 15 min after radionuclide administration. [See annotation for 182 and 183].)

182. Kelly JD, Forster AM, Higley B, et al. Technetium-99m-tetrofosmin as a new radiopharmaceutical for myocardial perfusion imaging. *J Nucl Med* 1993;34:222–227.
(The lower hepatic clearance of this new perfusion radiotracer and a simple freeze-dried kit formulation are emphasized in this review of the agent, which has been approved and already is used widely.)

183. Rossetti C, Vanoli G, Paganelli G, et al. Human biodistribution, dosimetry and clinical use of technetium (III)-99m-Q12. *J Nucl Med* 1994;35:1571–1580.
(The biodistribution and dosimetry of Q12 are assessed in 10 normal volunteers, and its clinical use was evaluated in 70 patients. There is good heart uptake [2.2%

after 1 hr] and absent washout after 5 hr. Rapid hepatobiliary clearance permits imaging in as little as 15 min. There are high heart-to-lung and heart-to-liver ratios at stress, independent of feeding. Hepatobiliary clearance is as short as 15 min, with heart-to-lung and heart-to-liver ratios greater at stress than at rest, regardless of time elapsed after injection or feeding. In this study, 46 of 47 patients with angiographic coronary disease show defects, a 97% sensitivity.)

184. Gerson MC, Millard RW, McGoron AJ, et al. Myocardial uptake and kinetic properties of technetium-99m-Q3 in dogs. *J Nucl Med* 1994;35:1698–1706.
(Technetium-99m Q3 distributed in parallel with regional perfusion from blood flows of 0–6.1 ml/min/g, with no evidence of redistribution after 4 hr.)

185. Gerson MC, Lukes J, Deutsch E, et al. Comparison of technetium-99m-Q3 and thallium-201 for detection of coronary artery disease in humans. *J Nucl Med* 1994;35:580–586.
(184,185: The authors of these articles review the properties of the new technetium-based perfusion imaging agents. To the extent that these agents monitor regional perfusion, persist in the myocardium with sufficient duration to perform SPECT studies and demonstrate reduced hepatobiliary excretion and gastrointestinal background, they will provide an advantage to the other available tracer, technetium-99m sestamibi.)

186. Glover DK, Ruiz M, Koplan BA, et al. Technetium-99m tetrofosmin assessment of myocardial perfusion in canine models of coronary occlusion and reperfusion. *J Nucl Med* 1999;40:142–149.
(In this animal study, tetrofosmin distribution parallels well that of thallium-201 and microspheres in occlusion and in reflow protocols. Tetrofosmin reflects flow heterogeneity well during coronary occlusion and, when given after reperfusion, reflects well viability and the degree of myocardial salvage and reperfusion flow. These studies validate the use of this agent for assessment of coronary occlusion, infarct size, and myocardial viability after reperfusion.)

187. Glover DK, Ruiz M, Yang JY, et al. Myocardial ^{99m}Tc-tetrofosmin uptake during adenosine-induced vasodilation with either a critical or mild coronary stenosis: comparison with ^{201}Tl and regional myocardial blood flow. *Circulation* 1997;96:2332–2338.
(In a canine model, relative myocardial underperfusion, induced pharmacologically, is seen better with thallium-201 [^{201}Tl] than with technetium-99m [^{99m}Tc] tetrofosmin. This could be explained by the reduced extraction fraction and reduced linearity with flow of the ^{99m}Tc-based agent. In the clinical setting, factors of attenuation and ^{201}Tl redistribution may blunt this difference.)

188. Hendel RC, Parker MA, Wackers FJTh, et al. Reduced variability of interpretation and improved image quality with a technetium 99m myocardial perfusion agent: comparison of thallium 201 and technetium 99m-labeled tetrofosmin. *J Nucl Cardiol* 1994;1:509–514.
(Tetrofosmin and thallium-201 [^{201}Tl] stress imaging are performed in the same 216 patients within a 2-wk period. More tetrofosmin images than ^{201}Tl images are of excellent quality [52% versus 38%, $P < 0.05$], and, when differences in image quality are noted, tetrofosmin images are generally superior [$P < 0.0001$]. Tetrofosmin demonstrates reduced interobserver variability and improved diagnostic accuracy compared with ^{201}Tl.)

189. Braat SH, Leclercq B, Itti R, et al. Myocardial imaging with technetium-99m tetrofosmin: comparison of one-day and two-day protocols. *J Nucl Med* 1994;35:1581–1585.
(A 1-day tetrofosmin protocol is compared to a 2-day protocol in 55 patients. The studies are comparable, except for defects in the inferior wall that appear to be more generally reversible on the 1-day and fixed on the 2-day protocol.)

190. Zaret BL, Rigo P, Wackers FJTh, et al. Myocardial perfusion imaging with ^{99m}Tc tetrofosmin: comparison to ^{201}Tl imaging and coronary angiography in a phase III multicenter trial. *Circulation* 1995;91:313–319.

(This comparative phase III multicenter study evaluates 252 patients with suspected coronary artery disease in 10 centers. The patients undergo exercise testing with technetium-99m tetrofosmin using 2 separate injections and have separate thallium-201 [^{201}Tl] stress and redistribution imaging. Tetrofosmin images are of high quality, with little extracardiac activity. Regional concordance between ^{201}Tl and tetrofosmin in normal or abnormal image findings vary from 81%–90%. When specific categories of abnormality [normal, ischemic, infarcted or mixed ischemic/infarcted segments] are demanded, concordance ranges from 64%–84%. When coronary angiography is used as the diagnostic criterion, sensitivity and positive and negative predictive values of the 2 methods are comparable, and tetrofosmin normalcy is 97%.)

191. Matsunari I, Fujino S, Taki J, et al. Myocardial viability assessment with technetium-99m tetrofosmin and thallium-201 reinjection in coronary artery disease. *J Nucl Med* 1995;36:1961–1967.

(Exercise and rest tetrofosmin images acquired in a 2-day protocol are compared with exercise-redistribution-reinjection SPECT thallium-201 [^{201}Tl] images for viability assessment. Eighty-three of 209 [40%] defects present after exercise on both tetrofosmin and ^{201}Tl imaging are discordant in subsequent behavior, in which 73 [88%] are reversible only on serial ^{201}Tl imaging. Thus, tetrofosmin is less sensitive than ^{201}Tl to the presence of regional viability, using reversibility as a marker. However, if quantitation of regional activity within irreversible defects is the yardstick of viability, the agents produce more comparable results.)

192. Miller DD. The growing flood of technetium-99m myocardial perfusion agents: more water... or more mud? *Circulation* 1995;91:555–558.

(Criticism is addressed to the method of evaluation and introduction of new radiotracers, with special reference to the multicenter trial of tetrofosmin [see reference 190]. The nature of the study suggests only a desire to demonstrate parity with current agents, most notably thallium-201, the Food and Drug Administration "gold standard." No SPECT images or gating are performed, nor is any attempt made to demonstrate superiority. This would appear to add to the "mud." However, those who sponsor these studies simply seek the data to gain recognition and approval of their agent. Demonstration of superiority must, ironically, await drug approval. However, the development of additional agents demonstrates the interest and capability of the field and will continue to add, albeit in a stuttering fashion, increments to its capabilities.)

193. Jain D, Wackers FJTh, Mattera J, et al. Biokinetics of technetium-99m tetrofosmin: myocardial perfusion imaging agent: implications for a one-day imaging protocol. *J Nucl Med* 1993;34:1254–1259.

(The agent remains where initially localized for ~8 hr. The second injection of a 1-day protocol must obscure the earlier dose. The second dose must be 4 times that of the first. The same principle applies with technetium-99m sestamibi.)

194. Matsunari I, Fujino S, Taki J, et al. Comparison of defect size between thallium-201 and technetium-99m tetrofosmin myocardial single-photon emission computed tomography in patients with single-vessel coronary artery disease. *Am J Cardiol* 1996;77:350–354.

(Defect size on exercise-rest technetium-99m tetrofosmin imaging is smaller than that on exercise thallium-201 [^{201}Tl] imaging. However, rest tetrofosmin images compare well to those of reinjection ^{201}Tl in 20 patients with single-vessel coronary disease. Such evaluation is important before clinical application of the new radionuclide.)

195. Gerson MC, Lakes J, Deutsch E, et al. Comparison of technetium 99m Q-12 and thallium 201 for detection of angiographically documented coronary artery disease in humans. *J Nucl Cardiol* 1994;1:499–508.

(Technetium-99m [^{99m}Tc] Q-12 employed in a rest–stress protocol completed in 100 min demonstrates overall and regional diagnostic accuracy similar to that of thallium-201 [^{201}Tl]. A 100-min rest–exercise Q12 protocol is applied in 20 patients with coronary artery disease and in 10 normal subjects. In this small study, there is no difference in sensitivity or specificity between the ^{99m}Tc Q-12 and ^{201}Tl, and there is good agreement in the localization of regional abnormalities [$\kappa = 0.88$].)

196. Matsunari I, Beoning G, Ziegler SI, et al. Attenuation-corrected 99m-Tc tetrofosmin single photon emission computed tomography in the detection of viable myocardium: comparison with positron emission tomography using ^{18}F-fluorodeoxyglucose. *J Am Coll Cardiol* 1998;32:927–935.

(Quantitative tetrofosmin analysis after attenuation correction demonstrates a good, albeit limited, correlation with viability measured by the PET fluorodeoxyglucose standard. Uptake >60% of peak activity correlates with PET viability in 93% of segments, whereas activity <30% correlates with PET scar in 100% of segments. Segments with activity between 30% and 60% correlate poorly, even with attenuation correction!)

197. van Dongen AJ, van Rijk. Minimizing liver, bowel, and gastric acidity in myocardial perfusion SPECT. *J Nucl Med* 2000;41:1315–1317.

(Direction is provided for acquisition of high-quality images.)

198. Liu Z, Johnson G III, Bej D, et al. Myocardial kinetics of ^{99m}Tc-sestamibi, ^{99m}Tc-tetrofosmin and ^{99m}Tc-Q12 in a severe model of ischemia with reperfusion injury [abstract]. *J Am Coll Cardiol* 1999;33:480A.

(Isolated perfused rat hearts are used to measure the kinetics of technetium-99m sestamibi, tetrofosmin and Q-12. All can distinguish infarcted from normal myocardium. However, sestamibi peak uptake and retention is greatest, suggesting that this radionuclide would better differentiate and more sensitively identify coronary lesions, especially those of lesser severity.)

199. Hendel R, Verani M, Miller DD, et al. Diagnostic utility of tomographic myocardial perfusion imaging with technetium-99m furifosmin (Q12) compared with thallium-201: results of the Phase III multicenter trial. *J Nucl Cardiol* 1996;3:291–300.

(This phase III study involves 7 sites, 150 patients and 30 volunteers. All patients have unequivocal thallium-201 [^{201}Tl] studies or a high pretest likelihood and are studied with a stress–rest same-day protocol. The furifosmin studies agree with those of ^{201}Tl in 86% [$\kappa = 0.87$]. The concordance with ^{201}Tl is 95% among those with prior myocardial infarction and 76% among those without prior infarction, with a normalcy rate for both agents of 100% in a small number of patients.)

200. Uccelli L, Giganti M, Duatti A, et al. Subcellular distribution of technetium-99m-N-NOET in rat myocardium. *J Nucl Med* 1995;36:2075–2079.

(This agent shows the greatest linear correlation with microsphere-determined coronary blood flow over the greatest range of flows among all perfusion agents. It maintains linearity to high flow rates and so has potentially great beneficial impact on perfusion imaging. It appears to localize by diffusion into myocardial cell membranes.)

201. Johnson III G, Allton IL, Nguyen KN, et al. Clearance of technetium-99m N-NOET in normal, ischemic-reperfused, and membrane-disrupted myocardium. *J Nucl Cardiol* 1996;3:42–54.

(Technetium-99m bis[N-ethoxy,N-ethyl dithiocarbamato] nitrido Tc[v] [^{99m}Tc-N-NOET] is a new, neutral cardiac perfusion imaging agent. This study again demonstrates the high uptake and retention of the radionuclide, far exceeding that of thallium-201 and proportional to regional perfusion to higher levels. Clearance is not affected by imposed ischemia or reperfusion injury. Clearance is increased dramatically with conditions of membrane disruption, supporting the concept that the agent is localized in cell membranes. These findings add to the potential of ^{99m}Tc-N-NOET as an improved myocardial perfusion imaging agent.)

202. Rumsey WL, Kuczynski B, Patel B, et al. SPECT imaging of ischemic myocardium using a technetium-99m-nitroimidazole ligand. *J Nucl Med* 1995;36:1445–1450.
(This new experimental agent, the technetium-99m–bound version of the long promising fluorine-18 fluoromisonidazole, appears capable of identifying oxygen-deprived, ischemic, but viable, myocardium.)

203. Ghezzi C, Fagret D, Arvieux CC, et al. Myocardial kinetics of TcN-NOET: a neutral lipophilic complex tracer of regional myocardial blood flow. *J Nucl Med* 1995;36:1069–1077.
(The kinetics of technetium-99m bis[N-ethoxy,N-ethyl dithiocarbamato] nitrido Tc[v] are described.)

204. Fagret D, Yves Marie P, Brunotte F, et al. Myocardial perfusion imaging with technetium-99m-Tc NOET: comparison with thallium-201 coronary angiography. *J Nucl Med* 1995;36:936–943.
(The authors study 25 patients with angiography by thallium-201 stress–reinjection protocol and compare the results with a technetium-99m bis[N-ethoxy,N-ethyl dithiocarbamato] nitrido Tc[v] stress–delayed protocol. The 2 studies agree in 88% of patients and in 93% of coronary regions and segments.)

205. Ghezzi C, Fagret D, Bricho P-Y, et al. Redistribution of Bis(N-ethoxy, N-ethyl dithiocarbamato) nitrido Tc-99m (V), a new myocardial perfusion imaging agent: comparison with Tl-201 redistribution [abstract]. *Circulation* 1996;94:I302.
(Technetium-99m bis[N-ethoxy,N-ethyl dithiocarbamato] nitrido Tc[v] has traits similar to thallium-201, including redistribution.)

206. Holly TA, Leppo JA, Gilmore MP, et al. The effect of ischemic injury on the cardiac transport of Tc-99m N-NOET in the isolated rabbit heart. *J Nucl Cardiol* 1999;6:633–640.
(The reduced extraction and retention of technetium-99m bis[N-ethoxy,N-ethyl dithiocarbamato] nitrido Tc[v] with severe ischemic injury make its uptake a potential viability marker.)

207. Germano G, Erel J, Kiat H, et al. Quantitative LVEF and qualitative regional function from gated thallium-201 perfusion SPECT. *J Nucl Med* 1997;38:749–754.
(This is a pivotal paper that presents a now common method for an automated left ventricular ejection fraction calculation with an evolving display of regional wall motion.)

208. DePuey EG, Nichols K, Dobansky C. Left ventricular ejection function in patients with coronary artery disease assessed by gated technetium-99m-sestamibi SPECT. *J Nucl Med* 1993;334:1871–1876.
(DePuey et al. validates a manual method to calculate left ventricular ejection fraction from gated sestamibi images, using studies in 30 patients with correlation coefficients ranging from 0.79–0.88 and with various operators and intra- and interobserver variability [r = 0.75].)

209. Williams KA, Kaillon LA. Left ventricular function in patients with coronary artery disease assessed by gated tomographic myocardial perfusion images: comparison with assessment by contrast ventriculography and first-pass radionuclide angiography. *J Am Coll Cardiol* 1996;27:173–181.

210. Germano G, Kiat H, Kavanagh PS, et al. Automatic quantification of ejection fraction from gated myocardial perfusion SPECT. *J Nucl Med* 1995;36:2138–2147.
(Presented are the methodology and results of a fully automated process to calculate left ventricular ejection fraction from gated myocardial perfusion scintigraphy.)

211. Smith WH, Kastner RJ, Calnon DA, et al. Quantitative gated single photon emission computed tomography imaging: a counts-based method for display and measurement of regional and global ventricular systolic function. *J Nucl Cardiol* 1997;4: 451–463.

(208–211: Left ventricular ejection fraction [LVEF] has been calculated by a number of workers by different methods. DePuey et al. base their method on the detection of endocardial boundaries. Williams et al. apply an inverted intensity display and a counts-based method. Germano et al. use a modified Simpson's Rule approach, and Smith et al. use the partial volume effect to calculate regional myocardial thickening and LVEF.)

212. Cooke CD, Garcia EV, Cullom J, et al. Determining the accuracy of calculating systolic wall thickening using a fast Fourier transform approximation: a simulation study based on canine and patient data. *J Nucl Med* 1994;35:1185–1192.

(This is an early study in the development of a method to measure systolic wall thickening on gated sestamibi perfusion images. A model is used to document the accuracy of the calculation of wall thickening from intensity variations with the cardiac cycle. Increasing regional intensity during systole is shown to parallel echocardiographic wall thickening. This paper validates the method of left ventricular ejection fraction calculation and demonstrates the reproducibility and stability of the calculation and its tolerance in the face of even markedly reduced data density.)

213. Adachi I, Morita K, Imran B, et al. Heterogeneity of myocardial wall motion and thickening in the left ventricle evaluated with quantitative gated SPECT. *J Nucl Cardiol* 2000;7:296–300.

(The presence of heterogeneous myocardial wall motion and thickening is demonstrated in 35 patients studied by gated SPECT, here using the Autoquant software, and suggests the need for segmental values for normal.)

214. Faber TL, Cooke CD, Folks RD, et al. An integrated processing program for analysis of left ventricular ejection fraction and perfusion. *Comput Cardiol* 1997;24:697–700.

(Faber et al. validate this method in 80 patients studied with first-pass technique [r = .82, SEE = 8.5%]. In addition, these same workers demonstrate the relative reproducibility of the left ventricular ejection fraction [LVEF] by this method and the stability of the calculation with varying assumed wall thickness, where the assumption of a 1.5-cm end-diastolic wall thickness brings only a 6% [relative] error in calculated LVEF. LVEF calculated from myocardial perfusion scintigraphy by this method is correlated with the first-pass LVEF in 80 patients [r = .82, SEE = 8.5%].)

215. Iskandrian AE, Germano G, VanDecker W, et al. Validation of left ventricular volume measurements by gated SPECT ^{99m}Tc-labeled sestamibi imaging. *J Nucl Cardiol* 1998;5:574–578.

(Among 24 patients, left ventricular volumes measured by gated SPECT myocardial perfusion scintigraphy compare well with values generated by the first-pass method and, as an automated method, have a high reproducibility [0.99].)

216. Faber TL, Cooke CD, Folks RD, et al. Left ventricular function and perfusion from gated SPECT perfusion images: an integrated method. *J Nucl Med* 1999;40:650–659.

(The method initially reported successfully completed automated localization of endocardial and epicardial surfaces with successful processing in 94% of 700 cases studied and, more recently, an 83% success rate in a prospective series. This study demonstrates the accuracy of the method compared with left ventricular ejection fraction [LVEF] with first-pass [r = 0.82] and MR imaging [r = .085] calculations. Volumes and mass correlate even better with those calculated by other methods. Using this method, LVEF, volumes and mass are well correlated with LVEF volumes and mass calculated from gated MR studies.)

217. Vansant JP, Faber TL, Folks RD, Rao JM, Garcia EV. Resting left ventricular volumes and ejection fraction from gated single-photon emission computed tomography (SPECT): correlation to first pass [abstract]. *Circulation* 1995;92: I11.

(The method also identifies the epicardium and contours the surfaces in 65 patients, with an $r = 0.91$ and SEE = 6.87%, when gated left ventricular ejection fraction [LVEF] values are compared in 65 patients with first-pass LVEF values.)

218. Faber TL, Cooke CD, Peifer JW, et al. Three-dimensional displays of the left ventricular epicardial surface from standard single-photon computed tomographic (SPECT) perfusion quantification techniques. *J Nucl Med* 1995;36:697–703.

(This is an early presentation of the 3-dimensional perfusion image display that is now so commonly applied in practice.)

219. Faber TL, Folks RD, Cooke CD, et al. Left ventricular mass from ungated perfusion images: comparison to MRI [abstract]. *J Nucl Med* 1997;38:20P.

(This method of left ventricular volume and mass calculation based in myocardial perfusion scintigraphy is well correlated with left ventricular volumes and mass calculated from gated MR studies.

The authors validate an automated method for left ventricular ejection fraction [LVEF] calculation in 75 patients, using a 34% peak-counts threshold. The method correlates well with gated equilibrium blood pool [$r = 0.87$] and first-pass studies performed in the same patients [$r = 0.87$]. This method of LVEF calculation correlates well with left ventricular volumes and mass calculated from gated MR studies.

220. Vallejo E, Dione SP, Sinusas AJ, et al. Assessment of left ventricular ejection fraction with quantitative gated SPECT: accuracy and correlation with first-pass radionuclide angiography. *J Nucl Cardiol* 2000;7:461–470.

(Left ventricular ejection fraction [LVEF] calculated from gated SPECT by the Autoquant processing software is compared with LVEF by the first-pass method in 400 patients. LV contours can not be fit in 35 cases, demonstrating a failure of the method. In those 365 cases in which adequate edges are detected, agreement with the first pass method is best in high-count SPECT studies, in normal studies and in large hearts, compared with those studies in low counts, normal perfusion and small hearts.)

221. Nichols K, Lefkowitz D, Faber T, et al. Echocardiographic validation of gated SPECT ventricular function measurements. *J Nucl Med* 2000;40:1308–1314.

(In 33 patients studied with both methods, all gated SPECT parameters of left ventricular size and function correlate well with those on echocardiography. Agreement is best when methods applied to calculate volumes by both modalities share the same underlying assumptions.)

222. Chua T, Yin LC, Thiang TH, et al. Accuracy of the automated assessment of left ventricular function with gated perfusion SPECT in the presence of perfusion defects and left ventricular dysfunction: correlation with equilibrium ventriculography and echocardiography. *J Nucl Cardiol* 2000;7:301–311.

(Left ventricular ejection fractions [LVEFs], volumes, and regional wall motion calculated in 84 patients by automated gated SPECT are compared with these values in the same patients with equilibrium blood pool scintigraphy (62 patients) and echocardiography (22 patients). Compared with these methods, automated gated SPECT provides an accurate assessment of global LVEF and regional function, even in the presence of an earlier myocardial infarction and LV dysfunction.)

223. Vallejo E, Dione DP, Bruni WL, et al. Reproducibility and accuracy of gated SPECT for determination of left ventricular volumes and ejection fraction: experimental validation using MRI. *J Nucl Med* 2000;41:874–882.

224. Udelson JE, Fares MA. Invited commentary: how accurate is quantitative gated SPECT? *J Nucl Med* 2000;41:883–886.

(223,224: The study by Vallejo et al., performed in 16 dogs, demonstrates highly reproducible measurements of left ventricular size and function using the Autoquant method. However, these results are significantly influenced by background activity, time of imaging and injected dose. In the presence of perfusion defects, this automated method overestimates volume relative to MRI, with a poor correlation between gated SPECT Autoquant and MRI-calculated left ventricular ejection fraction. The editorial by Udelson and Fares reviews the accuracy and reliability of left ventricular size and function measurements made by the method of gated SPECT sestamibi. It suggests reasons for the findings of Vallejo et al.)

225. Cullom SJ, Case JA, Bateman TM, et al. Electrocardiographically gated myocardial perfusion SPECT: technical principles and quality control considerations. *J Nucl Cardiol* 1998;5:418–425.

(The problem is that there are few quality control measures. After acquisition, we do not know the optimal number of frames per cycle, have no knowledge of the spectrum of beats accepted overall or in each projection or other factors.)

226. Paul AK, Hasegawa S, Yoshioka J, et al. Left ventricular volume and ejection fraction from quantitative gated SPECT: comparison with gated pool SPECT and contrast ventriculography [abstract]. *J Nucl Med* 1999;40:178P.

(End-diastolic, end-systolic and stroke volumes, as well as left ventricular ejection fraction calculated from gated tetrofosmin myocardial perfusion scintigraphy based on QGS software for volume determination correlate well with similar values calculated from 2 independent methods.)

227. Vaduganathan P, He ZX, Vick III W, et al. Evaluation of left ventricular wall motion, volumes and ejection fraction by gated tomography with technetium-99m-labeled tetrofosmin. A comparison with cine magnetic resonance imaging. *J Nucl Cardiol* 1999;6:3–10.

(An excellent correlation is seen among left ventricular [LV] ejection fraction, wall motion and LV volumes measured by gated SPECT myocardial perfusion scintigraphy and cine MR imaging in 25 patients with recent myocardial infarctions.)

228. Atsma DE, Croon C, Dibbets-Schneider P, et al. Good correlation between left ventricular ejection fraction and wall motion score assessed by gated SPECT as compared to left ventricular angiography [abstract]. *J Am Coll Cardiol* 1999;33: 409A.

(Left ventricular ejection fraction [LVEF] and regional wall motion on left ventriculography correlate well with these values calculated from gated technetium-99m tetrofosmin SPECT myocardial perfusion scintigraphy in 74 patients with widely varying LVEFs.)

229. Atsma DE, Kayser HWM, Croon C, et al. Good correlation between left ventricular ejection fraction, end-systolic and end-diastolic volume measured by gated SPECT as compared to magnetic resonance imaging [abstract]. *J Am Coll Cardiol* 1999; 33:436A.

(Left ventricular [LV] ejection fraction, regional wall motion and end-diastolic and end-systolic volumes calculated from gated technetium-99m tetrofosmin SPECT myocardial perfusion scintigraphy in 15 patients with coronary artery disease and widely varying LV function correlate well with these values calculated from 3-dimensional MR imaging.)

230. Nichols K, Lefkowitz D, Faber T, et al. Ventricular volumes compared among three gated SPECT methods and echocardiography [abstract]. *J Am Coll Cardiol* 1999;33:409A.

(Gated SPECT myocardial perfusion scintigraphy volumes compare well with echocardiographic volumes measured with a modified Simpson's rule approach, especially when the same analytic approach is applied to scintigraphy.)

231. Calnon DA, Kastner RJ, Smith WH, et al. Validation of a new counts-based gated single photon emission computed tomography method for quantifying left ventricular systolic function: comparison with equilibrium radionuclide angiography. *J Nucl Cardiol* 1997;4:464–471.

(As in references 217–230, this article validated a new method for calculation of left ventricular ejection fraction volumes or mass by comparison with an established method.)

232. Rozanski A, Nichols K, Siu-Sun Y, et al. Development and application of normal limits for left ventricular ejection fraction and volume measurements from ^{99m}Tc-sestamibi myocardial perfusion gated SPECT. *J Nucl Med* 2000;41:1445–1450.

(Gated SPECT with technetium-99m sestamibi presents a reproducible method for the evaluation of left ventricular ejection fraction [LVEF] and LV volumes. This article attempts to develop criteria for abnormal gated SPECT findings. Among 214 patients with a low Bayesian likelihood of coronary artery disease, sex-specific normal limits for LV volume and LVEF by gated SPECT sestamibi study are established. LVEF is higher and LV end-diastolic volume [LVEDV] is lower in women than men. In these findings, abnormal LVEF and LVEDV are evident among ~20% of hypertensive patients with LV hypertrophy. The lower limit of LVEF is lower than you might expect!)

233. DePuey EG, Nichols K, Dobrinsky C, et al. Left ventricular ejection fraction assessed from gated technetium-99m sestamibi SPECT. *J Nucl Med* 1993;34:1871–1876.

(The accuracy of left ventricular ejection fraction calculated from gated myocardial perfusion scintigraphy studies is reported.)

224. Chua T, Kiat H, Germano G, et al. Gated technetium-99m sestamibi for simultaneous assessment of stress myocardial perfusion, post-exercise regional ventricular function and myocardial viability: correlation with echocardiography and rest thallium-201 scintigraphy. *J Am Coll Cardiol* 1994;23:1107–1114.

(The paper supports the hypothesis that wall motion on gated poststress sestamibi images predicts viability and reversibility. Thus, there might be no need for rest or redistribution images to determine viability, because viability might be discerned from perfusion-related function. However, function or apparent function evaluation is imperfect and is influenced by other factors. Function may not be evaluated well in the presence of dense defects, although such evaluation is performed objectively and wall motion is, in fact, generally seen, even in the presence of many dense perfusion defects.)

235. Garcia EV, Faber TL, Cooke CD, et al. SPECT quantitative assessment of myocardial perfusion and function. In: *American Society of Nuclear Cardiology Categorical Program Course Syllabus.* Los Angeles, CA: American Society of Nuclear Cardiology; 1998:305–312.

(The authors review quantitative methods for analysis of myocardial perfusion and function by myocardial perfusion scintigraphy.)

236. DePuey EG, Rozanski A. Using gated technetium-99m sestamibi single photon emission computed tomography (SPECT) to characterize fixed myocardial defects as infarct or artifact. *J Nucl Med* 1995;36:952–955.

(Diaphragmatic and breast attenuation and apical thinning are common causes of fixed defects and are not related to perfusion. The differential diagnosis of fixed defects appears to be significantly aided by the findings in gated images. Increased detection of coronary artery disease is seen with end-diastolic images. In a study of 551 consecutive patients referred for clinical perfusion image evaluation, 78 patients have fixed defects in the absence of infarction history. Sixty of these have normal regional wall function, permitting their identification in relation to attenuation artifact rather than ischemic scar and reducing the incidence of unidentified fixed defects from 14% to 3%.)

237. Taillefer R, DePuey EG, Udelson JE, et al. Comparative diagnostic accuracy of Tl-201 and Tc-99m sestamibi SPECT imaging: perfusion and ECG-gated SPECT in detecting coronary disease in women. *J Am Coll Cardiol* 1997;29:69–77.

(This prospective study includes 85 consecutive female patients and 30 volunteers with a low likelihood of coronary disease. The overall sensitivities for the diagnosis of coronary stenoses >50% and >70% with stress imaging performed in the same patients with each radionuclide is uniformly high; 75% and 84% for thallium-201 [^{201}Tl] and 72% and 81% for technetium-99m [^{99m}Tc] sestamibi, respectively. In this study, sensitivity does not differ between agents and is not influenced by gating. However, specificities for stenoses >50% are 62% for ^{201}Tl and 86% for ^{99m}Tc sestamibi [$P < 0.03$], whereas specificities for stenoses >70% are 59% for ^{201}Tl and 83% for ^{99m}Tc sestamibi [$P < 0.02$]. When gated wall motion and thickening are added, the specificity of ^{99m}Tc sestamibi images is >92%.)

238. Yang L, Iwanochoko RM, Burke RJ, et al. Reconstruction of ECG-gated Tl-201 SPECT using only end-diastolic frames increases detection of CAD [abstract]. *J Nucl Med* 1999;40:170P.

(Among 75 SPECT stress thallium-201 myocardial perfusion scintigraphy studies, analysis of 2 summed diastolic slices yielded higher relative right ventricular counts, larger left ventricular volumes, larger defects and greater evidence of reversibility, compared with an 8-frame gated study. Analysis of end-diastolic frames may be of value, especially in patients with small ventricles.)

239. Taillefer R, DePuey EG, Udelson JE, et al. Comparison between the end-diastolic images and the summed images of gated Tc-99m sestamibi SPECT perfusion study in detection of coronary artery disease in women. *J Nucl Cardiol* 1999;6:169–176.

(Among 43 patients studied by exercise or pharmacologic stress myocardial perfusion scintigraphy, end-diastolic volume images show more ischemic [reversible] defects than summed images and may be of great diagnostic value in the interpretation of myocardial perfusion scintigraphy, particularly in patients with small hearts.

In another study, the authors choose 3 frames around end-diastole of a 16-frame acquisition. Fifty-three women with "smaller" hearts are studied in a 2-day protocol. Sensitivity is 73% for summed image [28/38] and 84% for end-diastolic images [32/38]. Four coronary patients are missed by the summed images, but all are seen on end-diastolic images, 3 with small hearts. Also, 106 defects are seen with summed images compared with 173 with end-diastolic images [$P < 0.001$].)

240. Mannting F, Morgan-Mannting MG. Gated SPECT with technetium-99m sestamibi for assessment of myocardial perfusion abnormalities. *J Nucl Med* 1993;34:601–608.

(The authors gate only stress studies and look at the value of end-diastolic images at stress compared with nongated rest and stress. They find that the right ventricle is more distinct and that the left ventricular cavity, not surprisingly, is larger in the end-diastolic image. Subtle defects and reversibility are more evident in the end-diastolic images, with increased sensitivity, better edge definition and increased resolution and improved detection of defects and reversibility. The authors recommend the comparison of end-diastolic stress with end-diastolic rest images and indicate the need to gate both rest and stress images. If we only gate stress studies, then sensitivity will be increased at the price of specificity. The method seems to be of greatest benefit in those with small, hypertrophied or hyperdynamic hearts.)

241. Ford PV, Chatzioannou SN, Moore WH, et al. The demonstration of overestimation of LVEF by quantitative gated SPECT in simulated left ventricles [abstract]. *J Nucl Med* 1999;40:5P.

(Limited image resolution is the likely reason for the over estimation of left ventricular ejection fraction in small ventricles. Because of the increased scatter, this should be a greater problem with gated ^{201}Tl myocardial perfusion scintigraphy. Alternatively, slow heart rates are associated with a prolonged diastolic phase and contracted systole, of which the latter may be undersampled at low sampling rates. This presents an increased possibility of missing end-systole and so overestimating end-systolic volume and counts.)

242. Bokhari S, Blood DK, Bergmann SR. Differences between stress and rest ejection fraction in gated perfusion SPECT imaging [abstract]. *J Nucl Med* 1999;40:45P.

(Fully 45% of 44 patient studies performed with the stress technetium-99m sestamibi/rest thallium-201 [^{201}Tl] protocol demonstrate a reduced left ventricular ejection fraction [LVEF] >5 EF units on poststress imaging compared with that on rest ^{201}Tl. No patients among 36 studied by a stress–redistribution ^{201}Tl protocol show this difference. Because this difference between rest- and stress-related LVEF has been said to relate to stunning, the incidence of stunning is low with the ^{201}Tl protocol. The differences in LVEF between rest and stress studies using the dual-isotope protocol may reflect intrinsic differences inherent in tracer and isotope characteristics, or methods of acquisition or analysis, rather than true stunning.)

243. Manrique A, Véra P, Hitzel An, et al. Sixteen-interval gating improves thallium-201 gated SPECT LVEF measurement in patients with large myocardial infarction [abstract]. *J Am Coll Cardiol* 1999;33:436A.

(Eight-frame gated SPECT myocardial perfusion scintigraphy underestimates left ventricular ejection fraction [LVEF] in patients with large defects. However, 16-frame gated acquisition and analysis impressively increases the correlation with gated equilibrium blood-pool values without underestimating the LVEF. Gated equilibrium blood-pool imaging was long ago demonstrated to underestimate LVEF when acquired with <14 frames.)

244. Nichols K, DePuey E G, Yao SS, et al. Clinical impact of gating errors on visual assessment of myocardial perfusion and ventricular function from SPECT data [abstract]. *J Am Coll Cardiol* 1999;33:435A.

(In a population of patients with atrial fibrillation and perfusion defects on stress myocardial perfusion scintigraphy, the study demonstrates that gating errors and irregularities alter the perfusion pattern minimally. However, wall thickening and wall motion are significantly affected.)

245. Nichols K, DePuey EG, Yoon J, et al. Relative influence of gating errors on myocardial perfusion and function computed QGS software [abstract]. *J Nucl Med* 1999; 40: 157P.

(The authors reprocess projection image data from gated SPECT myocardial perfusion scintigraphy studies acquired in sinus rhythm to simulate variable heart rate, atrial fibrillation and ectopic beats in 50 patients. Changes in volumes and left ventricular ejection fraction are small and perfusion defect alterations relatively minor. In only 2 of these 50 patients are changes in the polar map judged to be clinically important. Gating of myocardial perfusion scintigraphy is relatively tolerant to the artifacts of rhythm applied here. However, these do not necessarily span the limits seen in clinical application.)

246. Bruce A. Comparative prevalence of segment S-T depression after maximal exercise in healthy men in Seattle and Taipei. In: Simonson E, ed. *Physical Activity and the Heart.* Springfield, IL: Charles C. Thomas; 1967.

(The treadmill in this study, a moving platform with adjustable elevation and speed, permits the design of multiple protocols to accommodate patients over the spectrum of exercise capacity. The Bruce protocol, designed from gears available at the time, is best applied to vigorous individuals. The modification of the Bruce protocol inserts 6 min of limited stress before the standard Bruce protocol, to evaluate the cause of recent symptoms or electrocardiographic changes or reduce the anxiety in an otherwise vigorous individual. The Naughton protocol is designed for patients with limited exercise tolerance.)

247. Hambrecht RP, Schuler GC, Muth T, et al. Greater diagnostic sensitivity of treadmill versus cycle exercise testing of asymptomatic men with coronary disease. *Am J Cardiol* 1992;70:141–146.

(In the United States, the treadmill is generally used for dynamic stress testing. In Europe, the bicycle is more often applied. Some evidence suggests that the treadmill-based tests are more sensitive. However, this probably relates to the nature of the population studied.)

248. Ellestadt MH. *Stress Testing: Principles and Practice.* 4th ed. Philadelphia, PA: F.A. Davis Co.;1996.

(This is an excellent text in the field of stress testing.)

249. Chambers CE, Brown KA. Dipyridamole-induced ST segment depression during thallium-201 imaging in patients with coronary artery disease: angiographic and hemodynamic determinants. *J Am Coll Cardiol* 1988;12:37–41.

(The angiographic and hemodynamic correlates of dipyridamole-induced ST segment depression are presented. It appears that the presence of coronary collaterals is frequently associated with dipyridamole-induced ST segment depression, suggesting the background for the "steal" syndrome.)

250. Becker LC. Conditions for vasodilator-induced coronary steal in experimental myocardial ischemia. *Circulation* 1978;57:1103–1110.

(An early and important experimental study that defines the anatomic and hemodynamic conditions for vasodilator-related coronary steal.)

251. Demer LL, Goldstein R, Mullani L, et al. Coronary steal by noninvasive PET identifies collateralized myocardium. *J Nucl Med* 1986;27:977–983.

(An application of quantitative PET perfusion imaging to define the mechanism of "steal syndrome.")

(249–251: Coronary dilation induced by pharmacologic stress can occasionally cause ischemia. One mechanism for such induced ischemia is the "steal" syndrome, in which reduced resistance in the normal bed discourages flow through coronary collaterals, with possible absolute reduction in resting flow and related ischemia.)

252. Verani MS. Pharmacologic stress myocardial perfusion imaging. *Curr Prob Cardiol* 1993;18:481–528.

253. Botvinick EH, Dae MW. Dipyridamole perfusion scintigraphy in cardiovascular nuclear medicine: an update. *Semin Nucl Med* 1991;21:242–265.

(252,253: These review articles consider the theoretical, technical and clinical aspects of pharmacologic stress testing in its various combinations and permutations.)

254. Sharir T, Rabinowitz B, Livschitz S, et al. Underestimation of extent and severity of coronary artery disease by dipyridamole stress Tl-201 single photon emission computed tomographic myocardial perfusion imaging in patients taking antianginal drugs. *J Am Coll Cardiol* 1998;31:1540–1546.

(Contrary to previous and apparently established belief, continued use of anti-anginal drugs before dipyridamole [and low-level exercise] thallium-201 SPECT may reduce defect extent and severity of defects, potentially underestimating coronary artery disease and the extent of myocardium at ischemic risk.

One of the strong points of the pharmacologic method using direct coronary dilators, well supported in the literature, is that it can be performed while the patient is on anti-ischemic therapy without loss of sensitivity or ability to risk stratify! This seems to relate to the fact that these dilators act on the coronary flow supply rather than demands, whereas beta-blockers affect demands. This relationship recently has been brought into question. However, beta-blockers reduce myocardial oxygen demands at rest and reduce resting myocardial blood flow. With the subsequent administration of coronary dilators, there is an increase in the coronary flow reserve in areas supplied by stenotic vessels. Although a similar effect must occur in the bed of normal vessels, because of reduced baseline demands, this potentially could result in a relative reduction in the differential flow augmentation between stenotic and normal beds. In turn, this could result in an apparent reduction of the related induced defect with a potential underestimation of related disease and risk.)

255. Quinones MA, Verani MS, Haichin RM, et al. Exercise echocardiography versus Tl-201 single photon emission computed tomography in evaluation of coronary artery disease. *Circulation* 1992;85:1026–1031.

(This is an oft-quoted article that is cited as demonstrating the equality of results achieved with exercise stress echocardiography and perfusion scintigraphy. A careful analysis, performed in part by the authors of reference 242, however, demonstrates that this is not the case.)

256. Santiago P, Vacek JL, Rosamond TL. Dobutamine stress echocardiography: clinical utility and predictive value at various infusion rates. *Am Heart J* 1994;128:804–807.

(To assess the optimal infusion rate, 113 consecutive patients are studied in 3 patient groups of dobutamine infusion rate: 20, 30 and 40 μg/kg/min. The higher 30- and 40-μg/kg/min doses give the best sensitivity [85%], specificity [79%] and a positive predictive value of 88% and should be applied with dobutamine stress echocardiography for optimal evaluation.)

257. Botvinick EH. Stress imaging: current clinical options for the diagnosis, localization and evaluation of coronary artery disease. *Med Clin North Am* 1995;79:1025–1061.

(This critical review compares stress scintigraphic and stress echocardiographic methods. It includes an assessment of the article by Quinones et al. [*255*].)

258. Garcia E, ed. Imaging guidelines for nuclear cardiology procedures. *J Nucl Cardiol* 1996;3:G1–G46.

(Presented here are the detailed procedures related to nuclear cardiology imaging protocols.)

259. Johnstone D, Wackers FJTh, Berger H, et al. Effect of patient positioning on left lateral Tl-201 myocardial images. *J Nucl Med* 1979;20:183–188.

(To avoid diaphragmatic attenuation of the inferior left ventricular wall in planar imaging, this article suggests acquisition of the left lateral projection in the right decubitus position. Artifactual attenuation is also reduced by SPECT imaging and may be recognized with review of the projection images and objectified with reference to the polar coordinate map. A minor relative reduction in apparent inferior wall radioactivity on SPECT images is generally attenuation in origin.)

260. Cloninger KG, DePuey EG, Garcia EV, et al. Incomplete redistribution, in delayed thallium-201 single photon emission computed tomographic (SPECT) images: an overestimation of myocardial scarring. *J Am Coll Cardiol* 1988;12:955–963.

(This article documents the value of 24-hr delayed thallium-201 imaging to maximize redistribution and evaluation of viability. Reinjection technique is now established and reduces the need for 24-hr imaging.)

261. Dilsizian V, Rocco TP, Freedman M, et al. Enhanced detection of ischemic but viable myocardium by the reinjection of thallium after stress-redistribution imaging. *N Engl J Med* 1990;323:141–146.

(In this landmark study, the reinjection technique, previously considered and applied to a limited extent, is proven to yield reversibility in viable, stress-induced myocardial defects that is superior to even delayed redistribution. A subsequent study by Bonow et al. [*265*] compares the reinjection assessment of viability to PET perfusion and metabolism evaluation.)

262. Mori T, Minamiji K, Kurogane H, et al. Rest-injected thallium-201 imaging for assessing viability of severe asynergic regions. *J Nucl Med* 1991;32:1718–1724.

263. Ragosta M, Beller GA, Watson DD, et al. Quantitative planar rest-redistribution thallium-201 imaging in detection of myocardial viability and prediction of improvement in left ventricular function after bypass surgery in patients with severely depressed left ventricular function. *Circulation* 1993;87:1630–1641.

(262,263: Rest–redistribution imaging of thallium-201 is a well-accepted method to assess the presence of viable myocardium and “hibernation.” The mechanism is described in these articles.)

264. Favaro L, Masini F, Serra W, et al. Thallium-201 for detection of viable myocardium: comparison of different reinjection protocols. *J Nucl Cardiol* 1994;1: 515–521.

(Reinjection redistribution technique is evaluated in the same 27 patients with fixed defects after 3-hr redistribution. The separate-day protocol, in which reinjection is performed 48–96 hr later, is superior to the same-day protocol, with reinjection immediately after redistribution imaging and reimaging 15 min later. Reinjection after redistributed defects can reproduce the original defect, which can again be made to normalize with 24-hr delayed images.)

265. Bonow RO, Dilsizian V, Cuocolo A, et al. Identification of viable myocardium in patients with chronic coronary artery disease and left ventricular dysfunction: comparison of thallium scintigraphy with reinjection and PET imaging with ^{18}F-fluorodeoxyglucose. *Circulation* 1991;83:26–37.

(This classic article demonstrates that the reinjection technique maximizes thallium-201 "redistribution," reducing the need for 24-hr imaging, and that myocardial viability is identified by redistribution or a relatively high level of regional radioactivity, equal to 50% or more of the region with highest regional activity [assumed to be a normal region].)

266. Berman DS, Kiat H, Van Train KF, et al. Comparison of SPECT using technetium-99m agents and thallium-201 and PET for the assessment of myocardial perfusion and viability. A symposium: technetium-99m myocardial perfusion imaging agents and their relation to thallium-201. *Am J Cardiol* 1990;66:72E–79E.

(This is an excellent review of the factors and evidence relating the distribution of thallium-201 [^{201}Tl] and technetium-99m [^{99m}Tc] sestamibi to tissue viability. Although the evidence is growing in support of ^{99m}Tc sestamibi, ^{201}Tl remains the most sensitive viability agent among perfusion imaging agents.)

267. Dilsizian V, Bonow RO. Differential uptake and apparent ^{201}Tl washout after thallium reinjection: options regarding late redistribution imaging before reinjection or late redistribution imaging after reinjection. *Circulation* 1992;85: 1032–1038.

(Reinjection can actually induce a defect that would otherwise not have been evident, providing that defect would redistribute after 4 hr. A reinjection dose then could make it evident once again. However, if imaging is not performed at 4 hr, before reinjection, the defect may well appear fixed. Imaging again at 24 hr bears a high likelihood of renewed redistribution. Alternatively, SPECT imaging may be performed both before and after reinjection, after 4 hr. The latter would be arduous for both patients and staff. Therefore, 24-hr images are recommend after 4-hr reinjection, just as in the absence of reinjection, when further redistribution is both likely and clinically important.)

268. Bobba K, Botvinick EH, Dae MW, et al. Is there any advantage to the acquisition of 24-hour thallium images, in the presence of fixed defects at 4 hr after reinjection? *Eur J Nucl Med* 1998;25:509–514.

(The authors report on a clinical test of the observations noted in reference 267, in which 24-hr imaging is rarely necessary but is occasionally clinically critical. Twenty-four-hr delayed images should be acquired in unstable angina, after infarction or wherever the resolution of apparently fixed defects will make a clinical difference.)

269. Tartagni F, Fallani F, Corbelli C, et al. Detecting hibernated myocardium with SPECT and thallium-glucose-insulin infusion. *J Nucl Med* 1995;36:1377–1383.

(Possibly because thallium kinetics, like potassium kinetics, are influenced by insulin levels, a continuous thallium infusion with low-dose insulin in glucose/potassium chloride solution enhances thallium uptake in apparently severe ischemic regions. This is another method that may aid thallium viability recognition.)

270. Garcia MJ, Neumann D, Go RT, et al. Comparison of persistent thallium perfusion defects by quantitative washout analysis with thallium reinjection in patients with coronary artery disease. *Am J Cardiol* 1994;74:977–981.

(This study compares the quantitative washout of poststress thallium-201 with the distribution of activity after reinjection in 31 patients with fixed defects after 4-hr delayed images and reinjection thereafter. Thirty-eight of 39 segments that improve on reinjection also demonstrate normal washout ratios. This relationship holds at any segment location or severity. Washout predicts the results of reinjection and does not require an extra acquisition or added radionuclide administration.)

271. Maublant JC, Citron B, Lipiecki J, et al. Rest technetium 99m-sestamibi tomoscintigraphy in hibernating myocardium. *Am Heart J* 1995;129:306–313.

(Residual [62%] or normal [38%] technetium-99m sestamibi uptake is related to viability and restored regional function in 21 of 27 [78%] regions after revascularization in 25 patients studied at rest with the agent. The 4 dense "transmural" defects are functionally unchanged after revascularization.)

272. Verani MS, Jeroudi MO, Mahmarian JJ, et al. Quantification of myocardial infarction during coronary occlusion and myocardial salvage after reperfusion using cardiac imaging with technetium-99m hexakis 2-methoxyisobutyl isonitrile. *J Am Coll Cardiol* 1988;12:1573–1581.

(This thorough study using technetium-99m sestamibi demonstrates the correlation between pathologic and scintigraphic infarct size after 2 hr of coronary occlusion. Early injection demonstrates defect size proportional to the myocardium at risk. After 48 hr of reperfusion, image defect size is greatly reduced in correlation with the final infarct size.)

273. Wackers FJTh. Thrombolytic therapy for myocardial infarction: assessment of efficacy by myocardial perfusion imaging with technetium-99m sestamibi. A symposium: technetium-99m myocardial perfusion imaging agents and their relation to thallium-201. *Am J Cardiol* 1990;66:36E–41E.

(The long persistence of technetium-99m in the myocardium without significant redistribution permits injection before intervention, with subsequent imaging after intervention. This image, demonstrating the amount of myocardium at risk, may be compared with a post-intervention rest study to reveal the extent of myocardium salvaged. A subsequent stress study will then again reveal the extent of myocardium at risk post-intervention. This method has been used with thrombolysis, acute or rescue percutaneous transluminal coronary angioplasty and, when clinical doubts exist, also can be used to demonstrate indications for acute revascularization.)

274. Canby RC, Silber S, Pohost GM. Relations of the myocardial imaging agents ^{99m}Tc-MIBI and ^{201}Tl to myocardial blood flow in a canine model of myocardial ischemic insult. *Circulation* 1990;81:289–296.

(In low flow areas, relative myocardial uptake of sestamibi is greater than expected compared with microsphere-determined flow in normal flow areas. This is the result of increased extraction of the radiotracer at low flow rates, as is typical for diffusible and transported tracers, including thallium-201 [^{201}Tl] [see reference 151]. However, this article demonstrates that such evidence of increased extraction is not seen when flow is reduced and sustained at levels 0%–10% of normal due loss of viability. So, as with ^{201}Tl, evidence of increased technetium-99m sestamibi extraction in low flow areas relates to viability.)

275. Wackers FJTh, Gibbons RJ, Verani MS, et al. Serial quantitative planar technetium-99m isonitrile imaging in acute myocardial infarction: efficacy for noninvasive assessment of thrombolytic therapy. *J Am Coll Cardiol* 1989;14:861–873.

276. Gibbons RJ, Verani MS, Behrenbeck T, et al. Feasibility of tomographic ^{99m}Tc-hexakis-2-methoxy-2-methylpropyl-isonitrile imaging for the assessment of myocardial area at risk and the effect of treatment in acute myocardial infarction. *Circulation* 1989;80:1277–1286.

(275,276: These articles demonstrate the application of technetium-99m sestamibi to the evaluation of myocardium at risk before, and myocardium salvaged after, acute revascularization. It is the lack of sestamibi redistribution that permits the administration of the dose before intervention, with imaging of the agent and evaluation of the presenting region of myocardium at ischemic risk after revascularization. This, with the more general availability of the agent, provides a major logistic advantage over thallium-201 for this purpose.)

277. Maurea S, Cuocolo A, Soricelli A, et al. Enhanced detection of viable myocardium by technetium-99m-MIBI imaging after nitrate administration in chronic coronary artery disease. *J Nucl Med* 1995;36:1945–1952.

(Thirty-one patients with known coronary disease and chronic left ventricular dysfunction undergo technetium-99m sestamibi studies at rest and after nitroglycerine, followed by subsequent rest and redistribution thallium-201 [^{201}Tl] series. Among 302 segments with severely reduced activity at rest, 27% [54] improve after nitroglycerine and are viable on ^{201}Tl study. Among 8 patients studied after revascularization, 87% of those segments with reversible sestamibi defects demonstrate improved function, whereas 89% of those segments with irreversible defects demonstrate none.)

278. Bisi G, Sciagra R, Santoro G, et al. Technetium-99m sestamibi imaging with nitrate infusion to detect viable hibernating myocardium and predict postrevascularization recovery. *J Nucl Med* 1995;36:1994–2000.

(Sestamibi images are acquired at rest and with nitrate infusion in 28 patients with previous infarction. Nitrate-induced improvement in perfusion correlates well with postrevascularization functional changes, both on a global and regional basis. Postnitrate perfusion patterns may aid identification of viable hibernating myocardium and the prospect of functional recovery after revascularization.)

279. Lewin HC, Hachamovitch R, Harris AG, et al. Simultaneous reduction of exercise perfusion defect extent and severity with isosorbide mononitrate (Imdur) as demonstrated by means of technetium 99m sestabmibi. *J Nucl Cardiol* 2000;7:342–353.

(Patients with coronary disease and chronic stable angina treated with long-acting nitrates present an improvement in defect size and severity using both visual and quantitative methods of SPECT image analysis, when patients are studied serially and randomly by exercise perfusion imaging to the same achieved double product, on and off the drug.)

280. Haft JI, Hammoudeh AJ, Conte PJ. Assessing myocardial viability: correlation of myocardial wall motion abnormalities and pathologic Q waves with technetium-99m sestamibi single photon emission computed tomography. *Am Heart J* 1995;130:994–998.

(Although there is a correlation among Q waves, left ventricular wall motion abnormalities and stress sestamibi uptake in 201 patients studied, the high number of discordant segments suggests that nonviability cannot be established by wall motion and electrocardiogram findings alone but also requires metabolic, sestamibi or perfusion information.)

281. Maurea S, Cuocolo A, Soricelli A, et al. Myocardial viability index in chronic coronary artery disease: technetium-99m-methoxy isobutyl isonitrile redistribution. *J Nucl Med* 1995;36:1953–1960.

(This article tests the frequency and establishes the importance of technetium-99m sestamibi redistribution. The importance, suggested by a >10% increase compared with the initial data set, is demonstrated in 47 of 197 [24%] segments with severe reduction of radioactivity on rest imaging, when studied 5 hr later. These segments occur in 20 patients in whom thallium-201 reversibility is noted in the same segments. Sestamibi reversibility predicts functional reversibility late after revascularization in 83% of segments when seen. When absent, it is related to an absence of functional recovery in 96% of such segments.)

282. DePuey EG, Nichols KJ, Slowikowski JS, et al. Fast stress and rest acquisitions for technetium-99m-sestamibi separate-day SPECT. *J Nucl Med* 1995;36:569–574.

(Abbreviated SPECT acquisition is compared with the conventional protocol in 12 rest and 32 stress patient studies. The different protocols show no difference in image findings. Fast SPECT acquisition may increase patient tolerance as well as laboratory throughput. It will add to the efficiency of acquisition with multihead detectors.)

283. Milan E, Giubbini R, Gioia G, et al. A cost-effective sestamibi protocol in the managed health care era. *J Nucl Cardiol* 1997;4:509–514.

(A stress–rest sestamibi protocol is applied in 200 patients with known or suspected coronary artery disease but without histories of infarction, revascularization or ventricular dysfunction. The findings demonstrate that the analysis of a normal stress study is rarely affected by the subsequent rest study. Rest studies are most useful with abnormal or equivocal stress studies. The elimination of the rest study in the absence of prior infarction, left ventricular dysfunction or prior revascularization appears cost effective.)

284. Maddahi J, Kiat H, Van Train KF, et al. Myocardial perfusion imaging with technetium-99m sestamibi SPECT in the evaluation of coronary artery disease. *Am J Cardiol* 1990;66:55E–62E.

(Sestamibi is rarely acquired in the planar manner and is ideal for SPECT imaging. This is an excellent review of methods and results of sestamibi imaging.)

285. Taillefer R, Gagnon A, Laflamme L, et al. Same day injections of Tc-99m methoxyisobutyl isonitrile (hexamibi) for myocardial tomographic imaging: comparison between rest-stress and stress-rest injection sequences. *Eur J Nucl Med* 1989;15:113–117.

(The stress-first protocol results in an overestimation of infarction with an underestimation of viable myocardium at ischemic risk. A rest image acquired after an abnormal stress image may yet reveal apparent radiotracer heterogeneity deriving from the background distribution of the earlier stress image. A 1-day protocol should be employed with rest first to avoid overestimating infarction. In addition, because a lower dose is injected with the first of the 1-day imaging studies, rest-first imaging employs the high dose for the more informative stress study. Here, the results of a 1-day protocol agree well with results of the 2-day protocol and with conventional thallium-201 protocols.)

286. Berman DS, Kiat H, Friedman JD, et al. Separate acquisition rest thallium-201/stress technetium-99m sestamibi dual isotope myocardial perfusion SPECT. A clinical validation study. *J Am Coll Cardiol* 1993;22:1455–1464.

(This article validates the accuracy of the sequential, dual-isotope thallium-201 rest/technetium-99m sestamibi stress protocol in a population with known anatomy. A subsequent rest sestamibi study is read with the stress sestamibi study, and little difference is found from the excellent diagnostic ability of the dual-isotope images.)

287. Berman DS, Kiat H, Van Train K, et al. Dual isotope myocardial perfusion SPECT with rest thallium-201 and stress Tc-99m sestamibi. *Clin Cardiol* 1994;12:261–270.

(The authors discuss the new and somewhat controversial thallium-201 [^{201}Tl] rest/technetium-99m sestamibi stress protocol. Primarily advantageous for its rapid patient throughput, it presents both the potential for sestamibi stress function analysis and ^{201}Tl viability analysis. However, this protocol could be more expensive in association with low patient volumes and provides some ambiguities in interpretation, as a result of the necessary comparison of different imaging agents. It is now one of several possible protocols that may be applied according to the patient's clinical needs, laboratory schedules and physician preferences.)

288. Botvinick E, O'Connell JW, Dae M, et al. Analysis of thallium-201 "washout" from color-coded images. *J Nucl Med* 1988;29:302–311.

(This analysis of regional planar washout uses parametric imaging to identify regional washout and to gain insight into the meaning and content of the ventricular cavity and cavitary dilation.)

289. Weiss AT, Berman DS, Lew AS, et al. Transient ischemic dilation of the left ventricle on stress thallium-201 scintigraphy: a marker of severe and extensive coronary artery disease. *J Am Coll Cardiol* 1987;9:752–758.

(This is a specific analysis of the phenomenon of cavitary dilation, a nonperfusion indicator [see ref. 98] of extensive coronary disease. With planar methods, apparent "cavitary dilation" may be seen and are associated not with a dilated cavity but with reduced radioactivity [ischemia] in the overlying wall. Because of the apparently larger cavity on technetium-99m [^{99m}Tc] sestamibi compared with that on thallium-201 [^{201}Tl] images, this phenomenon may be diagnosed too frequently when applying the dual-isotope ^{201}Tl rest/^{99m}Tc sestamibi stress protocol.)

290. Lucas JR, Pounds TR, Ratzlaff NW, et al. Differentiation of myocardial perfusion abnormalities from attenuation effects in combined Tl-201/Tc-99m sestamibi studies using relative regional activity profiles [abstract]. *J Nucl Med* 1993;34: 65P.

(This initial study suggests that the differing energies of the radionuclides employed in the sequential-acquisition dual-isotope protocol and their differential attenuation could be analyzed to determine the cause of a regional defect. That is, assuming a similar distribution of thallium-201 [^{201}Tl] at rest and technetium-99m [^{99m}Tc] with stress, the relationship between the high-energy ^{99m}Tc 140-keV gamma rays and the low-energy 68–80-keV ^{201}Tl x-rays should be constant and based on their relative abundance and the injected doses. With increasing attenuation, relatively less evident low-energy ^{201}Tl photons would be expected. Practically, this would make an attenuation-related defect appear more severe on ^{201}Tl than on ^{99m}Tc images. This study evaluates the relative regional radioactivity of high- and low-energy photons in superimposed dual-isotope images and finds an increased ability and accuracy in coronary disease diagnosis based on this information. This method does not account for scatter or differences in agent distribution. More satisfactory would be a similar analysis dealing with high- and low-energy photons of ^{201}Tl. The low abundance of the high-energy protons makes such analysis problematic.)

291. Maddahi J, Kiat H, Berman DS. Myocardial perfusion imaging with technetium-99m-labeled agents. A symposium: advances in nuclear cardiac imaging. *Am J Cardiol* 1991;67:27D–34D.

(This is a thorough review of the physical properties and clinical applications of current technetium-99m-based myocardial perfusion agents.)

292. Matzer L, Kiat H, Wang FP, et al. Pharmacologic stress dual-isotope myocardial perfusion SPECT. *Am Heart J* 1994;128:1067–1076.

(In this analysis, the dual-isotope rest thallium-201/stress sestamibi protocol is successfully applied with high diagnostic accuracy for coronary disease diagnosis in a pharmacologic stress protocol using a direct coronary dilator.)

293. Kiat H, Germano G, Friedman JD, et al. Comparative feasibility of separate or simultaneous rest thallium-201–stress technetium-99m sestamibi dual isotope myocardial perfusion SPECT. *J Nucl Med* 1994;35:542–548.

(Simultaneous acquisition of the dual-isotope, rest thallium-201 [^{201}Tl]/stress-technetium-99m [^{99m}Tc] sestamibi protocol would confine acquisition of rest and stress studies to a single sitting. This would cut considerably the time of acquisition and increase patient tolerance, method responsivity and laboratory throughput. It would also provide images in registry for possible analysis of differential attenuation. Currently, such a protocol is not possible because of contamination of the ^{201}Tl image with downscattered photons from the ^{99m}Tc study.)

294. Kiat H, Friedman J, Van Train K, et al. Simultaneous rest Tl-201/stress Tc-99m sestamibi dual isotope myocardial perfusion SPECT: a pilot study. *J Nucl Med* 1991;32:1006–1009.

295. Case A, Bateman TM, Cullom SJ, et al. Validation of Tl-201 LVEF measurements using simultaneous acquired Tc-99m sestamibi/Tl-201 ECG-gated SPECT perfusion scintigraphy [abstract]. *J Nucl Med* 1999;40:159P.

(294,295: Subtraction of a Compton scatter photopeak from the thallium-201 [^{201}Tl] data permits the calculation of left ventricular ejection fraction [LVEF] from simultaneously acquired gated ^{201}Tl and technetium-99m sestamibi SPECT myocardial perfusion scintigraphy studies in 20 patients. A strong correlation is noted between LVEF [r = 0.94] and end-systolic [r = 0.95] and end-diastolic [r = 0.97] volumes by the same method acquired using different tracers.)

296. Hannequin P, Mas J, Germano G. Photon energy recovery for crosstalk correction in simultaneous ^{99m}Tc/^{201}Tl imaging. *J Nucl Med* 2000;41:728–736.

(Photon energy recovery is efficient in removing technetium-99m [^{99m}Tc] crosstalk photons from thallium-201 [^{201}Tl] images for ^{99m}Tc/^{201}Tl ratios ranging from 5:1 to 2:1. Accurate photon recovery for crosstalk could make possible simultaneous ^{99m}Tc/^{201}Tl imaging.)

297. Bateman T, Case JA, Moutra KL, et al. Clinical evaluation of a novel dual-simultaneous SPECT myocardial perfusion protocol: blinded comparison to dual-sequential images [abstract]. *J Am Coll Cardiol* 1999;33:418A.

(Adenosine stress myocardial perfusion images acquired by a unique simultaneous thallium-201 rest/technetium-99m sestamibi dual-isotope protocol in 30 patients are compared with the same data acquired by the standard sequential dual-isotope protocol. Blinded readings of the 2 data sets reveal concordance for any abnormality at 100%; for abnormalities of the left anterior descending artery, 97%; of the right coronary artery, 93%; and of the left cirumflex coronary artery, 97%! When segmental scoring is considered, 545 of 600 [91%] segments are scored identically. The simultaneous acquisition protocol requires acquisition of and correction for photons seen in a window for "scatter" radiation. The protocol appears to be accurate, with reproducible results that are comparable with the standard protocol. If confirmed, the method will make a major impact on laboratory throughput, efficiency and cost effectiveness.)

298. Fukuchi K, Katafuchi T, Fukushima K, et al. Estimation of myocardial perfusion and viability using simultaneous ^{99m}Tc-tetrofosmin-FDG collimated SPECT. *J Nucl Med* 2000;41:1318–1323.

(In this article based on evaluation of images in 18 patients, simultaneous acquisition dual-isotope technetium-99m [^{99m}Tc] tetrofosmin and fluorodeoxyglucose imaging is shown to be feasible for the assessment of regional myocardial perfusion and viability with 3-channel acquisition and weighted scatter correction of crosstalk from the fluorine-18 photopeak to the ^{99m}Tc photopeak.)

299. DePuey EG, Rozanski A. Gated Tc-99m sestamibi SPECT to characterize fixed defects as infarct or artifact. *J Nucl Med* 1992;33:927–934.

(Gated sestamibi images and related regional systolic function are shown to be valuable in the differentiation of fixed defects resulting from prior infarction and attenuation artifact.)

300. Vacearino RA, Johnson LL, Antunes ML, et al. Thallium-201 lung uptake and peak treadmill exercise first pass ejection fraction. *Am Heart J* 1995;129:320–329.

(Seventy consecutive patients with similar angiographic anatomy are studied with exercise stress thallium-201 perfusion imaging and technetium-99m [^{99m}Tc] sestamibi. The incremental diagnostic value of first-pass ejection fraction acquired during dynamic exercise with ^{99m}Tc sestamibi is demonstrated.)

301. Chin BB, Zukerberg BW, Buchpiquel C, et al. Thallium-201 uptake in lung cancer. *J Nucl Med* 1995;36:1514–1519.

(Never overlook extracardiac localization of the perfusion radiotracer.)

302. Bax JJ, Visser FC, van Lingen A, et al. Comparison between 180° and 360° data sampling in thallium-201 rest-redistribution single photon emission tomography to predict functional recovery after revascularization. *Eur J Nucl Med* 1997;24:516–522.

(Thirty-two patients with left ventricular dysfunction who are scheduled for revascularization are studied with rest–redistribution imaging using 360° acquisition. The studies are then reformatted using the appropriate 180° data, from 45° right anterior oblique to 45° left posterior oblique. Both 360° and 180° acquisition methods bring accurate assessment of viability [sensitivity, 82% and 89%, respectively; specificity 51% and 55%, respectively] and predict well-postrevascularization functional restoration.)

303. Friedman J, Van Train K, Maddahi J, et al. "Upward creep" of the heart: a frequent source of false-positive reversible defects during thallium-201 stress-redistribution SPECT. *J Nucl Med* 1989;30:1718–1722.

304. Kiat H, Van Train K, Friedman JD, et al. Quantitative stress-redistribution thallium-201 SPECT using prone imaging: methodologic development and validation. *J Nucl Med* 1992;33:1509–1515.

(303,304: Upward creep [*303*] is a well-understood source of motion-related SPECT artifact. It probably results from altered and changing respiratory patterns and consequent cardiac displacement when imaging relatively soon after exercise. Reduced by prone positioning [*304*], it is seen less often with an extended period of recovery after exercise and before image acquisition. In addition to its ability to reduce patient motion, prone imaging is also of value in removing attenuation artifacts and intense and proximate subdiaphragmatic radioactivity. However, prone imaging also may introduce anterior wall artifacts!)

305. Jain AK. *Fundamentals of Digital Image Processing.* Englewood Cliffs, NJ: Prentice Hall; 1989.

(This is an excellent presentation of value to all in the field.)

306. Faber TL, Folks RD. Computer processing methods for nuclear medicine images. *J Nucl Med Tech* 1994;22:145–164.

(An overview of image processing methods.)

307. Wackers FJTh, Fetterman RC, Mettera JA, et al. Quantitative planar thallium-201 stress scintigraphy: a critical evaluation of the method. *Semin Nucl Med* 1985;15:46–66.

(Quantitative methods are applied to analysis of planar perfusion images.)

308. Goris ML, Daspit SG, McLaughlin P, et al. Interpolative background subtraction. *J Nucl Med* 1976;17:744–747.

(The authors describe the most common forms of planar image data processing. This background correction method seeks to account for the irregular nature of cardiac background activity. The authors' method of interpolative background subtraction attempts, with some success, to model background on the basis of regional extramyocardial sampling of a rectangular boundary. The activity filling this region, the ventricular background, is modeled as a linear transition from border to border. Problems arise when an area of intense extracardiac radioactivity is presumed erroneously to extend to the opposite border in gradually decreasing intensity. Background is overestimated, and a dense artifactual defect is created.)

309. Koster K, Wackers FJTh, Mattera JA, et al. Quantitative analysis of planar technetium-99m-sestamibi myocardial perfusion images using modified background subtraction. *J Nucl Med* 1990;31:1400–1408.

(This study documents the imperfection of interpolative background subtraction and the varying nature of related errors when applied to images acquired with different radionuclides.)

310. Segall GM, Atwood JE, Botvinick EH, et al. Variability of normal coronary anatomy: implications for the interpretation of thallium SPECT myocardial perfusion images in patients with single vessel disease. *J Nucl Med* 1994;36:944–951.

(This careful study correlates the location of stress-induced scintigraphic defects with angiographic anatomy in patients with single-vessel coronary disease. The findings reveal the spectrum of possible induced image abnormalities resulting from disease in a given distribution.)

311. Watson DD, Campbell NP, Read EK, et al. Spatial and temporal quantitation of planar thallium myocardial scans. *J Nucl Med* 1981;22:577–584.

(This method for the quantitative analysis of planar perfusion images should be compared with that discussed in reference 61.)

312. Garcia EV, Cooke CD, Van Train KF, et al. A symposium: technical aspects of myocardial SPECT imaging with technetium-99m sestamibi. *Am J Cardiol* 1990;66: 23E–31E.

(This is an early review of the proper parameters to apply in the processing of SPECT technetium-99m sestamibi studies.)

313. Beller GA. Instrumentation in nuclear cardiology. In: Beller GA, ed. *Clinical Nuclear Cardiology*. Philadelphia, PA: W.B. Saunders Co.; 1995:1–36.

(This is an excellent review of technical aspects and instrumentation in nuclear cardiology. Attenuation and methods to reduce attentuation are considered.)

314. Strauss HW, Miller DD, Wittry MD, et al. Procedure guideline for myocardial perfusion imaging. *J Nucl Med* 1998;39:918–923.

(The authors present a current review of acquisition and processing methods for all perfusion imaging protocols.)

315. American College of Cardiology, American Hospital Association, and Society of Nuclear Medicine. ACC/AHA/SNM policy statement: standardization of cardiac tomographic imaging. *J Nucl Cardiol* 1994;1:117–119.

(This statement recommends a standard format for presentation of SPECT perfusion image data. This is necessary to avoid confusion and to aid comparison of studies performed in different institutions.)

316. Brundage BH, Massie BM, Botvinick EH. Improved regional ventricular function after successful revascularization. *J Am Coll Cardiol* 1984;3:902–908.

(This study analyzes serial changes of regional wall motion on left ventriculograms performed pre- and postsurgical coronary revascularization in patients with resting dysynergy [wall motion abnormalities] and related reversible perfusion abnormalities. The authors find that the presence of a reversible perfusion defect predicts normalization of regional function in a high percentage of cases and so stands as a marker for viability and hibernating myocardium. Although this study is supported by substantial additional data, it does not analyze segments with fixed defects for evidence of scar, nor the relative regional radioactivity in the absence of reversibility, as independent evidence of viability.)

317. Foster E, O'Kelly B, LaPidus A, et al. Segmental myocardial viability can be inferred from combined analysis of echocardiographic function and scintigraphic perfusion: implications for 24-hour redistribution and PET scanning. *Am Heart J* 1994;129:7–14.

(Echocardiographic function correlates imperfectly but surprisingly well with regional scintigraphic perfusion. A logical analysis of regional perfusion and function can do much to determine regional viability. This now can be performed entirely on a single perfusion image.)

318. Gallik DM, Obermueller SD, Swarna US, et al. Simultaneous assessment of myocardial perfusion and left ventricular function during transient coronary occlusion. *J Am Coll Cardiol* 1995;25:1529–1538.

(Decremental perfusion and reduced left ventricular ejection fraction are measured by technetium-99m sestamibi first-pass radioangiography during clinically indicated angioplasty balloon occlusion of the designated vessel in 35 patients with single-vessel disease. Both perfusion and functional decrements are greatest with left anterior descending artery occlusion and are well correlated generally, although with significant individual variations. No measurement is made of regional wall motion abnormalities induced or of the correlation in association with narrowing but not occlusion.)

319. Borges-Neto S, Coleman RE, Potts JM, et al. Combined exercise radionuclide angiocardiography and single-photon emission computed tomography perfusion studies for assessment of coronary artery disease. *Semin Nucl Med* 1991;21:223–241.

320. Port SC. Recent advances in first-pass radionuclide angiography. *Nucl Cardiol Symp Clin Cardiol* 1994;12:359–372.

(319,320: A special, highly sensitive, multicrystal camera is applied to the acquisition and analysis of first-pass blood-pool studies on the stress sestamibi dose with determination of the exercise left ventricular ejection fraction. This value and regional wall motion may be compared with stress regional perfusion and rest function in an effort to better risk-stratify coronary patients. Reference 319 is 1 of a small number of studies that suggest an added independent prognostic value of first-pass function evaluation. The article by Port is an excellent review of the field he helped popularize.)

321. Iskandrian AS, Chae SC, Heo J, et al. Independent and incremental prognostic value of exercise single-photon emission computed tomographic (SPECT) thallium imaging in coronary artery disease. *J Am Coll Cardiol* 1993;22:665–670.

322. Berman DS, Hachamovitich R, Kiat H, et al. Incremental value of prognostic testing in patients with known or suspected ischemic heart disease: a basis for optimal utilization of exercise technetium-99m sestamibi myocardial perfusion single-photon emission computed tomography. *J Am Coll Cardiol* 1995;26:639–647.

(321,322: The full value of the myocardial perfusion scintigraphy method is only now being revealed, with its application as a quantitative parameter of coronary risk. It is quantitation that demonstrates the variability in myocardium infarcted or at risk in relation to coronary angiography.)

323. DePuey EG. How to detect and avoid myocardial perfusion SPECT artifacts. *J Nucl Med* 1994;35:699–702.

(Along with reference 350, this is one of the few classic reviews of literature on image artifacts, their avoidance and recognition. These articles are a "must" for the image reader and reveal the possible causes of perfusion image artifacts. Although the causes are diverse, those that are attenuation related are clearly the most frequent and most damaging: thus the current focus on attenuation correction methods.)

324. Burns RJ, Galligan L, Wright LM, et al. Improved specificity of myocardial thallium-201 single-photon emission computed tomography in patients with left bundle branch block by dipyridamole. *Am J Cardiol* 1991;68:504–508.

(Although exercise stress myocardial perfusion scintigraphy [MPS] demonstrates reduced specificity and specificity for left anterior descending coronary artery disease, pharmacologic, dipyridamole MPS is associated with specificities equal to those without left bundle branch block.)

325. Krishnan R, Lu J, Zhu YY, et al. Myocardial perfusion scintigraphy in left bundle branch block: a perspective on the issue from image analysis in a clinical context. *Am Heart J* 1993;126:578–586.

(Stress myocardial perfusion scintigraphy is evaluated in 69 consecutive patients with left bundle branch block [LBBB]. Among 32 who underwent coronary angiography, the overall and per-vessel sensitivity and specificity for right coronary arteries and left circumflex coronary arteries are similar to those studied without LBBB. However, overall specificity and specificity for left anterior descending [LAD] coronary artery disease are reduced. Nonetheless, the predictive value of a positive test remains high [83%] because of the relatively low angiography rate in patients with minimally abnormal scans. Specificity may also be adversely affected by the presence of cardiomyopathy in some patients with LBBB and the bias toward catheterization for those with LAD disease. This diagnostic difficulty is associated with studies performed with exercise stress. Pharmacologic, dipyridamole myocardial perfusion scintigraphy is associated with specificities equal to those without LBBB.)

326. Wagdy HM, Hodge D, Christian TF, et al. Prognostic value of vasodilator myocardial perfusion imaging in patients with left bundle-branch block. *Circulation* 1998;97:1563–1570.

(The diagnostic [*324,325*] and prognostic [*326*] value of stress myocardial perfusion scintigraphy in the setting of left bundle branch block [LBBB] is demonstrated. Prognostic value is demonstrated among 245 patients with LBBB studied with dipyridamole [n = 173] or adenosine [n = 92]. Those with normal images have a 1-yr [soft] event rate of 3%, with no myocardial infarctions [MIs] or deaths, whereas an abnormal image is associated with a 1-yr event rate of 42%, with 11% having MIs and 8% dying.)

327. Johnston DL, Scanlon PD, Hodge DO, et al. Pulmonary function monitoring during adenosine myocardial perfusion scintigraphy in patients with chronic obstructive pulmonary disease. *Mayo Clin Proc* 1999;74:339–346.

(Vasodilator stress testing is generally safe in patients with chronic obstructive pulmonary disease [COPD] in the absence of bronchospasm. It is also safe in the presence of historic but medically controlled bronchospasm. It presents increased risks when performed in the presence of active bronchospasm. This article examines pulmonary function in patients with COPD during adenosine infusion.)

328. Chikamori T, Doi YL, Yonezawa Y, et al. Value of dipyridamole thallium-201 imaging in noninvasive differentiation of idiopathic dilated cardiomyopathy from coronary artery disease with left ventricular dysfunction. *Am J Cardiol* 1992;69:650–653.

329. Tauberg SG, Orie JE, Bartlett BE, et al. Usefulness of thallium-201 for distinction of ischemic from idiopathic dilated cardiomyopathy. *Am J Cardiol* 1993;71:674–680.

(328,329: The perfusion pattern, the presence of reversibility and the relationship with left ventricular function help determine the origin of a congestive, dilated cardiomyopathy. The presence of segmental defects with a reversible component and wall motion abnormalities, which generally relate to perfusion defects, suggests an ischemic etiology.)

330. Ritchie JL, Bateman TM, Bonow RO, et al. Guidelines for clinical use of cardiac radionuclide imaging. Report of the American College of Cardiology/American Heart Association Task Force on Assessment of Diagnostic and Therapeutic Cardiovascular Procedures (Committee on Radionuclide Imaging), developed in collaboration with the American Society of Nuclear Cardiology. *J Am Coll Cardiol* 1995;125:521–547.

(Presented are the guidelines for use of radionuclide imaging. These are just that—guidelines—and are not without controversy and flaws. The decision of the appropriateness or value of application of myocardial perfusion scintigraphy [or any scintigraphic method] and its superiority to other methods rests entirely with the physician in charge. This obvious statement sometimes may need a vigorous defense, and knowledgeable physicians must not shrink from it.)

331. Reisman S, Maddahi J, Van Train K, et al. Quantitation of extent, depth, and severity of planar thallium defects in patients undergoing exercise thallium-201 scintigraphy. *J Nucl Med* 1986;27:1273–1281.

(Presented is the quantitative method of circumferential profile analysis of planar images. [See also reference 317.])

332. Van Train KF, Maddahi J, Berman DS, et al. Quantitative analysis of tomographic stress thallium-201 myocardial scintigrams: a multicenter trial. *J Nucl Med* 1990;31:1168–1179.

333. Garcia EV, DePuey EG, Sonnemaker RE, et al. Quantification of the reversibility of stress-induced thallium-201 myocardial perfusion defects: a multicenter trial using bull's-eye polar maps and normal limits. *J Nucl Med* 1990;31:1761–1765.

(95,311,332,333: These articles present methods for the quantitation of SPECT perfusion images employing circumferential profiles translated into polar maps. These are never to be read in a vacuum but serve as objective and quantitative guidelines to SPECT image interpretation.)

334. Nuyts J, Mortelmans L, Suetens P, et al. Model-based quantification of myocardial perfusion images from SPECT. *J Nucl Med* 1989;30:1992–2001.

(The method of polar map analysis is presented.)

335. Germano G, Kavanagh PB, Su HT, et al. Automatic reorientation of 3-dimensional transaxial myocardial perfusion SPECT images. *J Nucl Med* 1995;36:1107–1114.

(Processing algorithms recently have become fully automated, rapid and reliable [see reference 344].)

336. Bieszk JA, Hawman EG. Evaluation of SPECT angular sampling effects: continuous versus step-and-shoot acquisition. *J Nucl Med* 1987;28:1308–1314.

(Acquisition protocols affect the accurate measurement of image parameters, including regional brightening, wall motion and wall thickening.)

337. Wackers FJTh. Artifacts in planar and SPECT myocardial perfusion imaging. *Am J Cardiol Imaging* 1992;6:42–58.

(This is another well-illustrated review of image artifacts and ways to recognize and avoid them.)

338. Galt JR, Garcia EV, Robbins W. Effects of myocardial wall thickness on SPECT quantification. *IEEE Trans Med Imaging* 1990;9:144–150.

(Brightening has been shown to relate to wall thickening, resulting from an interaction of partial volume effects and camera resolution properties.)

339. Shen MYH, Liu YH, Sinusas AJ. Quantification of regional myocardial wall thickening on electrocardiogram-gated SPECT imaging. *J Nucl Cardiol* 1999;6:538–595.

(The authors describes a new computer algorithm for the objective quantitation of regional wall thickening from variations in regional count-density changes during the cardiac cycle.)

340. Eisner R, Tamas MJ, Cloninger K, et al. Normal SPECT thallium-201 bull's-eye display: gender differences. *J Nucl Med* 1988;29:1901–1909.

(Normal, sex-matched distributions of sestamibi and thallium have been determined and incorporated into myocardial perfusion polar map analysis programs.)

341. Van Train KF, Areeda J, Garcia EV, et al. Quantitative same-day rest-stress technetium-99m sestamibi SPECT: definition and validation of stress normal limits and criteria for abnormality. *J Nucl Med* 1993;34:1494–1502.

(Presented are the normal limits for quantitative SPECT image analysis. A certain amount of regional heterogeneity is within normal limits, when compared with a sex-matched normal population.)

342. Lucas JR, Ratzlaff NW, O'Connell JW, et al. The Tl-201–Tc-99m difference bull's-eye: an objective method to identify perfusion abnormalities and attenuation artifacts in dual Tl-201 rest/Tc-99m stress perfusion scans [abstract]. *Clin Res* 1994;42: 37A.

(Generally, but with rare exceptions, stress-induced perfusion defects will be more evident on the stress technetium-99m [^{99m}Tc] images, whereas attenuation will be most evident on the lower-energy thallium-201 rest images. Areas such as the thin apex will be better resolved on ^{99m}Tc-based images and so some areas of reduced activity that are more prominent on the stress ^{99m}Tc-based images may simply represent normal anatomy.)

343. Wallis JW, Miller TR. Three-dimensional display in nuclear medicine and radiology. *J Nucl Med* 1991;32:534–546.

(Three-dimensional displays of myocardial perfusion scintigraphy data are now commonplace. With added layovers of individualized coronary anatomy, they promise a unique and clinically valuable technique, permitting even more accurate correlations of image and anatomical data.)

344. Mullick R, Ezquerra NF. Automatic determination of left ventricular orientation from single-photon emission computed tomography (SPECT) data. *IEEE Trans Nucl Med* 1995;14:88–99.

(See reference 335.)

345. Germano G, Kavanaugh PB, Waechter P, et al. A new algorithm for the quantitation of myocardial perfusion SPECT: I. Technical principles and reproducibility. *J Nucl Med* 2000;41:712–719.

346. Sharir T, Germano G, Waechter P, et al. A new algorithm for the quantitation of myocardial perfusion SPECT: II. Validation and diagnostic yield. *J Nucl Med* 2000;41:720–727.

(345,346: A new algorithm is presented for automatic 3-dimensional quantitation of perfusion from SPECT thallium-201 and technetium-99m sestamibi images [*345*]. A second article applies the method in 195 patients in a 131 validation set, with the finding that the method is highly sensitive and specific for the detection and localization of coronary artery disease, with accurate and automated quantitation of regional perfusion. Its high reproducibility suggests its clinical value for the accurate assessment of serial changes in quantitative regional perfusion.)

347. Van Train KF, Garcia EV, Maddahi J, et al. Multicenter trial validation for quantitative analysis of same-day rest-stress technetium-99m-sestamibi myocardial tomograms. *J Nucl Med* 1994;35:609–618.

(296,330: A collaborative effort develops a now widely disseminated quantitative program called CEQual [for Cedars-Emory Quantitative Analysis], with software that permits near-total automation of the processing phase. Better but not perfect, this method still does not resolve all problems of the method and continues to need a critical reader.)

348. Dunn R, Botvinick E, Hattner R, et al. A consideration of factors affecting the diagnostic accuracy of thallium-201 myocardial perfusion scintigraphy in detecting coronary artery disease. *Semin Nucl Med* 1980;5:245–271.

349. Watson DD, Smith WH. SPECT: current and future developments. *J Nucl Biol Med* 1992;36:108–112.

(348,349: See annotation for reference 321.)

350. DePuey EG, Garcia EV. Optimal specificity of thallium-201 SPECT through recognition of imaging artifacts. *J Nucl Med* 1989;30:441–449.

(This is an excellent review of potential artifacts on SPECT perfusion imaging.)

351. Eisner RI, Martin SE, Leon AR, et al. Inhomogeneity of gated and ungated SPECT technetium-99m-sestamibi bull's-eyes in normal dogs: comparison with thallium-201. *J Nucl Med* 1993;34;281–287.

(The distribution of thalliium-201 and technetium-99m sestamibi within the myocardium is one consideration, but the way in which we perceive this distribution, given attenuation, scatter and other causes of heterogeneity, is another important clinical factor that will aid image interpretation. The factors noted, as well as any differences in actual myocardial perfusion, may vary in relation to the energy, other characteristics or distribution of the different perfusion agents.)

352. Botvinick EH, Zhu YY, O'Connell JW, et al. A quantitative assessment of patient motion and its effect on myocardial perfusion SPECT images. *J Nucl Med* 1993;34: 303–312.

(This article analyzes the resultant intensity and extent of induced SPECT perfusion image defect when the projection images of a normal study are selectively and variably moved in a vertical plane by specially designed software. Also evaluated are the effects of rotary motion and the potential for correcting any derived artifacts by realigning the projection images. The extent of motion and its duration are compounded in their artifactual effect on the final SPECT slices. Limited and returning vertical motion has little effect on the processed image. Motion greater than 3–4 pixels and at least 3 frames in duration causes image artifact. Any, even gross, motion in a single frame is not likely to cause a defect. Vertical motion potentially could be corrected on projection images and reprocessed. Rotary motion, which introduces artifacts, have to be reacquired.)

353. Maublant JC, Peycelon P, Kwiatkowski F, et al. Comparison between 180° and 360° data collection in technetium-99m MIBI SPECT of the myocardium. *J Nucl Med* 1989;30:295–300.

354. Knesaurek K, King MA, Glick SJ, et al. Investigation of causes of geometric distortion in 180° and 360° angular sampling in SPECT. *J Nucl Med* 1989;30:1666–1675.

(353,354: The authors of both articles consider the importance of uniform sensitivity across the entire detector field of view.)

355. Hoffman EJ. 180° compared with 360° sampling in SPECT [teaching editorial]. *J Nucl Med* 1982;23:745–747.

356. Tamaki N, Mukai T, Ishii Y, et al. Comparative study of thallium emission myocardial tomography with 180° and 360° data collection. *J Nucl Med* 1982;23:661–666.

(355,356: Because the center of rotation is rarely in the center of the field of view, images must be shifted so that the center of the acquisition matrix matches the center of rotation.)

357. Cooper JA, McCandless BK. Preventing patient motion during tomographic myocardial perfusion imaging. *J Nucl Med* 1995;36:2001–2005.

(The application of a device that positions and supports the upper extremities and back during SPECT acquisition reduces both the incidence [from 38% to 26%] and the amount [by 5.3 mm] of motion. This reduces the incidence of reconstruction artifacts by one-third.)

358. Toma DM, White MP, Mann A, et al. Influence of arm positioning on rest/stress technetium-99m-labeled sestamibi tomographic myocardial perfusion imaging. *J Nucl Cardiol* 1999;6:163–168.

(Arm positioning, whether above the head or at the patient's side, yields the same SPECT image data. There is no influence on image quality or alteration of defect size or location. The overhead arm position is conventional but can be changed to one in which the arms are at the patient's side, if necessary.)

359. Kang X, Berman DS, Lewin HC, et al. Comparative localization of myocardial ischemia by exercise electrocardiography and myocardial perfusion SPECT. *J Nucl Card* 2000;7:140–145.

(In 552 consecutive patients studied by exercise myocardial perfusion imaging, the site of maximal ST depression does not identify the localization of stress-induced perfusion defects. However, ST elevation does localize related perfusion defects, confirming prior findings.)

360. Dae M, Canhasi B, Botvinick E, et al. The etiology and implications of dense cavitary "photopenia" on myocardial perfusion scintigraphy. *Invest Radiol* 1985;20: 388–392.

361. Sciagraa R, Bisi G, Buonamici P, et al. Left ventricular cavity to myocardial count ratio in technetium-99m sestamibi SPECT in the detection of resting left ventricular dysfunction. *J Nucl Med* 1997;38:766–770.

(360,361: "Dense cavitary photopenia"[*360*] or a high myocardial-to-cavity count ratio[*361*] may be seen with planar or SPECT imaging. The imperfectly tomographic SPECT image may demonstrate photopenia because of a lack of activity or motion in the overlying wall. It is a property of the overlying wall—not of the cavity! However, when fixed, as is often the case, it indicates scar; if induced by stress, it suggests a tight, high-risk lesion.)

362. Corbett JR, Ficaro EP. Clinical review of attenuation-corrected cardiac SPECT. *J Nucl Cardiol* 1999;6:54–68.

(This is an in-depth review of the subject of SPECT attenuation correction, current methods and their clinical utility.)

363. DePuey EG, Nichols K, Salensky H, et al. Gated sestamibi correlates of myocardial viability assessed with rest/delayed Tl-201 SPECT [abstract]. *J Nucl Med* 1995;36:56P.

(Regional function parallels viability. However, dysfunction is itself often ambiguous. In seeking to determine regional viability of a dysfunctional segment, gated perfusion images will add to the clarity with which perfusion data can be related to the dysfunctional segment.)

364. Chuttani K, Metherall J, Griffith J, et al. Enhanced hepatic uptake of thallium-20l in patients with severe narrowing of the right coronary artery. *Am J Cardiol* 1995;76:1020–1024.

(Liver-to-heart and stress-to-rest radioactivity demonstrates increased hepatic uptake in those with right coronary artery disease.)

365. Segall GM, Davis MJ. Prone versus supine thallium myocardial SPECT: a method to decrease artifactual inferior wall defects. *J Nucl Med* 1989;30:548–555.

(The nature and cause of diaphragmatic attenuation is carefully analyzed and demonstrated. MR images in varying patient positions demonstrate the varying anatomic relationships that contribute to the structural overlap intrinsic to attenuation abnormalities and their solution.)

366. Beller GA. Detection of coronary disease. In: Beller GA, ed. *Clinical Nuclear Cardiology.* Philadelphia, PA: W.B. Saunders Co.;1995:82–136.

(This is a thorough review of the method of perfusion scintigraphy and its clinical applications. Considered are methods of image display and interpretation and the recognition of image artifacts.)

367. Nuyts J, Dupont P, Van den Maegdenbergh V, et al. A study of the liver-heart artifact in emission tomography. *J Nucl Med* 1995;36:133–139.

(When high levels of hepatic uptake of perfusion tracers are evident, lower than expected counts values are recognized in the adjacent inferior myocardial wall. This phenomenon is studied in simulations and found to be the result of photon attenuation effects during reconstruction, distorting liver reconstruction and influencing inferior wall activity. The phenomenon can be eliminated by attenuation correction.)

368. Maddahi J, Prigent F ,Garcia E, et al. Validation of newly developed attenuation and scatter correction methods for quantitating myocardial perfusion by Tc-99mm sestamibi SPECT [abstract]. *Circulation* 1990;82:III64.

(This is an early effort attempting attenuation correction and, apparently, claiming success prematurely.)

369. Cullom SJ, Galt JR, Maddahi J, et al. Scatter and attenuation correction of SPECT Tc-99m sestamibi myocardial distributions: experimental validation of the effect on uniformity and contrast. *J Nucl Med* 1991;32:1067–1073.

(368,369: These are 2 preliminary reports of the effects of the attenuation and scatter correction method applied to perfusion imaging. The development of such a method that could be applied routinely to clinical studies would represent a major advance and would favorably affect diagnostic accuracy. In this and other studies, Cullom et al. apply the method in 40 coronary patients and 10 healthy individuals undergoing stress–reinjection–redistribution thallium-201 studies. The attenuation method demonstrates its ability to correct for attenuation in phantoms and in 6 specific patient studies. The authors find increased homogeneity in attenuation-corrected normal studies. Improved specificity is also demonstrated when the method is applied to technetium-99m sestamibi studies. However, the findings are not confirmed elsewhere, and there are no prospective studies.)

370. Gregoriou GK, Tsui BMW, Gullberg GT. Effect of truncated projections on defect detection in attenuation-compensated fanbeam cardiac SPECT. *J Nucl Med* 1998;39:166–175.

371. Ficaro EP, Fessler JA, Shreve PD, et al. Simultaneous transmission/emission myocardial perfusion tomography: diagnostic accuracy of attenuation corrected ^{99m}Tc-sestamibi single-photon emission computed tomography. *Circulation* 1996;93:463–473.

372. Case JA, Pan TS, King MA, et al. Reduction of truncation artifacts in fan beam transmission imaging using a spatially varying gamma camera. *IEEE Trans Nucl Sci* 1995;42:2660–2265.

(370–372: Several authors have presented methods to gain true attenuation correction and reduce the error of truncation artifacts by excluding aspects of the patient from the field of view. Ficaro et al. use a triple-head detector with an americium-241 transmission source.)

373. Bacharach SL, Buvat R. Attenuation correction in cardiac positron emission tomography and single-photon emission computed tomography. *J Nucl Cardiol* 1995;2:246–253.

(Attenuation correction is reviewed in this article.)

374. Frey EC, Tsui BMW, Perry JR. Simultaneous acquisition of emission and transmission data for improved thallium-201 cardiac SPECT imaging using a technetium-99m transmission source. *J Nucl Med* 1992;33:2238–2245.

375. Fleming J. A technique for using CT images in attenuation correction and quantification in SPECT. *Nucl Med Commun* 1989;10:83–88.

(374,375: The current method of choice and the most easily available is a scanning line source for transmission-image generation on a dual-head camera with a 90° configuration and parallel-hole collimation, applied over 180° from the right anterior oblique to the left posterior oblique, as described in these articles.)

376. Kluge R, Sattler B, Seese A, et al. Attenuation corrected by simultaneous emission-transmission myocardial single-photon emission tomography using a technetium-99m-labeled radiotracer: impact on diagnostic accuracy. *Eur J Nucl Med* 1997;24: 1107–1114.

(The authors study 50 males, 25 with 1- and 2-vessel disease of the right coronary artery and/or left circumflex coronary artery and 25 with a low likelihood of coronary artery disease. All undergo stress–rest technetium-99m [^{99m}Tc] tetrofosmin imaging. The study demonstrates enhanced contrast between normal and abnormal areas and increased homogeneity in normal studies. However, the study population is select, and the authors do not evaluate the method in left anterior descending artery disease or in women.)

377. Hendel RC, Berman DS, Cullom SJ, et al. Multicenter clinical trial to evaluate the efficacy of correction for photon attenuation and scatter in SPECT myocardial perfusion imaging. *Circulation* 1999;99:2742–2749.

(The authors evaluate technetium-99m sestamibi in dual-isotope and 1-day stress–rest protocols with attenuation and scatter correction using gadolinium-153 line sources. The effort results in an improved normalcy but not in improved sensitivity.)

(373–377: The accuracy of attenuation-corrected myocardial perfusion scintigraphy is analyzed and presented in these papers. Although some authors have reported increased homogeneity in attenuation-corrected normal studies and improved specificity, when the method is applied to ^{99m}Tc sestamibi studies the findings are not confirmed elsewhere, are inconsistent at best and there are no prospective studies. The method has yet to be proven clinically.)

378. Links JM, Becker L, Rigo PM, et al. Combined corrections for attenuation, depth-dependent blur and motion in SPECT: a multicenter trial. *J Nucl Cardiol* 2000;7:414–425.

(This multicenter trial demonstrates that attenuation correction, when combined with motion- and depth-dependent loss of spatial resolution, provides greater diagnostic accuracy than conventional reconstruction of myocardial SPECT studies in both men and women. Exercise or dipyridamole stress is applied with thallium-201 or technetium-99m tracers. Attenuation is corrected with an iterative, nonuniform Chang algorithm, using a transmission-scan–generated attenuation map. Sensitivity and specificity rise from 86% and 73% to 91% and 94%, respectively, for men, and from 75% and 64% to 75% and 89%, respectively, for women.)

379. Duvernoy CS, Ficaro EP, Karabajakian MZ, et al. Improved detection of left main coronary artery disease with attenuation corrected SPECT. *J Nucl Cardiol* 2000;7:639–648.

(Attenuation correction with application of the algorithm applied here improves diagnostic accuracy for the identification of left main coronary artery disease.)

380. Stone CD, McCormick JW, Gilliland DR, et al. Effect of registration errors between transmission and emission scans on a SPECT system using sequential scanning. *J Nucl Med* 1998;39:365–373.

(Patient motion within and between transmission and emission scans is also a likely source of gross error in the method but has yet to be characterized. This article evaluates the effect of such registration errors.)

381. Beller GA, Radiopharmaceuticals in nuclear cardiology. In Beller GA, ed. *Clinical Nuclear Cardiology.* Philadelphia, PA: W.B. Saunders Co.;1995:37–81.

(The author reviews the pertinent aspects of radiopharmaceuticals employed in nuclear cardiology and considers methods of scatter correction employing off-peak imaging data. A similar approach might employ the evaluation of differential attenuation of multiple peaks of the same radiopharmaceutical.)

382. O'Connor MK, Caiati C, Christian TF, Gibbon RJ. Effects of scatter correction on the measurements of infarct size from SPECT cardiac phantom studies. *J Nucl Med* 1995;36:2080–2086.

(Both thallium-201 [^{201}Tl] and technetium-99m [^{99m}Tc] sestamibi cardiac images are degraded by their contained scattered radiation. This phantom experiment seeks to determine the beneficial effect of scatter correction methods contained in current scintillation cameras. The study demonstrates that scatter correction reduces the error resulting from measurement of infarct size and increases image contrast and quality in both ^{201}Tl and ^{99m}Tc sestamibi images.)

383. Boning G, Ziegler S, Ficaro EP, et al. Attenuation correction of gated SPECT: influence of length of transmission scan [abstract]. *J Nucl Med* 1997;38:64P.

(The contribution from noise in the transmission scan increases with decreasing acquisition time and causes errors in the "corrected" emission scan. This statistical problem increases as the transmission source deteriorates.)

384. Brown JK, Tang HR, Hattner RS, et al. Intrinsic dual energy processing (IDEP) of myocardial perfusion images. *J Nucl Med* 2000;41:1287–1297.

(An effort is made to recognize and differentiate the effects of decreased perfusion from attenuation, based on the differential regional attenuation of the varying emission energies of thallium-201.)

385. Chang LT. A method for attenuation correction in radionuclide computed tomography. *IEEE Trans Nucl Sci* 1978;25:638–643.

386. Hansen CL, Siegel JA. Attenuation correction of thallium SPECT using differential attenuation of thallium photons. *J Nucl Med* 1992;33:1574–1577.

(385,386: These 2 articles present common attenuation correction algorithms that are often applied.)

387. Esquerre JP, Coca FJ, Martinez SJ, et al. Prone decubitus: a solution to inferior wall attenuation in thallium-201 myocardial tomography. *J Nucl Med* 1989;30: 398–401.

(Imaging in varying patient positions often aids recognition of attenuation and motion artifact.)

388. King MA, Tsui BMW, Pan TS, et al. Attenuation compensation for cardiac single-photon emission computed tomographic imaging: Part 1. Impact of attenuation and methods of estimating attenuation maps. *J Nucl Cardiol* 1995;2:513–524.

389. King MA, Tsui BMW, Pan TS, et al. Attenuation compensation for cardiac single-photon emission computed tomographic imaging: Part 2. Attenuation compensation algorithms. *J Nucl Cardiol* 1996;3:55–64.

(388,389: These articles review the field of attenuation correction in SPECT.)

390. LaCroix K, Tsui BMW, Frey EC, et al. Receiver operator characteristic evaluation of iterative reconstruction with attenuation correction in ^{99m}Tc-sestamibi myocardial SPECT images. *J Nucl Med* 2000;41:502–513.

(In this phantom study, an improvement in defect detection is evident among myocardial SPECT images using maximum likelihood expectation maximization with nonuniform attenuation correction in comparison with images using filtered backprojection without attenuation correction. This is most noticeable among phantoms with large simulated breasts or high diaphragms.)

391. El Fakhri G, Buvat I, Benali H, et al. Relative impact of scatter, collimator response, attenuation, and finite spatial resolution corrections in cardiac SPECT. *J Nucl Med* 2000;41:1400–1408.

(This study uses computer simulation and phantom studies to assess the respective effects of correction for scatter, depth-dependent collimator response, attenuation and finite spatial resolution on different image features in cardiac SPECT, when quantified for a specific acquisition configuration.)

392. Blue, PW. Accuracy of center of rotation determination for SPECT imaging. *J Nucl Med Technol* 1989;17:61–65.

393. Cerqueira MD, Matsuoka D, Ritchie JL, et al. The influence of collimators on SPECT center of rotation measurements: artifact generation and acceptance testing. *J Nucl Med* 1988;29:1393–1397.

(392,393: The importance of the center of rotation to the generation of accurate SPECT data and methods of quality control and assurance is considered in this article.)

394. O'Conner MK. Instrument and computer-related problems and artifacts in nuclear medicine. *Semin Nucl Med* 1996;26:256–277.

(This is an excellent and well-illustrated review of nuclear medicine image artifacts associated with camera or computer errors in camera.)

395. Maddahi J, Kiat H, Friedman JP, et al. Tc-99m sestamibi myocardial perfusion imaging for evaluation of coronary disease: results of the North American Phase III Multicenter Clinical Trial. In Zaret B, Beller G, eds. *Nuclear Cardiology.* St Louis, MO: C.V. Mosby;1992:191–200.

(The results of a multicenter trial of the accuracy of stress planar and SPECT myocardial perfusion scintigraphy are presented. The shape of the orbit is not specifically built into quantitative algorithms of image interpretation.)

396. Eisner RL. Sensitivity of SPECT thallium-201 myocardial perfusion imaging to patient motion [editorial]. *J Nucl Med* 1992;33:1571–1573.

397. Brust KD, Graham MM. Aspects of patient imaging with SPECT. *J Nucl Med Technol* 1987;15:133–137.

398. Chen Q, Franken PR, Defrise M, et al. Detection and correction of patient motion in SPECT imaging. *J Nucl Med Technol* 1993;21:198–205.

399. Feldkamp MJ. SPECT quality improvement. *J Nucl Med Technol* 1994;22:35–38.

400. Prigent FM, Hyun M, Berman DS, et al. Effect of motion on thallium-201 SPECT studies: a simulation and clinical study. *J Nucl Med* 1993;34:1845–1850.

401. Eisner R, Churchwell A, Noever T, et al. Quantitative analysis of the tomographic thallium-201 myocardial bullseye display: critical role of correcting for patient motion. *J Nucl Med* 1988;29:91–97.

402. Cooper JA, Neumann PH, McCandless BK. Effect of patient motion on tomographic myocardial perfusion imaging. *J Nucl Med* 1992;33:1566–1571.

403. Cooper JA, Neumann PH, McCandless BK. Detection of patient motion during tomographic myocardial perfusion imaging. *J Nucl Med* 1993;34:1341–1348.

(397–403: These articles represent a body of work on the recognition and analysis of the effects of patient motion on SPECT myocardial perfusion scintigraphy. Little has been published on the effects of respiratory motion, which is both largely ignored and pervasive. The relatively poor image resolution of the scintigraphic method makes it more tolerant than other methods to slight motion variations.)

404. Cooper JA. Detection of patient motion during tomographic myocardial perfusion imaging. *J Nucl Med* 1993;34:1349–1355.

(See reference 357.)

405. Sorrell V, Figueroa B, Hansen CL. The "hurricane sign": evidence of patient motion artifact on cardiac single-photon emission computed tomographic imaging. *J Nucl Cardiol* 3:86–88.

(The hurricane sign presents a graphic representation of the comma-shaped artifacts extending from the myocardium at opposite sides of the short-axis perfusion scintigram slices processed from projection images in the presence of motion artifact.)

406. Germano G, Kavanagh PB, Kiat H, et al. Temporal image fractionation: rejection of motion artifacts in myocardial SPECT. *J Nucl Med* 1994;35:1193–1197.

(Static myocardial perfusion SPECT studies are acquired as 3-interval dynamic studies, with continuous alternating detector rotation of a multidetector camera. The method permits extraction of data from frames with patient motion without degrading the data set, minimizes upward creep by the alternating rotation and enlarges the angular range, which reduces the effect of motion.)

407. Germano G, Chua T, Kavanaugh P, et al. Detection and correction of patient motion in dynamic and static myocardial SPECT using a multi-detector camera. *J Nucl Med* 1993;34:1349–1355.

(406,407: These articles present methods to recognize and correct SPECT motion artifact. Generally, only vertical motion can be corrected. The relatively stable distribution of technetium-99m sestamibi permits reacquisition without losing data. Images should always be processed and reviewed before the patient is dismissed, so that reacquisition is possible and delayed imaging can be arranged as needed.)

408. DePuey EG. Artifacts in SPECT myocardial perfusion imaging. In: DePuey EG, Berman DS, Garcia EV, eds. *Cardiac SPECT Imaging.* New York, NY: Raven Press Ltd.;1995:169–200.

(The problem of recognition of pathologic cavitary dilation in single-isotope and dual-isotope protocols and artifacts of the SPECT method in general are considered.)

409. Kelly BJ, O'Conner MK. Comparison of the gray scale characteristics of analog and video (digital) formatters. *J Nucl Med Technol* 1992;20:62–67.
(Gray scale and the instrumentation to display it are considered.)

410. Rigo P, Leclercq B, Itti R, et al. Technetium-99m tetrofosmin myocardial imaging: a comparison with thallium-201 and angiography. *J Nucl Med* 1994;35:587–593.
(The problem of extracardiac activity may be somewhat alleviated with the introduction of technetium-99m–based tetrofosmin, which has reduced biliary excretion.)

411. Gabor FV, Datz FL, Christian PE, et al. Computer-assisted diagnosis of cardiac perfusion studies. *J Nucl Med Technol* 1991;19:238–244.

412. Siegel HJ, Chen DCP, Jacobs L, et al. The impact of operator decision on quantitative circumferential profile analysis of myocardial thallium-201 scintigraphy: a systematic evaluation. *J Nucl Med Technol* 1989;17:58–60.
(335,344,411,412: The commercial normal database provides a polar map of usual coronary artery perfusion areas. Sometimes the defect will be misrepresented in its angular location because of the application of a different reference point in its formulation.)

413. Starksen NF, O'Connell JW, Dae MW, et al. Basal interventricular septal thallium-201 defects: real or artifact? *Clin Nucl Med* 1993;18:291–296.
(The article presents the formulation of a well-known artifact related to the application of variable axes of SPECT reconstruction at rest and with stress.)

414. Ratzlaff NW, Brown PH, Cox DJ, Krishnamurthy GT. The effects of collimator malpositioning in seven-pinhole tomography. *J Nucl Med Technol* 1984;12:51–55.

415. Barrett HH. Limited-angle tomography for the nineties [editorial]. *J Nucl Med* 1990;31:1688–1692.
(414,415: The importance of the axis of reconstruction and factors that influence its selection and reproducibility are demonstrated in these papers.)

416. Desmarais R, Kaul D, Watson D, et al. Do false-positive thallium scans lead to unnecessary catheterization? Outcome of patients with perfusion defects on quantitative planar thallium-201 scintigraphy. *J Am Coll Cardiol* 1993;21:1058–1063..
(The problem of the false-positive perfusion scintigram is considered and its clinical impact assessed, as are methods to reduce its frequency. It should be remembered that a normal or "probably normal" image is associated with an excellent prognosis and low event rate. Images that demonstrate defects of an artifactual nature, or most likely of an artifactual nature, should not be called positive nor lead to intervention. Instead, the nature of the defect should be identified with the comment that there is no evidence of perfusion defect, and such studies should be placed in the normal category. This approach will reduce significantly the frequency and impact of false-positive studies.)

417. Bax JJ, Visser FC, Blanksma PK, et al. Comparison of myocardial uptake of fluorine-18 fluorodeoxyglucose imaged with PET and SPECT in dysynergic myocardium. *J Nucl Med* 1996;37:1631–1636.
(Here 20 patients with prior infarction and wall motion abnormalities are studied by fluorodeoxyglucose [FDG] metabolic imaging with both SPECT and PET methods under conditions of hyperinsulinemic glucose clamping. Each is also studied by rest thallium-201 [^{201}Tl] SPECT and nitrogen-13 [^{13}N] ammonia PET for regional perfusion evaluation. The agreement between [^{201}Tl]/FDG SPECT and ^{13}N ammonia/FDG PET for detection of viable dysynergic segments is 76%. Among those 12 patients with left ventricular ejection fraction <35%, all SPECT and PET data are identical.)

418. Burt RW, Perkins OW, Oppenheim BE, et al. Direct comparison of fluorine-18 FDG SPECT, fluorine-18 FDG PET and rest thallium-201 SPECT for detection of myocardial viability. *J Nucl Med* 1995;36:176–179.
(The authors compare the accuracy of fluorodeoxyglucose [FDG] SPECT, FDG PET and rest thallium-201 [^{201}Tl] imaging methods in 20 patients with left

ventricular dysfunction and fixed ^{201}Tl defects at rest. Although FDG metabolic imaging is found to identify 13 additional viable segments among 60 dysfunctional segments with fixed defects on rest ^{201}Tl imaging, both SPECT and PET FDG imaging are equally accurate. It is important to note that roughly 4 of 5 dysfunctional segments are correctly classified by ^{201}Tl rest imaging if, indeed, FDG is the "gold standard" and is always correct and the criterion for lack of viability on perfusion images is a measure of the relative radiotracer uptake! Evaluation of function after revascularization is not included.)

419. Delbeke D, Videlesky S, Patton JA, et al. Rest myocardial perfusion/metabolism imaging using simultaneous dual-isotope acquisition SPECT with technetium-99m-mibi/fluorine-18-FDG. *J Nucl Med* 1995;36:2110–2119.

(Simultaneous evaluation of rest myocardial perfusion/metabolism with a multihead SPECT camera and an ultrahigh energy collimator is possible using technetium-99m sestamibi/fluorodeoxyglucoise with a dual-isotope simultaneous acquisition.)

420. Sandler MP, Patton JA. Fluorine 18-labeled fluorodeoxyglucose myocardial single-photon emission computed tomography: an alternative for determining myocardial viability. *J Nucl Cardiol* 1996;3:342–349.

(This review article presents evidence that fluorodeoxyglucose PET with conventional perfusion agents might provide an acceptable alternative to PET imaging for the detection of hibernating myocardium.)

421. Srinivasan G, Kitsiou AN, Bacharach SL, et al. [F-18] fluorodeoxyglucose single photon emission computed tomography: can it replace PET and thallium SPECT for the assessment of myocardial tomography? *Circulation* 1998;97:843–850.

(In order to compare SPECT and PET technologies, as well as to assess viability by perfusion and metabolism tracers, the authors evaluate 28 patients with chronic coronary artery disease using fluorine-18 [^{18}F] fluorodeoxyglucose [FDG] SPECT, ^{18}F FDG PET and thallium-201 [^{201}Tl] SPECT. Although SPECT and FDG PET yield similar results, as do ^{201}Tl and FDG distributions, ^{201}Tl underestimates viability among those with left ventricular ejection fraction $<$25% and in the inferior wall, the latter probably because of attenuation. Rarely, FDG SPECT may falsely indicate viability where other methods correctly find scar.)

422. Valkema R, Poldermans D, Reijs AEM, et al. Evaluation of myocardial viability using dual isotope simultaneous acquisition (DISA) with Tc-99m-tetrofosmin and 18-FDG and a three-head SPECT camera [abstract]. *J Nucl Med* 1996;37:231.

(417–422: Much effort has been made to image fluorodeoxyglucose with conventional scintillation cameras, and much progress has been made. These articles present the method and its current capabilities.)

423. Sandler MP, Bax JI, Patton JA. et al. Fluorine-18-fluorodeoxyglucose cardiac imaging using a modified scintillation camera: state of the art. *J Nucl Med* 1998;39: 2035–2043.

(Collimated acquisition with a modified camera presents a superior imaging result.)

424. Sandler MP, Videlefsky S, Delbeke D, et al. Evaluation of myocardial ischemia using a rest metabolism/stress perfusion protocol with ^{18}FDG/^{99m}Tc-MIBI and dual isotope simultaneous acquisition SPECT. *J Am Coll Cardiol* 1995; 26: 870–878.

(The authors seek to establish a dual-isotope single-acquisition SPECT protocol with an ultra-high-energy collimator to evaluate rest metabolism and stress perfusion with fluorine-18 [^{18}F] fluorodeoxyglucose [FDG] and technetium-99m [^{99m}Tc] sestamibi. After glucose loading, ^{18}F FDG is given intravenously. After a 35-minute distribution phase, stress–perfusion imaging is performed. A 20% window for both photopeaks and a ^{99m}Tc/^{18}F concentration of 3.2/1 gives a 6% spillover of ^{18}F into the ^{99m}Tc window. With a 70% lesion considered diagnostic of coronary disease, SPECT sensitivity is 100%, specificity is 88%, positive predictive value is 93% and negative predictive value is 100%. Dual-isotope SPECT with FDG as the rest–perfusion surrogate may provide a cost-effective alternative to conventional PET flow-metabolism imaging or thallium-201 reinjection technique and provide state of the art data regarding both myocardium at ischemic risk and viability.)

425. Chen EQ, MacIntyre WJ, Go RT, et al. Myocardial viability studies using fluorine-18 FDG SPECT: a comparison with fluorine-18 FDG PET. *J Nucl Med* 1997;38:582–586.
(The physical and imaging characteristics of SPECT, acquired using either a high-energy [HE], general-purpose collimator or a special, ultrahigh [UH] energy, 511-keV, collimator and PET, methods for fluorodexoyglucose [FDG] evaluation are analyzed and compared among 18 patients. PET is superior to SPECT in all physical imaging characteristics, especially sensitivity and contrast resolution, regardless of the collimator applied. Nonetheless, application of the UH collimator reduces septal penetration, significantly improves both spatial and contrast resolution and reduces sensitivity. Although there is a high concordance in segmental viability information between PET and SPECT using either collimator, the agreement between PET and SPECT is statistically better when the UH collimator is employed. SPECT with special 511-keV collimation appears to serve as an alternative to PET FDG imaging for viability evaluation.)

426. Yamaguchi H, Hasegawa S, Yoshioka J, et al. Myocardial viability assessment by FDG uptake with coincidence detection and 511 keV collimator by gamma camera imaging: comparison with conventional PET imaging [abstract]. *J Nucl Med* 40:155P.
(Fifteen patients with prior infarction and 5 with none are studied with fluorodeoxyglucose [FDG] by both coincidence detection and with a 511-keV collimator on the gamma camera and by FDG PET. Collimator FDG imaging overestimates regional viability compared with PET, whereas coincidence gamma camera FDG imaging compares well with PET but is more affected by attenuation. Gamma-camera coincidence FDG imaging may well assess viability with application of an accurate attenuation method.)

427. Bax JJ, Comeil JH. Visser FC, et al. Prediction of improvement of contractile function in patients with ischemic ventricular dysfunction after revascularization by F18-fluorodeoxyglucose SPECT. *J Am Coll Cardiol* 1997;39:377–384.

428. Bax JJ, Comeil JH, Visser FC, et al. Prediction of recovery of myocardial dysfunction after revascularization: comparison of fluorine-18 fluorodeoxyglucose/thallium-201 SPECT, thallium-20I stress-reinjection SPECT and dobutamine echocardiography. *J Am Coll Cardiol* 1996;28:558–564.

429. Srinivasan G, Kitsiou AN, Bacharach SL, et al. ^{18}F-deoxyglucose SPECT: can it replace PET and thallium SPECT for the assessment of myocardial liability? *Circulation* 1998;97:843–850.
(427–429: References 427 and 428, from the same group, are the only 2 studies currently in print that evaluate the ability of fluorodeoxyglucose SPECT to determine viability and restoration of function with revascularization. The results are promising and seem to mirror the value of standard perfusion-metabolism PET imaging. This raises the question posed in reference 429.)

430. Stollfuss J, Haas F, Neverve J, et al. Gated Tc-99m tetrofosmin SPECT for assessment of viability in patients with severe left ventricular dysfunction [abstract]. *J Nucl Med* 1997;38(suppl):97.
(The ability to evaluate images that at once display both regional perfusion and function in registry permits the ready and accurate identification of the state of perfusion in dysfunctional segments. This proves most valuable when determining the state of viability in the setting of severe left ventoricular dysfunction. This has been aided further by the application of attenuation correction.)

431. Levine MG, McGill CC, Ahlberg AW, et al. Functional assessment with electrocardiographic gated single-photon emission computed tomography improves the ability of technetium-99m sestamibi myocardial perfusion imaging to predict myocardial viability in patients undergoing revascularization. *Am J Cardiol* 1999;83:1–5.

(This study demonstrates the value of gated SPECT wall motion and thickening as markers of viability before revascularization and as markers of functional improvement after revascularization.)

432. TMG Technology Marketing Group. *1996 Nuclear Medicine Database Summary Report Analysis.* Author's personal copy of private report.

(Report of the marketing group hired to analyze current uses of nuclear cardiology methods.)

433. Field M. *Telemedicine: A Guide to Assessing Telecommunications in Healthcare.* Washington, DC: National Academy Press; 1996.

(The benefits of teleradiogy are great, and its use will increase dramatically.)

434. Gerson MC, Leppo J, Corbett JR, et al. Symposium: new tracers and new approaches. *J Nucl Cardiol* 1999;6:112–121.

(This is an excellent, in-depth review of the new tracers and related protocols now available and in development.)

435. Iskandrian AS. Is quantification necessary in SPECT perfusion imaging? *Am J Cardiol* 1995;75:1175–1176.

(This editorial asks whether routine quantitation of perfusion images is necessary for good results. Although quantitation is not absolutely necessary, prognostic, if not diagnostic, measures, as well as serial assessment to determine regression and progression and the benefits of related medical or interventional therapies, rely on the extent and depth of myocardial involvement. It is quantitation that demonstrates the variability in myocardium infarcted or at risk in relation to coronary angiography presented in several studies. It is quantitation that now tests the value of new anti-ischemic methods [See *Self Study Program III. Nuclear Medicine: Cardiology.* Topic 6. Myocardial Perfusion Scintigraphy. Clinical Aspects.] Quantitative measures likely form the basis of scintigraphic prognostic value. Parameters of relative defect intensity also need evaluation for viability assessment, and quantitative polar maps aid the objective comparison of clinical data with a population of normals. Each of these aspects of quantitation elevate the method and increase its reliability and clinical value. PET quantitative methods, when applied to metabolic measures, coronary flow or flow reserve, will add even more to their clinical value.)

Questions and Case Examples

1. Shown in Figure 86 are exercise (Ex) and redistribution (R) thallium-201 (^{201}Tl) planar images in the anterior projection in a normal subject. There are no obvious defects. However, 2 "hot spots"(small arrows) are noted near the anterior papillary muscle. The bottom panel shows the circumferential counts distribution profiles of the exercise (large dots) and redistribution (small dots) images. The solid black line represents the "lower-limit-of-normal" curve. The patient circumferential profile is normalized to the most intense area in the heart, the anterior papillary muscle. The exercise profile dips below the limits of normal in the region of the high anterior basal wall (AB; large arrow). This presents a quantitative defect. However, visually, no defect exists. How would you read this study?

   a. Normal
   b. Abnormal
   c. Grossly abnormal with the only normal region being the intense area near the papillary muscles

2. Shown in Figure 87 are several SPECT short-axis images that were acquired in the same healthy patient, applying a noncircular or "body contour" orbit. The latter applies the camera closely to the body. What is the explanation(s) for the evident defects in the body contour orbit acquisition? Choose all correct answers.

   a. They are the result of varying intensity and resolution related to the orbital effects of varying camera distance from the myocardium.
   b. The finding is caused by attenuation effects, which vary with the different orbits.
   c. The abnormality could be exaggerated with varying body habitus.
   d. Longer acquisition time with the body contour acquisition makes patient motion and related defects more likely.
   e. The findings are caused by an unrelated technical factor.

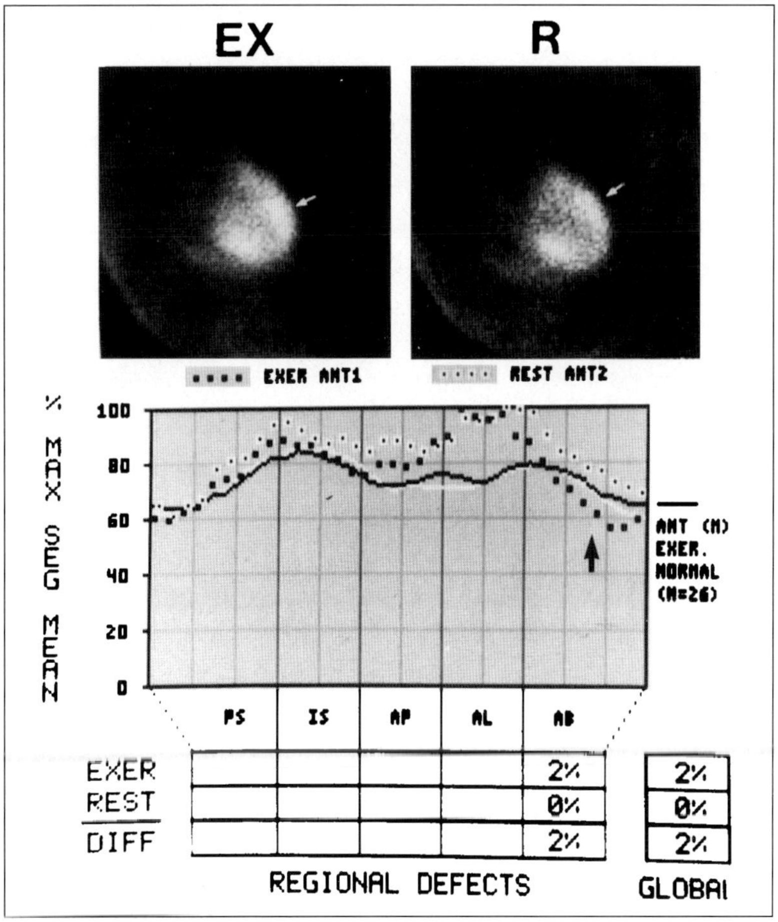

Figure 86

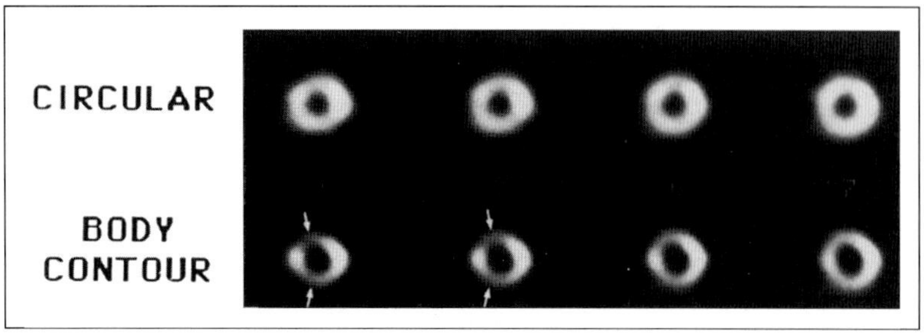

Figure 87

3. **Again, regarding the orbit for SPECT acquisitions, which of the following is (are) true?**

   a. Generally, 180° acquisitions relate to higher contrast and spatial resolution than 360° acquisition.
   b. Generally, 360° acquisitions relate to higher contrast and spatial resolution than 180° acquisition.
   c. Acquisitions in 180° elliptical orbits have been more commonly related to image artifacts.
   d. Artifacts in 180° orbits are most common in elliptical rather than circular orbits.
   e. Elliptical 360° orbits are less problematic and relate to fewer artifacts than elliptical 180° orbits.

4. **Shown in Figure 88 are several short-axis tomographic slices of a cardiac phantom without true defects. The normal slice is shown at upper left. A technical artifact has been imposed in increasing magnitude during the acquisition, from upper right to lower left to lower right, to produce the findings shown. Which of the following has (have) been done?**

   a. The effects of a blown photomultiplier tube are evident.
   b. An attenuation artifact of increasing severity in serial acquisitions was superimposed on the homogeneous phantom.
   c. A heterogeneous flood field was employed in imaging.
   d. The findings relate to a progressively irregular orbit.
   e. The findings relate to progressive alteration in the applied filter and cutoff frequency.
   f. Center of rotation (COR) errors of 1, 2 and 3 pixels have been simulated.

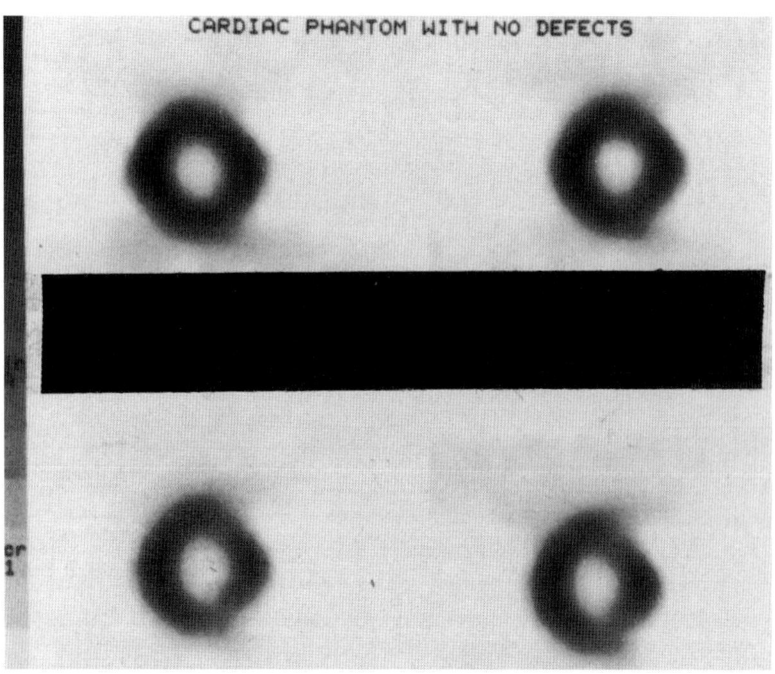

Figure 88

5. **Shown in Figure 90 are short-axis (top), horizontal-long-axis (middle) and vertical (bottom) long-axis SPECT slices from exercise (E) and rest (R) ^{201}Tl perfusion images acquired in a female patient with atypical chest pain. Noted with arrows are abnormalities in the anterior and distal lateral walls. The cause of these findings is most likely related to:**

   a. Induced ischemia in the left anterior descending coronary artery region.
   b. Vertical patient motion.

c. A COR artifact.
d. Attenuation artifact.
e. A flood field artifact.

6. **Shown in Figure 91 are horizontal long-axis slices from a rest perfusion image acquired in a patient with normal coronary arteries. An artifact is evident here, seen primarily in the background, adjacent to the left ventricular myocardium. The artifact best relates to:**

a. Horizontal patient motion.
b. Vertical patient motion.
c. A COR artifact.
d. Attenuation artifact.
e. A flood field artifact.

7. **Shown previously in Figures 59–62 and here in Figures 92 and 93 are 6 examples of the effects of image artifacts on the polar map display. (Figure reprinted with permission from DePuey EG, Garcia EV. Optimal specificity of thallium-201 SPECT through recognition of image artifacts. *J Nucl Med* 1989;30:444–449.) Without reviewing the figure legends in those images already presented, match the findings in these figures with the description of their causes in a–f.**

a. Immediate postexercise ^{201}Tl polar plot (left) and related standard deviation (SD) blackout plot demonstrating regional abnormalities >2.5 SD from the normal sex-matched database (right), acquired in an obese man with normal coronary arteries. He has a broad chest diameter, with high activity in adipose tissue in the lateral chest wall. In the related image, 45° left anterior oblique (LAO) (left) and left lateral (right) planar projection images show marked attenuation of the

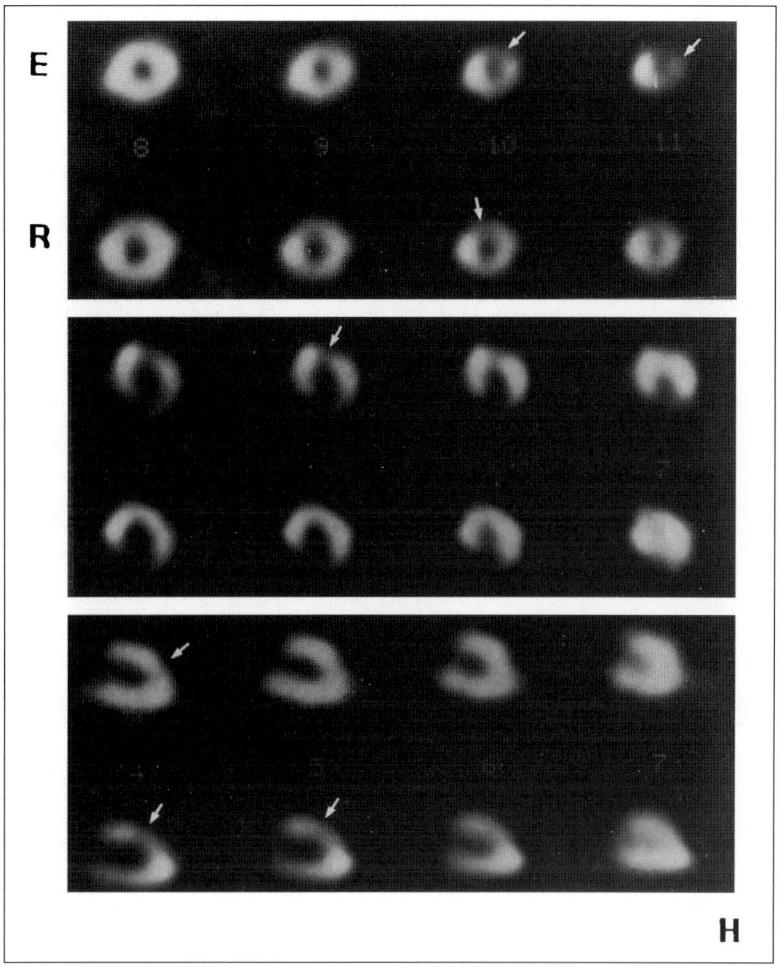

Figure 90

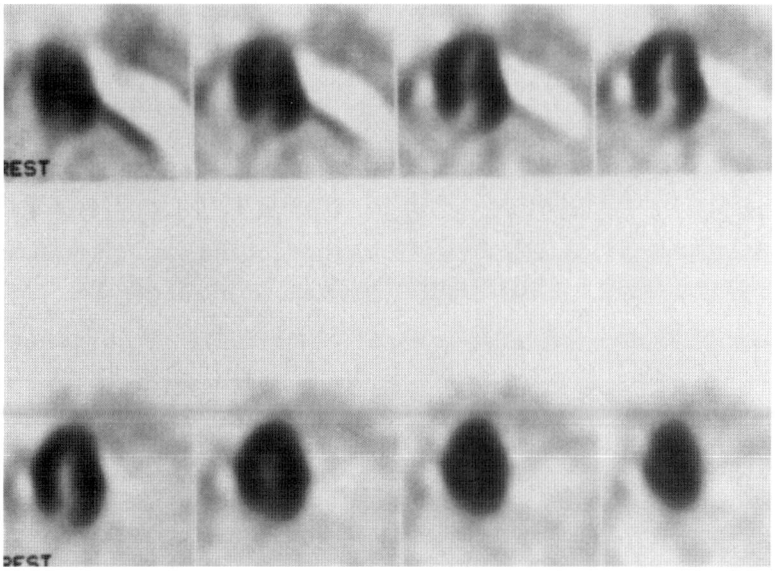

Figure 91

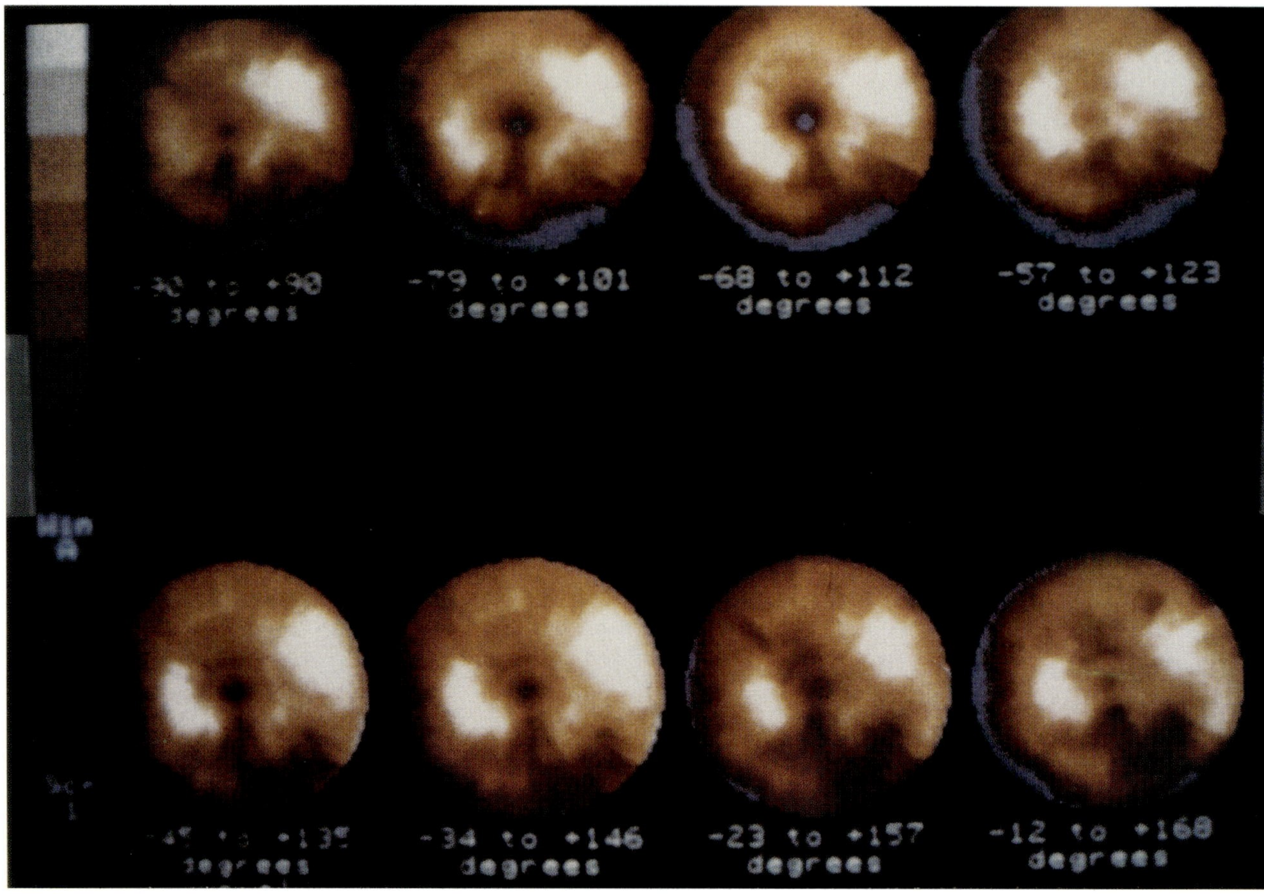

Figure 92

myocardium in the left lateral projection as a result of interposed soft tissue of the lateral wall.

b. Thallium-201 polar plots (left) and related SD blackout plot acquired immediately postdipyridamole infusion (above) and after 4-hr delay. In the early plots is an apparent marked increase in tracer concentration in the inferior left ventricular wall. Because the image is normalized to the "hottest" pixel, the remainder of the ventricle remains counts poor and is identified as abnormal in the SD blackout map. Actually, this intense region represents extracardiac activity in the spleen, which was included in the regional polar analysis of myocardial activity. At 4 hr, the tracer is no longer resident in the spleen, the inferior artifact is no longer present and the polar map is more homogeneous and normal. Generation of a polar map with boundaries excluding the spleen could have normalized the immediate poststress polar map. Review of the poststress projection images in the same figure reveals a normal or low-intensity inferior wall and more intense anterior wall with obvious splenic activity.

c. Thallium-201 polar plots acquired in a man with normal coronary arteries and a normal polar map at the lower left. Polar maps (top) are formulated with progressive cardiac levorotation made by altering the rotational arc used for acquisition (top) and with increasing dextrorotation (bottom). Similar rotation may be introduced by the erroneous setting of landmarks used for polar map reconstruction.

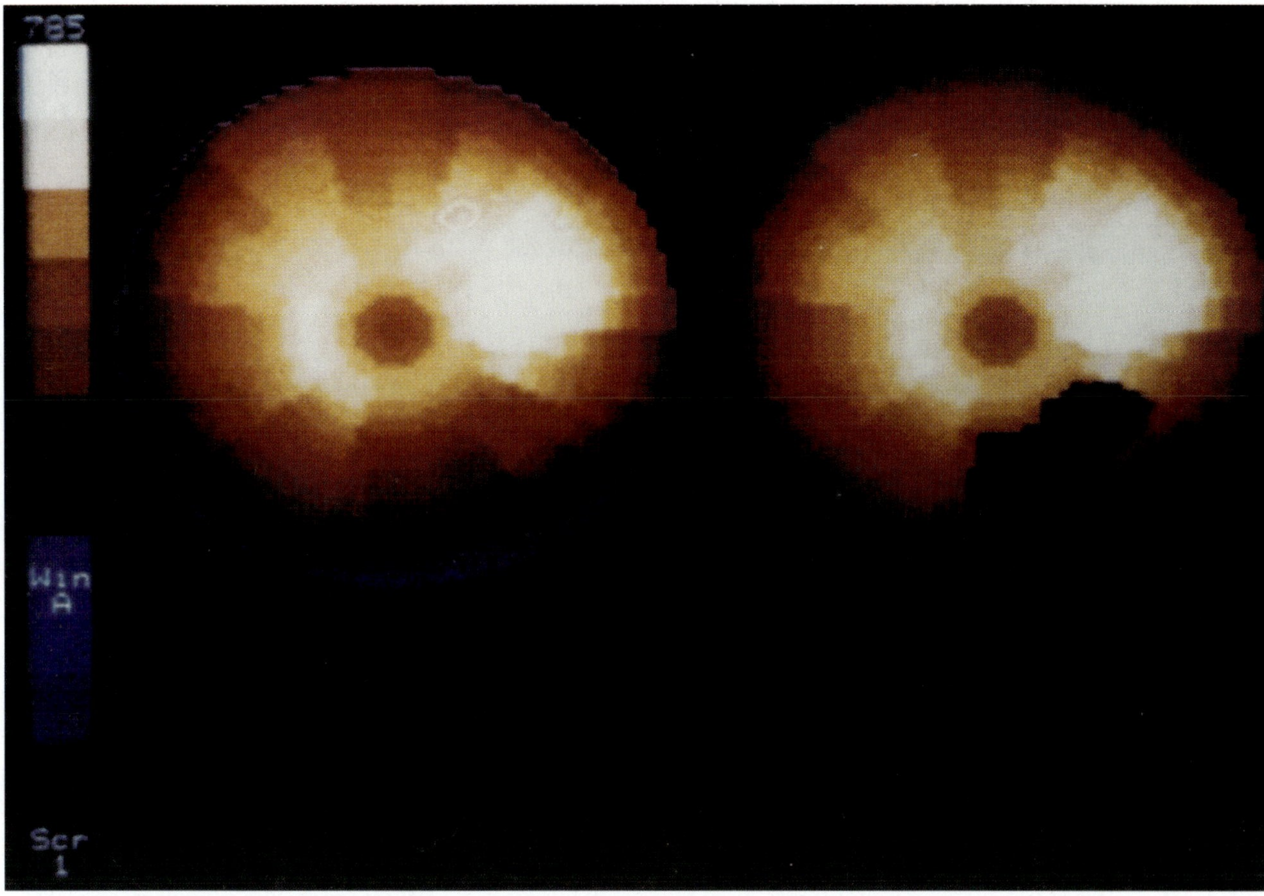

Figure 93

d. Midventricular short-axis (left) and vertical long-axis (right) ^{201}Tl SPECT slices demonstrating increased activity in the anterior wall region of the anterior papillary muscle. By default, the remainder of the ventricle appears relatively counts poor, because the image sets are normalized to the hottest pixel. The corresponding polar map (left) and its SD blackout map (right) demonstrate the artifactual effect in this apparent comparison to the normal database.

e. Polar maps reconstructed from ^{201}Tl SPECT images acquired 3 hr after exercise in a woman with normal coronary arteries and large breasts imaged with bra off (bottom left) and bra on (top left). Blackout polar maps (right) show the artifactual abnormality with bra on, resulting from the concentration of breast tissue anteriorly. It is best to image women without their bras and without binding the breasts. Most important is reproducible breast position between stress and rest studies.

f. Polar map reconstructed from ^{201}Tl SPECT images (left) acquired immediately after exercise in a woman with normal coronary arteries after bilateral mastectomies. When this distribution is compared with the normal female database at right, the related SD blackout map demonstrates an inferior wall abnormality as a result of its comparison with the relatively unattenuated anterior wall.

8. Illustrated in Figure 44 are short-axis SPECT ^{201}Tl slices at stress and rest, acquired in a female patient with atypical chest pain. Noted are apparent

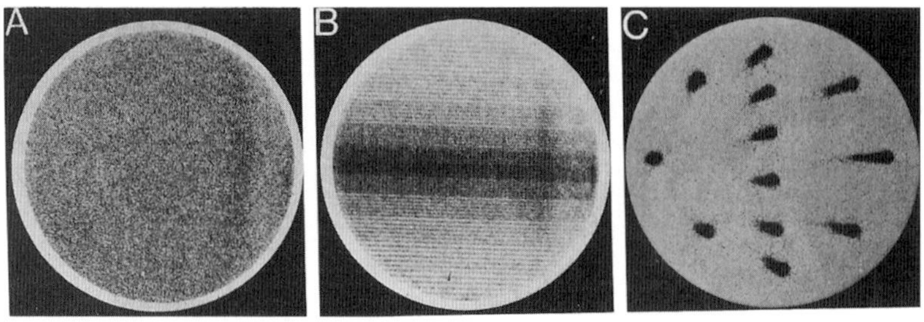

Figure 94

fixed abnormalities and a possible method to distinguish attenuation artifact from true perfusion defects. Which among the following features can help differentiate attenuation artifact from perfusion defect? Choose all correct answers.

a. Wall motion and "thickening" on gated evaluation
b. The effects of prone imaging
c. Review of projection images
d. Repositioning the patient and reacquiring the study
e. Evidence of differential attenuation on dual-isotope imaging

9. **Figures 94–104 show several examples of image artifacts and technical errors that could cause image artifacts. Match each of these figures with the appropriate description. (Figure 94 reprinted with permission from Oswald MK, O'Conner MK. A noisy photomultiplier tube: its unusual effect on gamma camera image uniformity. *J Nucl Med* 1987;15:157–163; Figures 95–103 reprinted with permission from O'Conner MK. Instrument and computer-related problems and artifacts in nuclear medicine. *Semin Nucl Med* 1996;26:256–277; Figure 104 reprinted, with permission, from Wackers FJTh. Artifacts in planar and SPECT myocardial perfusion imaging. *Am J Cardiol Imaging* 1992;6:42–58.)**

a. Multiple scores on the underside of a collimator caused by failure to clear a locating pin on the detector head during collimator change
b. Effects on the flood image of a scored, traumatized collimator
c. A noisy photomultiplier tube resulted in a nonuniform band on the right side of the field of view (A). This brought a reduction in image resolution on a line phantom (B) and distortion of point sources imaged with this flawed system (C)
d. Image of an orthogonal-hole phantom acquired without linearity correction with resultant deterioration in image uniformity and spatial linearity with generally preserved resolution
e. Cold defect in a flood image caused by a small dent in the collimator
f. Flood image showing loss of signal from a large number of photomultiplier tubes caused by a loose circuit board in the detector head
g. Short-axis slices of the heart before (left) and after (right) correction

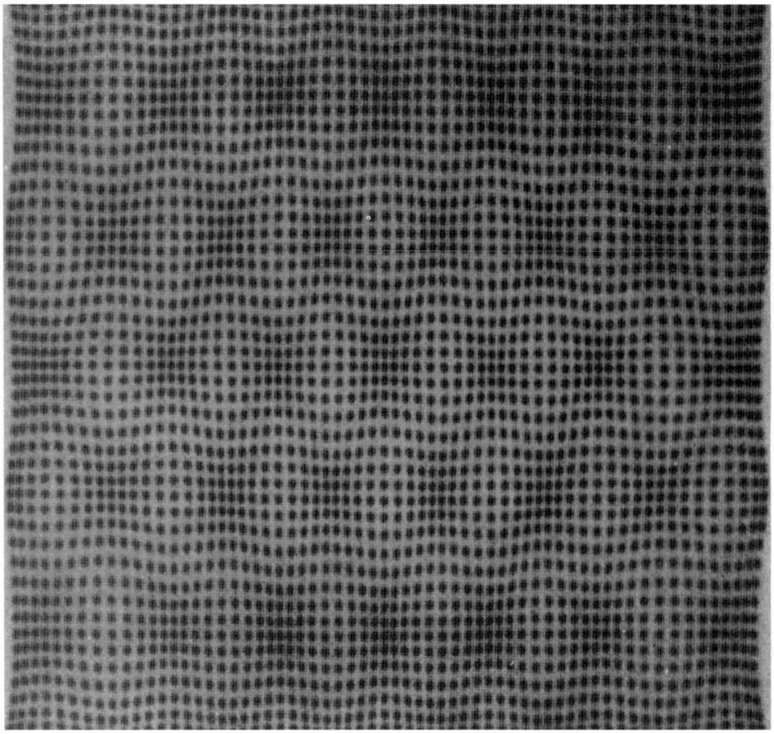

Figure 95

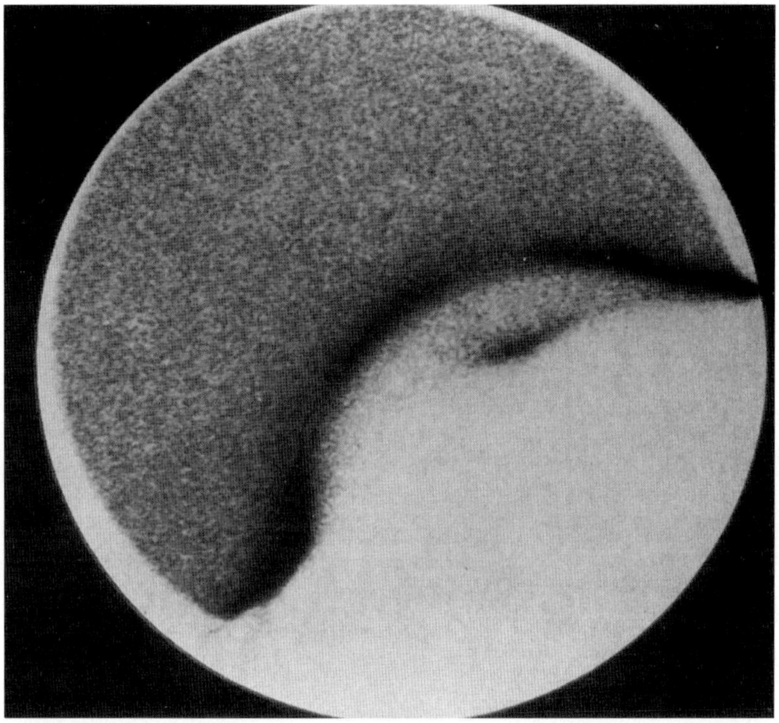

Figure 96

for a ring artifact caused by a software error in the application of the uniformity correction map. The artifact caused an apparent reduction in septal wall activity.

h. Flood images from a small-field-of-view gamma camera system before (A) and after (B) application of a corrupted uniformity correction map

i. An extrinsic flood image showing increased activity at the edges of the field of view, caused by poor mating of the collimator to the detector head

j. Transaxial images from the study shown in i. The artifact (arrow) now is easily identified, and placement of cross-hairs shows the ring to be concentric with the center of the transaxial image slice, demonstrating this to be a ring artifact. Ring artifacts are always concentric with the COR and, therefore, concentric with the center of the transaxial slice.

k. Transaxial SPECT images of a cardiac phantom acquired on a single-head camera in which the head was aligned properly, set at 0° at onset of rotation with the gantry (A) and with misalignment of 5° (B). Here, a 1° gantry misalignment with the detector operating at a 20-cm radius of rotation will bring a 3.5-mm displacement of image data along the axis of rotation.

l. Transaxial images with evidence of an incremental COR artifact identified by the characteristic "tail"(arrows) that originates from the apex of the heart. COR artifacts often cause apical defects. The typical overriding of walls is seen in the image at right.

10. Which of the following is (are) true regarding the parameter of the COR?

a. The SPECT camera gantry has a COR determined by both mechanical and electronic factors.

b. Ideally, the COR should be exactly in the center of the field, between pixels 32 and 33 in a 64 × 64 matrix.

c. Changes in tuning and gains of the photomultiplier tubes change the location of detected counts.

d. The camera detector changes its orbit with wear of the mechanical components.

e. COR errors violate the basic underlying principle of SPECT reconstruction: that all contributing projections see the same point in space at the same location.

f. It is important to apply the correct value of the COR and also that this value remain constant as a function of angle.

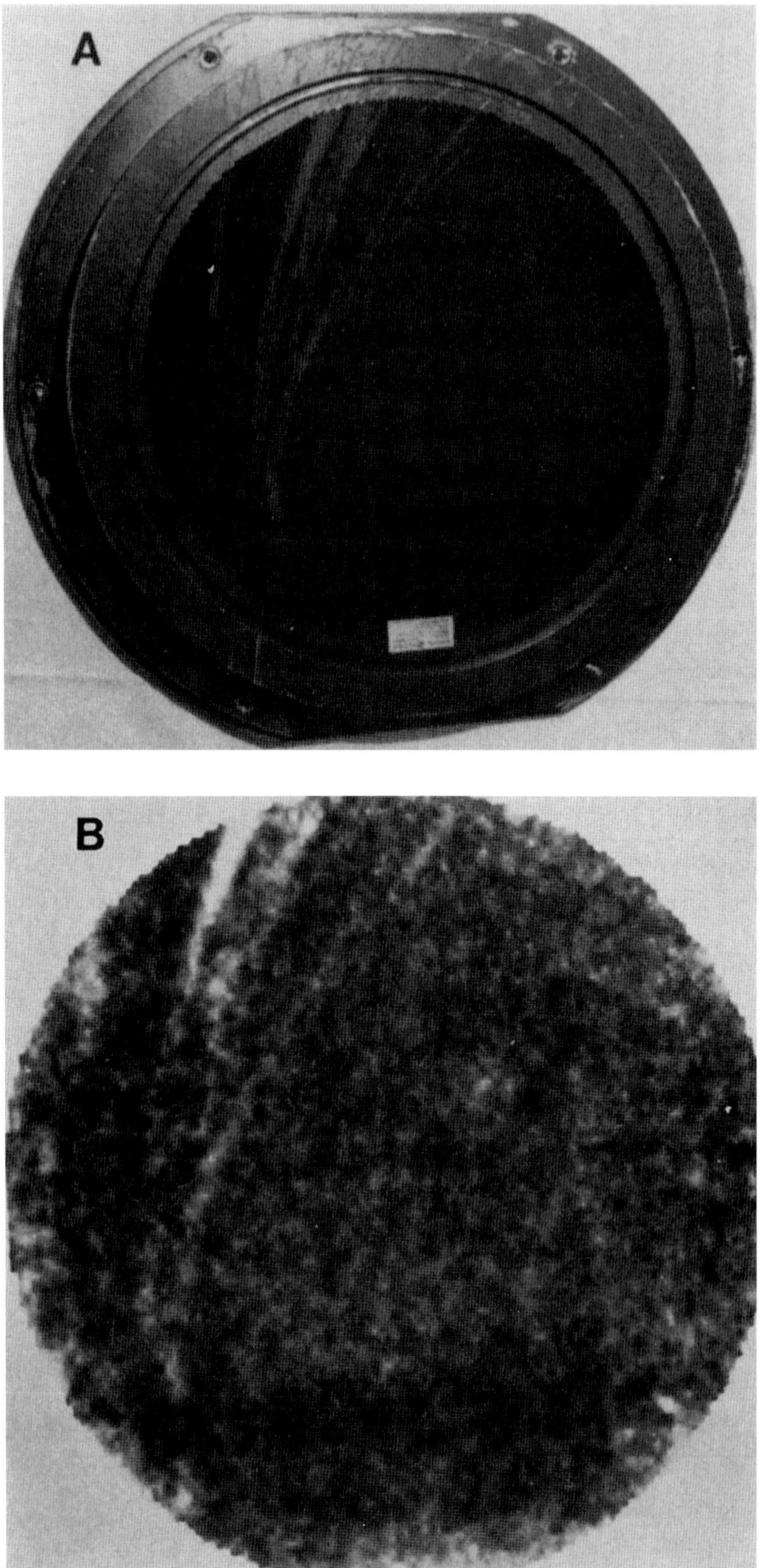

Figure 97

g. When measured on a gamma camera at a rotation radius of 20 cm, both x and y values for the COR should show <2 mm variation over a 360° orbit.
h. The COR usually is very stable, and a weekly check is adequate to ensure proper correction.

11. **SPECT image defects may be related to artifacts, rather than to true perfusion abnormalities. The following are image patterns that have been observed in your laboratory in stress–rest (redistribution) studies performed today. Your associate has seen them but calls you for advice and to consider the possibility of artifact. Review the patterns listed and describe the likelihood of image artifact versus true perfusion defect as: likely artifact, likely perfusion defect or ambiguous.**

a. Seen in the ^{201}Tl stress–redistribution study of a large 55-yr-old woman is a fixed defect of moderate intensity that involves the anterior wall but spares the septum and apex. Examination of both projection image sets demonstrates an anterior curvilinear area of reduced activity overlying the superior aspect of the heart.
b. Seen in the ^{201}Tl stress–redistribution study of a large 55-yr-old woman is a reversible defect of moderate intensity that involves the anterior wall but spares the septum and apex. Examination of the stress projection images demonstrates an anterior curvilinear area of reduced activity overlying the anterior aspect of the heart but which surrounds the entire heart on rest projection images.
c. Seen in the stress–redistribution study of a man weighing 60 kg

is a reversible anterior septal and apical defect. The projection images are unimpressive.

d. Seen in a technetium-99m (^{99m}Tc) sestamibi stress study is a dense inferior and inferolateral defect in the presence of intense hepatic uptake. At rest, neither the defect nor the intense extracardiac activity is evident with ^{99m}Tc.

e. Seen in a sestamibi stress study is a moderately dense inferior defect. The defect is no longer evident in the presence of intense hepatic uptake at rest with ^{99m}Tc.

12. **What are the advantages/disadvantages of acquiring limited planar with SPECT images? Choose all correct answers.**

a. Limited planar ^{201}Tl images, acquired in the anterior projection, permit evaluation of lung uptake.

b. Limited planar images, acquired in a "mid" LAO projection corresponding to the left ventricular long axis, permit identification of the phenomenon of "apparent cavitary dilation," not easily seen on SPECT images.

c. Limited planar images acquired before SPECT, in association with a ^{201}Tl stress–reinjection imaging protocol, permit analysis of "washout."

d. Limited planar images acquired before SPECT, in association with a ^{201}Tl stress–4-hr redistribution imaging protocol, permit analysis of "washout."

e. Limited planar images acquired before SPECT, in association with a ^{201}Tl rest/stress ^{99m}Tc sestamibi imaging protocol, permit analysis of "washout."

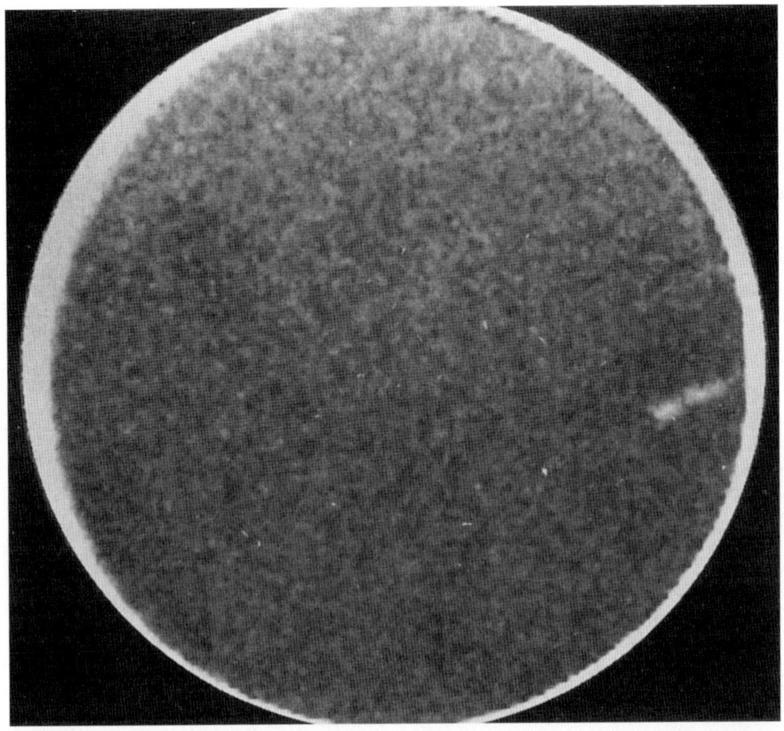

Figure 98

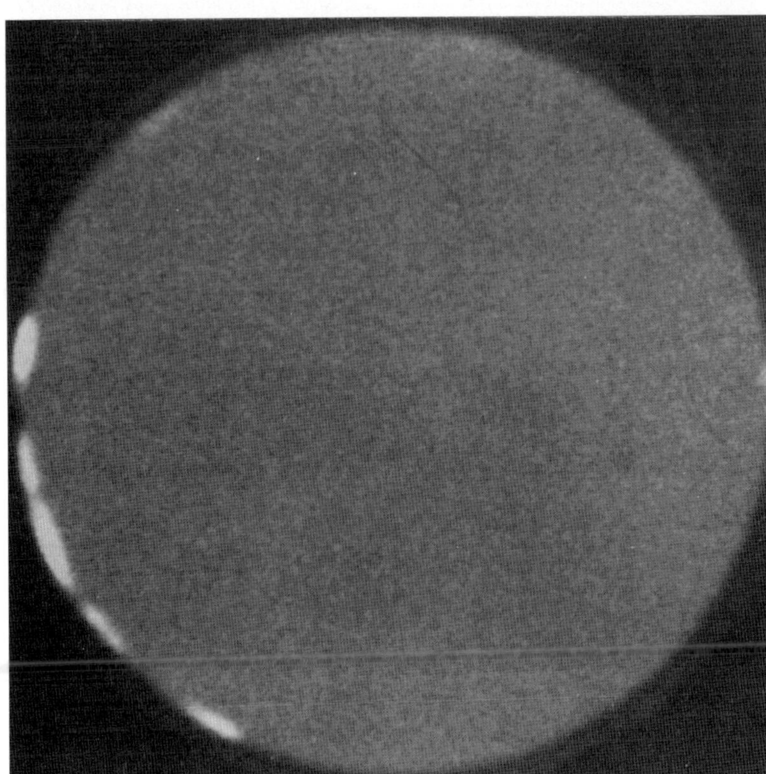

Figure 99

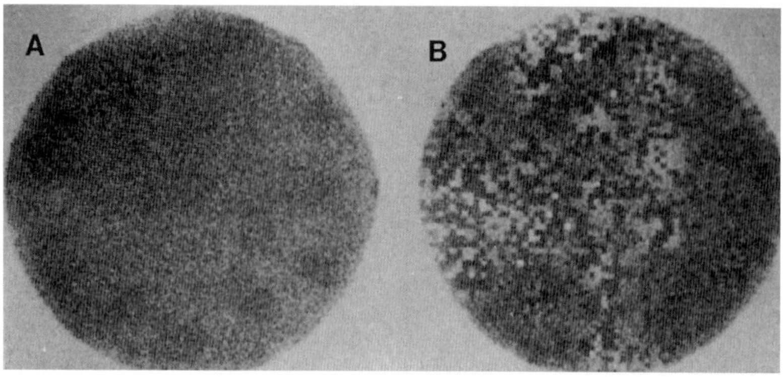

Figure 100

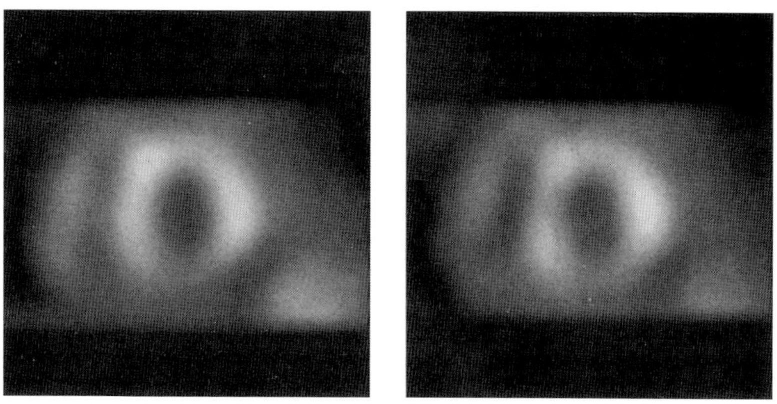

Figure 101

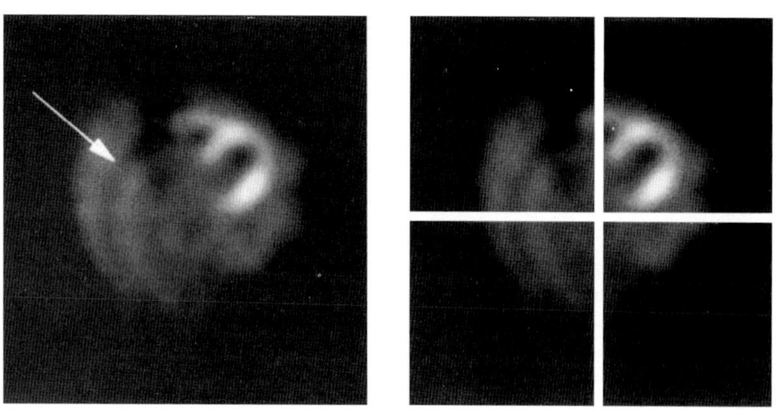

Figure 102

13. **Consider the possible advantages of the dual-isotope sequential rest ^{201}Tl/stress ^{99m}Tc sestamibi protocol. Choose all correct answers.**

    a. It is the most rapidly executed of all protocols.
    b. With 24-hr ^{201}Tl imaging, it combines the advantages of both ^{99m}Tc sestamibi (tetrofosmin) and ^{201}Tl.
    c. With in-house fabrication of ^{99m}Tc sestamibi, the protocol is more economical than other protocols when the daily study volume is exceeds 5.
    d. It is a less expensive protocol than others under all circumstances.
    e. It is the most efficient in conserving time for the patient and technologist and increases laboratory throughput.
    f. Patients are stressed first, so that the physician can start the day with several stress tests and then attend to other duties.
    g. Diagnostic accuracy is maintained.

14. **Consider the possible disadvantages of the dual-isotope sequential rest ^{201}Tl/stress ^{99m}Tc sestamibi protocol. Choose all correct answers.**

    a. It tends to be more expensive at low patient volumes.
    b. If ^{201}Tl stress–reinjection–redistribution is the optimal protocol for viability evaluation, this protocol may sacrifice some sensitivity.
    c. The different characteristics of the radionuclides produce imaging differences that may adversely influence image interpretation.
    d. To best assure 1-day completion, the protocol requires initial rest evaluation, when rest study may be unnecessary.
    e. It spreads physician responsibility for test performance throughout the day.

15. **Which statements are true regarding the choice and number of projections when acquiring planar ^{201}Tl perfusion images? Choose all correct answers.**

a. One LAO projection in the left ventricular long axis will suffice
b. One LAO projection in the left ventricular long axis and 2 additional projections 30°–45° right and left of that projection are needed to gain data for circumferential profile and washout analysis.
c. An anterior and "hard" LAO or left lateral projection helps to best identify inferior wall perfusion and avoid diaphragmatic attenuation.
d. A series of 3 and generally 4 or 5 images progressing from anterior to LAO 60° or left lateral projections best helps resolve varying regional intensities based on cardiac rotation.
e. The left lateral projection is often most attenuated. However, a well-visualized inferior wall, seen clearly here, supports the normal evaluation of the right coronary region.

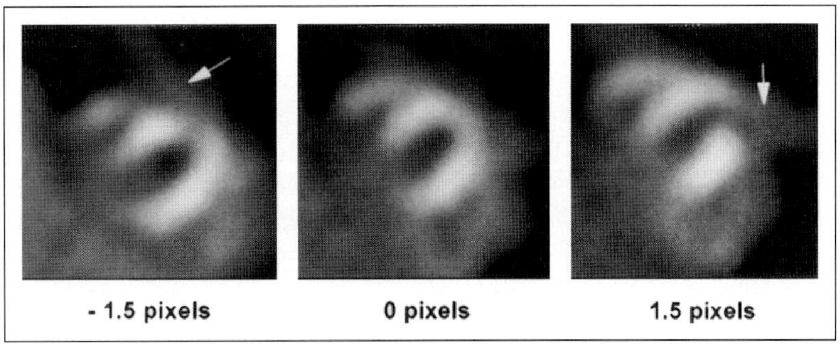

Figure 103

16. A patient is evaluated for coronary disease, using a ^{201}Tl stress image, followed in 4 hr by reinjection of an additional 1-mCi dose, with delayed imaging 10–15 min later. A persistent defect is noted on completion of the delayed image. What can correctly be said about the defect noted? Choose all correct answers.

a. It most likely represents scar.
b. It may yet be viable, because reinjection may actually enhance a defect that redistributes at imaging later than 4 hr before reinjection. This 4-hr preinjection image was not performed here.
c. The defect may resolve on 24-hr delayed imaging.
d. The defect may not have been there on 4-hr imaging before reinjection.
e. The washout characteristics of the defect cannot be evaluated after reinjection.

17. Is there anything additional that can be done to increase defect reversibility in the study presented in question 16? Choose all correct answers.

a. Give a second reinjection dose.
b. Perform 48-hr imaging.
c. Add 1 mCi ^{99m}Tc sestamibi.
d. Image the patient prone.
e. Repeat the study on another day using a higher ^{201}Tl dose.
f. Repeat the image 24 hr later.

18. Which is (are) true regarding background gastrointestinal radioactivity on ^{99m}Tc sestamibi studies?

a. It must be discouraged or large amounts of the agent, absorbed from the gut, will adversely alter images.

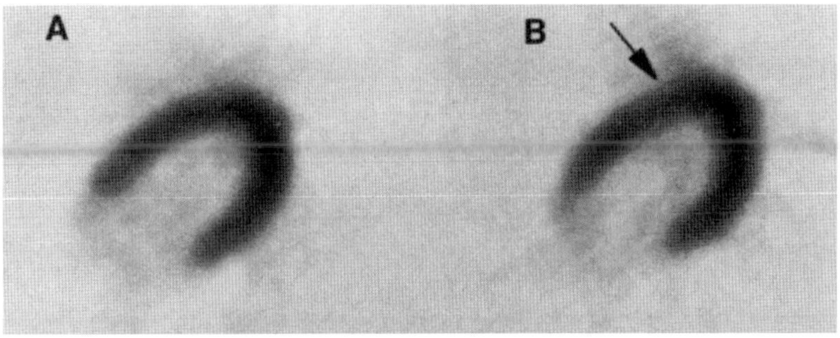

Figure 104

b. It should be discouraged, because it obscures the myocardium.
c. It may actually be reduced by imaging early.
d. A milk or high-fat drink is given before imaging, to reduce such background by encouraging gallbladder emptying and excretion.
e. Gallbladder emptying, with high-intensity bowel labeling, may actually worsen paracardiac background.
f. High background radioactivity can produce artifactual abnormalities of high or low intensity.

19. If we assume that all other parameters of the acquisition (frame duration, frame number, etc.) are the same, which is (are) true regarding the relationships of the number of camera heads, their relative orientation and the orbital configuration?

a. Double-head cameras with heads configured at 90° or 180° take half the time to image a study acquired at 360° as a single-head camera.
b. Double-head cameras with heads configured at 90° or 180° take the same time to image a study acquired at 360° as a single-head camera.
c. A triple-head camera, with heads at 120°, can acquire both 180° and 360° studies in the same time and each in half the time of a single-head camera.
d. A triple-head camera, with heads at 120°, can acquire a 180° study in two-thirds and a 360° study in one-third the time of a single-head camera.
e. A triple-head camera, with heads at 120°, can acquire a 180° study in one-third and a 360° study in two-thirds the time of a single-head camera.

20. Shown in Figure 24 are poststress and redistribution planar images in anterior (ANT) and multiple LAO projections in a patient with suspected coronary disease. Evident in the images are lung uptake, cavitary dilation and "basal uptake." What is (are) true regarding the origin and implications of these "nonperfusion indicators"?

a. Basal uptake reflects increased relative perfusion in a region not generally so well visualized, indicating widespread distal underperfusion.
b. Lung uptake is not specific for coronary disease.
c. Lung uptake relates to slowed transpulmonary transit with increased extraction and may be seen with mitral stenosis.
d. In association with coronary disease, lung uptake indicates severe disease and a high prognostic risk of subsequent events.
e. Unlike apparent cavitary dilation, true dilation indicates a general effect resulting from induced ischemia.
f. In Figure 24, the epicardial dimension as well as the internal cavitary size are increased, indicating true cavitary dilation and an ischemic cause.
g. Apparent cavitary dilation on planar imaging relates to reduced perfusion in one wall overlying the cavity, making that wall more "transparent" and suggesting an increased cavitary size only in projections looking through this local ischemic wall. For the same reason, a hypertrophied ventricle shows a reduced cavitary size.

21. Shown in Figure 23A is the radial distribution of ^{201}Tl counts in the visually normal planar anterior projection of a patient with documented coronary disease. Radial distribution of washout data in this same image is

presented in Figure 23B. What is (are) the implications of the washout data?

a. It, too, is normal
b. It demonstrates generalized abnormalities consistent with extensive 3-vessel disease.
c. It is abnormal but would be expected to add little to SPECT evaluation.
d. Such widespread washout abnormalities are commonly seen and a practical concern when performing SPECT perfusion scintigraphy.
e. Although not needed frequently, access to washout data analysis might be an advantage to preserve in this age of reinjection studies.
f. Washout analysis cannot be applied to ^{99m}Tc sestamibi studies.

22. **Shown in Figure 73 are ^{201}Tl planar perfusion scintigrams in anterior (ANT), 45° and 60° LAO projections in a patient with a large apical aneurysm. There is an area of reduced radioactivity (arrows). Appropriate descriptions of the finding, its cause and implications include:**

a. This minor defect is of little clinical significance.
b. The region demonstrates reduced radioactivity even when compared with background, demonstrating the contribution of the overlying wall to apparent "cavitary" activity.
c. The region of reduced radioactivity extends beyond the apparent wall and into the region of the cavity, demonstrating the contribution of the overlying wall to apparent "cavitary" activity.
d. The findings are classic for an apical thrombus displacing cavitary radioactivity.
e. The findings are typical for dense, fixed or reversible perfusion defect.

23. **Shown in Figure 105 are selected slices from a dipyridamole pharmacologic stress ^{99m}Tc sestamibi perfusion scintigram performed for coronary screening and acquired 45 min after tracer administration and before vascular surgery in a 58-yr-old man who was obese and who had hypertension, diabetes and severe claudication. Which of the following is (are) true?**

a. A dense anterior wall perfusion abnormality is evident.
b. A dense inferior wall defect is evident.
c. An intense area of hepatic background is evident adjacent to the inferior defect
d. The intense extracardiac collection may be the cause of the apparent inferior myocardial defect.
e. The acquisition of sestamibi images in the presence of such gross background activity presents a handicap to interpretation, because of the possibility of related artifactual reduction of inferior wall activity.

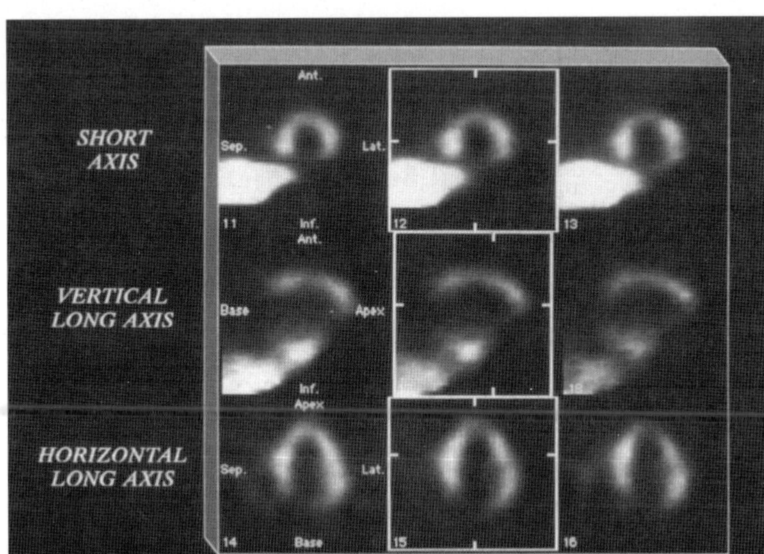

Figure 105

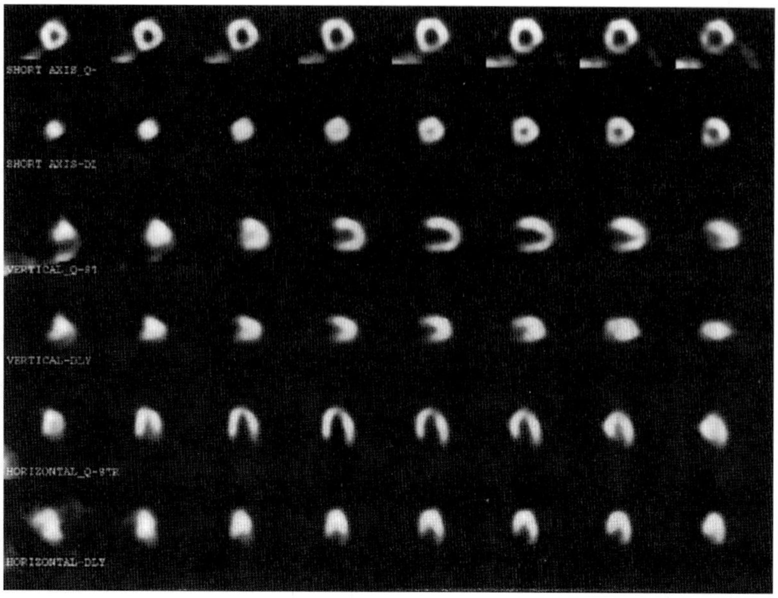

Figure 107

23B. How could this artifact be avoided?

a. These artifacts are not seen with dynamic exercise stress.
b. This artifact is unusual with ^{201}Tl.
c. The artifact can be avoided by acquisition early, in the absence of intense hepatic uptake.
d. The artifact can be avoided by acquisition late, in the absence of intense hepatic uptake
e. This artifact probably will be less evident when applying some of the new technetium-based perfusion agents that are primarily excreted in the urine.

24. Shown in Figure 107 according to the standard format are the technically optimal stress (above) and rest (below) ^{99m}Tc sestamibi perfusion images of a 76-yr-old man being screened for coronary disease and evaluation of left ventricular function. Note specifically the difference in apparent ventricular size. Among the following explanations for this varying ventricular size, which make(s) clinical and scientific sense?

a. Cavitary dilation seen here is representative of severe ischemic dilation.
b. The finding is an artifact resulting from misalignment of slices.
c. The finding relates to an abnormal zoom factor applied with the larger image.
d. The finding relates to severe volume depletion on the rest study.
e. The finding relates to the tachycardia associated with stress.
f. The finding relates to tachycardia at the time of rest acquisition.

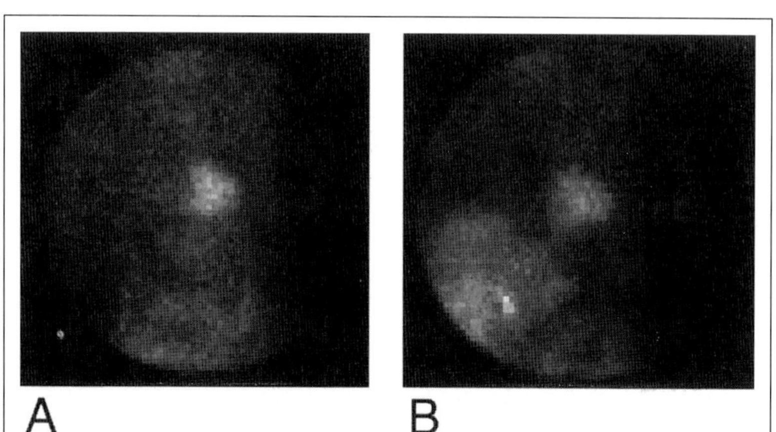

Figure 109

25. Shown in Figures 109A and B are individual, 20-sec frames from the 64-frame SPECT projection set acquired over 180° in the conventional manner in 2 different patients: an abnormal study, A, and a normal study, B. Each frame had approximately 100,000 counts when acquired about 1 hr after administration of 20 mCi ^{99m}Tc sestamibi. What was the indication for study A? (A clue is clearly present [or absent] on the image.)

a. The study was performed to assess viability in this patient with a dilated cardiomyopathy.
b. The study was a screening evaluation to exclude coronary disease.
c. The study was a preoperative evaluation before liver transplantation.
d. The study was performed to evaluate the cause of a small heart.
e. The study was performed to exclude congenital heart disease and a large left-to-right shunt.

26. **Shown in Figure 110A is a dual-isotope (rest ^{201}Tl/exercise ^{99m}Tc tetrofosmin) study performed in a 78-yr-old man with multiple risk factors for coronary disease. The stress test was normal. The raw projection images revealed a small amount of axial and lateral motion that was corrected with a widely available motion correction algorithm. True or false:**

    The image is definitely abnormal.

27. **Shown in Figures 111A and B are single-projection frames from the raw acquisition data of exercise (left) and redistribution (right) SPECT studies acquired in a 65-yr-old woman being evaluated for chest pain. The intense spotty activity seen above and below the heart is the result of:**

    a. Lymph nodes indicating active, disseminated malignancy.
    b. Atrial activity.
    c. Breast activity suggesting cancer.
    d. Extracorporeal activity, probably gown contamination.
    e. Extracardiac concentration in another internal organ.

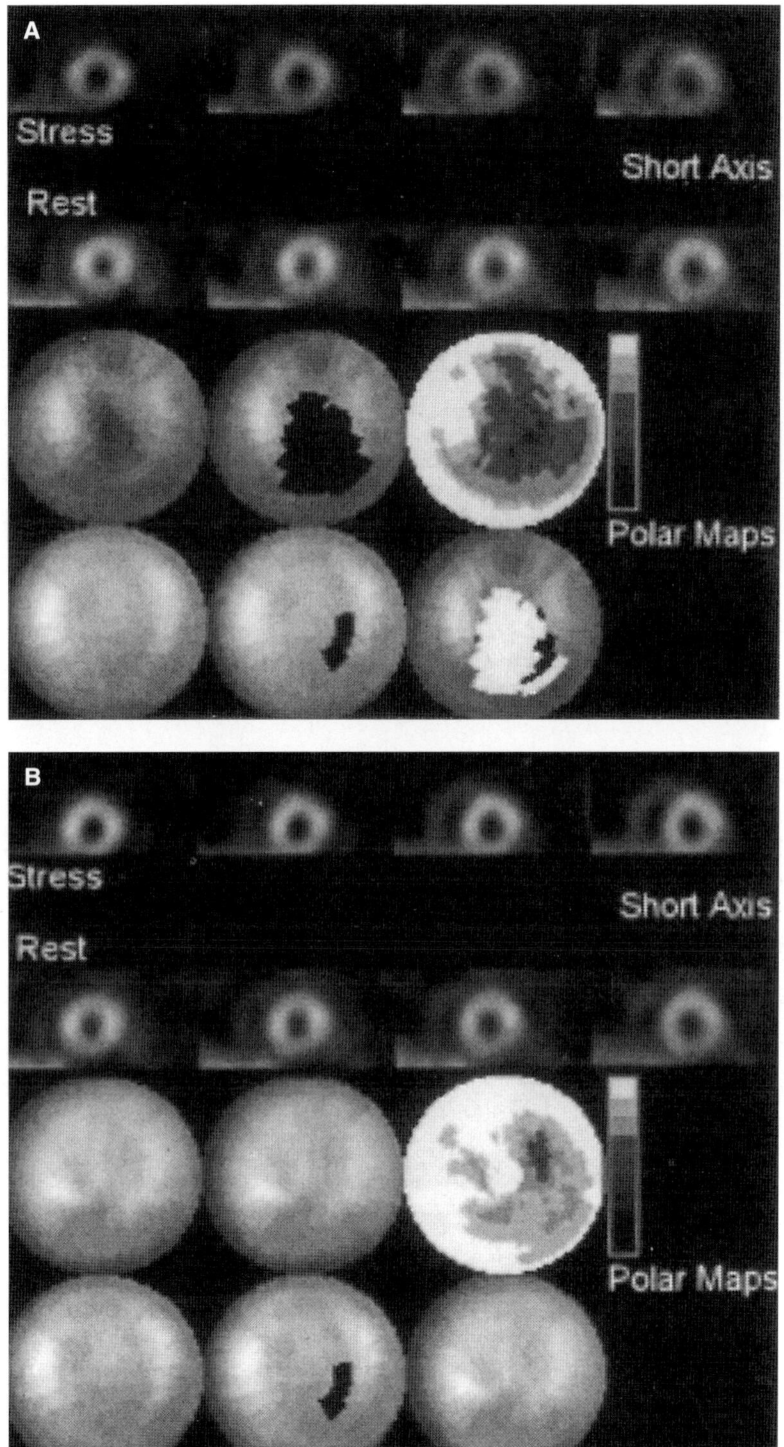

Figure 110

28. **Shown in alternating panels of Figure 112 are supine exercise (above) and rest (below) sets of ^{99m}Tc sestamibi SPECT slices, displayed according to**

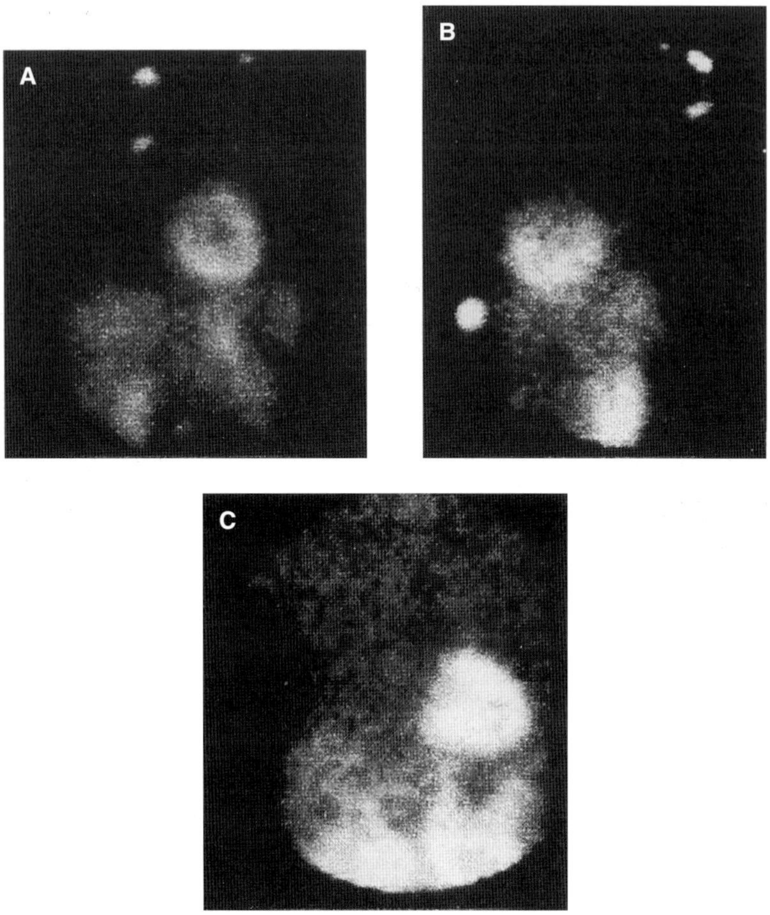

Figure 111

the standard format from above downward in short, horizontal and vertical long axes. They reveal a dilated left ventricle with a clear and essentially fixed inferior defect. The study was acquired in a 48-yr-old man with heart failure, grossly reduced left ventricular ejection fraction, and a congestive cardiomyopathy, who was being evaluated for possible ischemia. However, complicating the study was a factor that could reduce image sensitivity to induced ischemia. Which statement(s) identifies a possible cause of such reduced image sensitivity during exercise or pharmacologic stress?

a. Submaximal exercise fails to test the coronary flow reserve.
b. An infiltrated exercise-related ^{99m}Tc sestamibi (or tetrofosmin) dose provides continuous infusion of radionuclide poststress testing.
c. Adherence of the stress-administered radiopharmaceutical to the venous endothelium reduces the stress-related dose and could provide continued radionuclide infusion poststress.
d. An infiltrated dipyridamole dose will reduce related coronary dilation and blunt the related test of the coronary flow reserve.
e. Administration of aminophylline, the dipyridamole antidote, before myocardial localization of the radiotracer, would result in reduced coronary dilation at the time of radionuclide localization and reduced test sensitivity.
f. An infiltrated exercise-related ^{201}Tl dose provides continuous infusion of radionuclide poststress.

29. **The same patient discussed in quesion 28 is now imaged in the prone position. Figure 115 presents alternating rows of supine (above) and prone (below) SPECT slices according to the same format shown in Figure 112. Which statement(s) is (are) true about this study?**

a. Prone positioning moves the heart away from the diaphragm and subdiaphragmatic structures, reducing their attenuation of the inferior wall and exposing its full intensity.
b. The evident improvement of inferior wall uptake on prone imaging indicates the likely origin of the defect in attenuation.
c. The evident improved inferior uptake on prone imaging is an artifact of positioning at stress.
d. The apparent improved inferior uptake on prone imaging indicates normal regional perfusion.

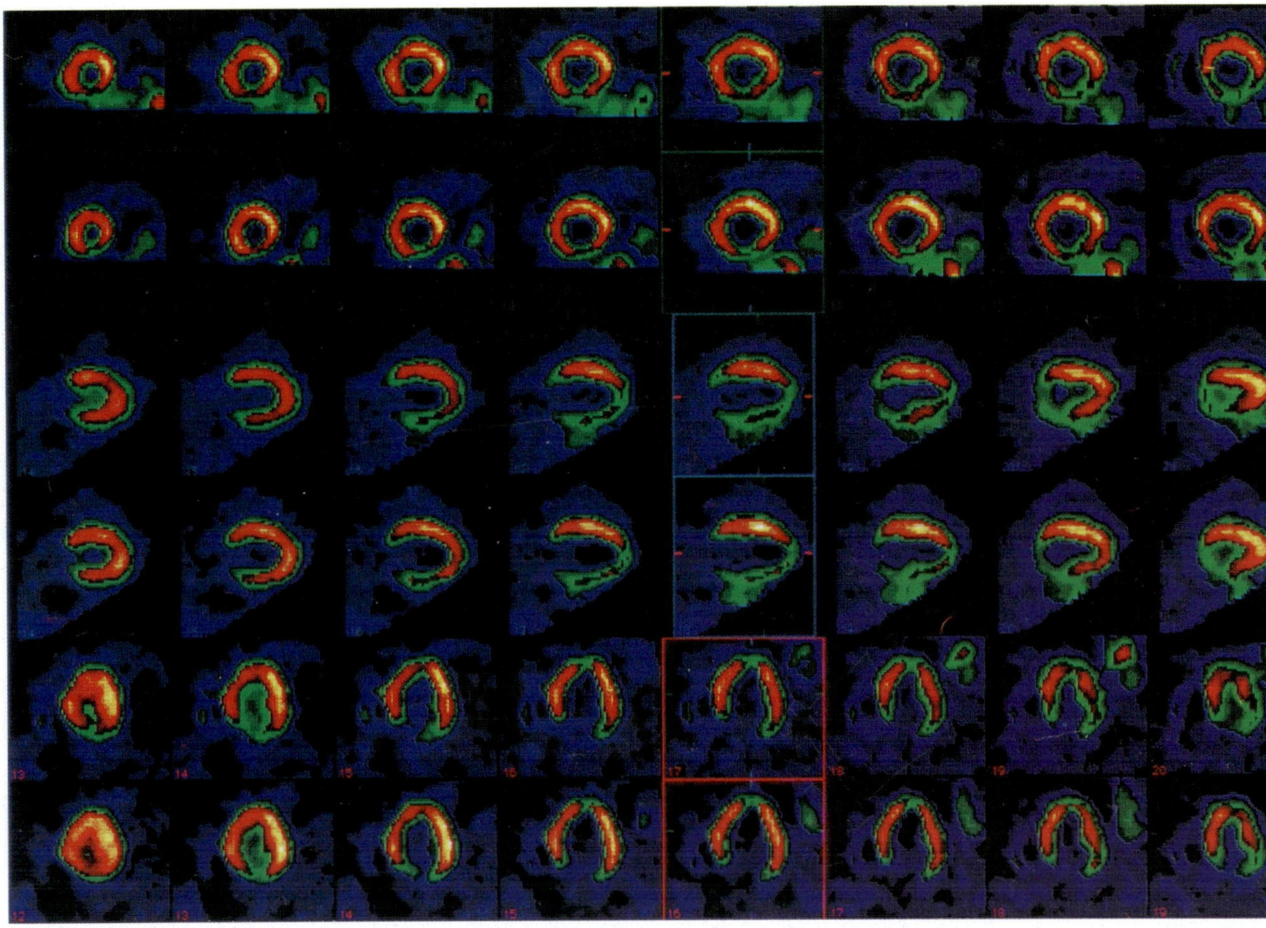

Figure 112

e. Taken in full context, and assuming optimal technique, the improved inferior uptake on prone imaging suggests the presence of a noncoronary cardiomyopathy.
f. The findings on prone imaging do not overcome the effects of factors reducing test sensitivity enumerated in question 28.

30. **Figures 116–118 present a stress SPECT ^{99m}Tc sestamibi study in the standard format. Here, the lower image set in each panel is processed optimally, whereas the same image set in the upper row of each panel is influenced by a technical factor or artifact. Match the image with its artifact. Which is (are) correct?**

a. Figure 116 shows the result of application of a bad flood field; Figure 117 is affected by upward creep; and Figure 118 shows the same image sets processed by different filter cut-offs.
b. Figure 118 is affected by upward creep; Figure 117 shows the result of application of a bad flood field; and Figure 116 shows the same image sets processed by different filter cut-offs.
c. Figure 116 reveals the effects of breast attenuation artifact.
d. Figure 117 shows the same image sets processed by different filter cut-offs; Figure 116 is affected by upward creep; and Figure 118 shows the result of application of a bad flood field.
e. Figure 117 demonstrates a form of motion artifact.

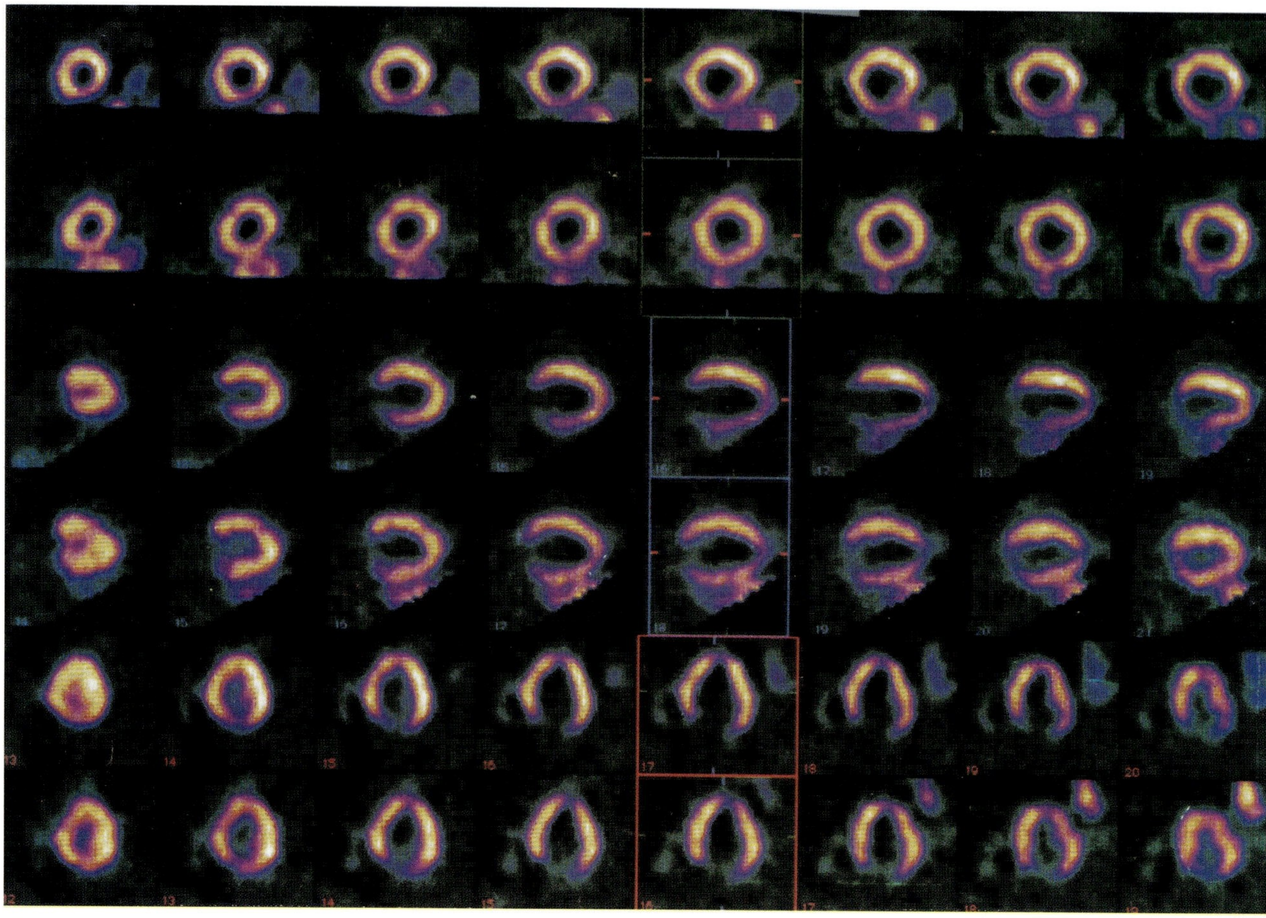

Figure 115

31. **Shown in Figures 119 and 120 are the same stress (top) and rest (bottom) SPECT perfusion images, processed in different ways. True or false:**

    The diffence in the 2 figures relates to the fact that in Figure 119 the rest image has been normalized to the full screen rather than to the peak myocardial counts in each image set as in Figure 120.

32. **This 73-yr-old woman with hypertension, left ventricular hypertrophy and other coronary risk factors undergoes an exercise-only ^{99m}Tc sestamibi perfusion scintigraphic study for coronary screening. She is asymptomatic from a coronary standpoint. The patient has no chest pain or induced ST changes in completing 6.5 min of a standard Bruce protocol, achieving a high double product. Shown in Figure 122 are the supine poststress images initially sent for evaluation. They employed a newly purchased, Food and Drug Administration–approved method for attenuation correction applied to acquisition and processing. The top 2 panels present the short-axis slices from apex (left) to base (right). The third row presents the vertical long-axis slices from septum to lateral wall, and the bottom row presents horizontal long-axis slices from inferior to anterior walls. You interpret the study. It is clearly and widely**

abnormal. Be analytical and choose all correct answers that describe your next steps.

a. The image is abnormal and is supported by the abnormal segmental score at lower right. Obtain a rest study to seek defect reversibility.
b. The area of abnormality suggests disease in a part of the left anterior descending coronary region, possibly in a diagonal branch.
c. The defect is limited in size and, even if it is fully reversible, medical treatment would be advised.
d. The defect may be artifactual in nature, and the projection images must be reviewed for technical problems.
e. Review the nonattenuation-corrected image set.
f. The defect is anterior and lateral and relates to a dilated left ventricle, suggesting a significant related risk. The patient should be referred immediately to coronary angiography.
g. Evaluate related gated images for regional wall motion.

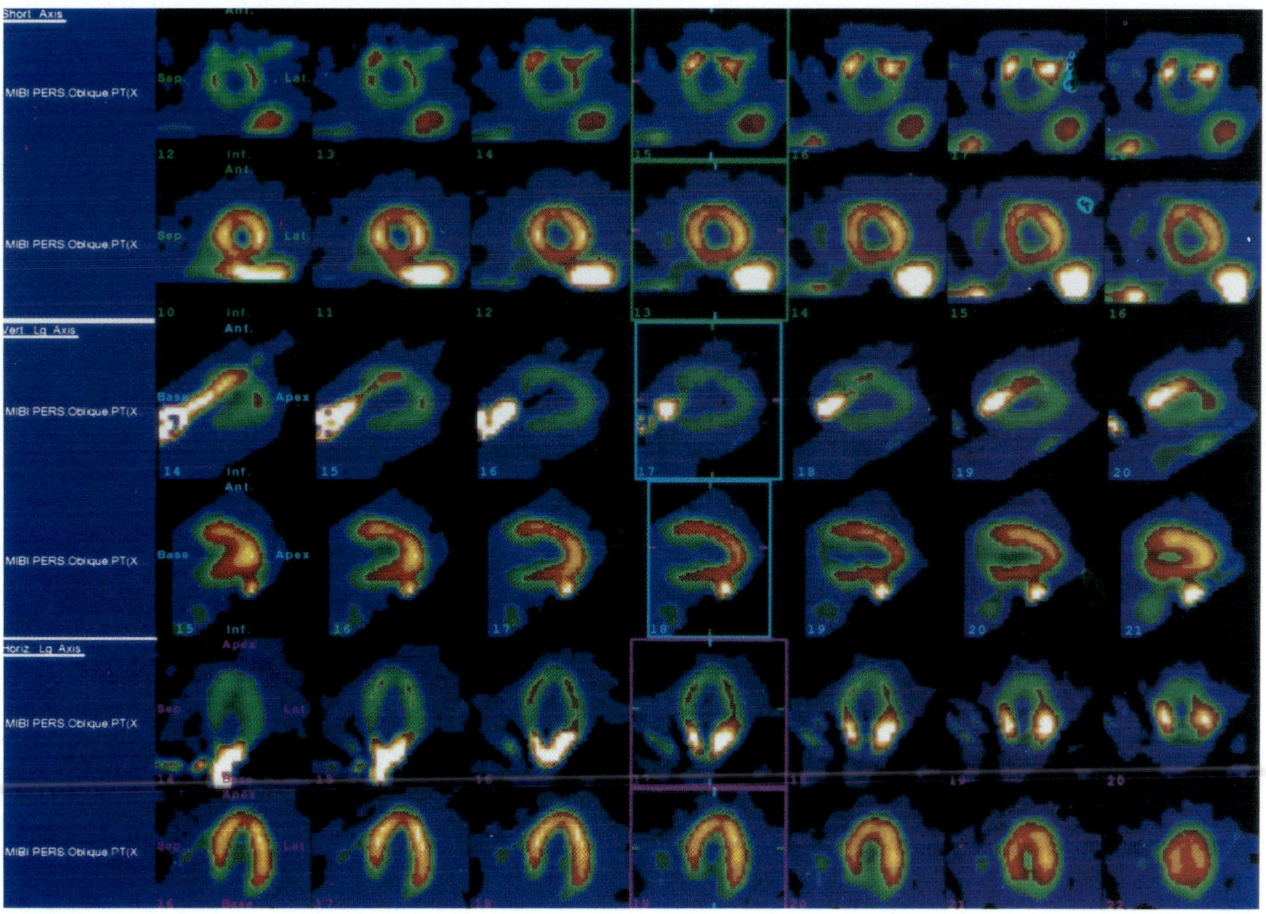

Figure 116

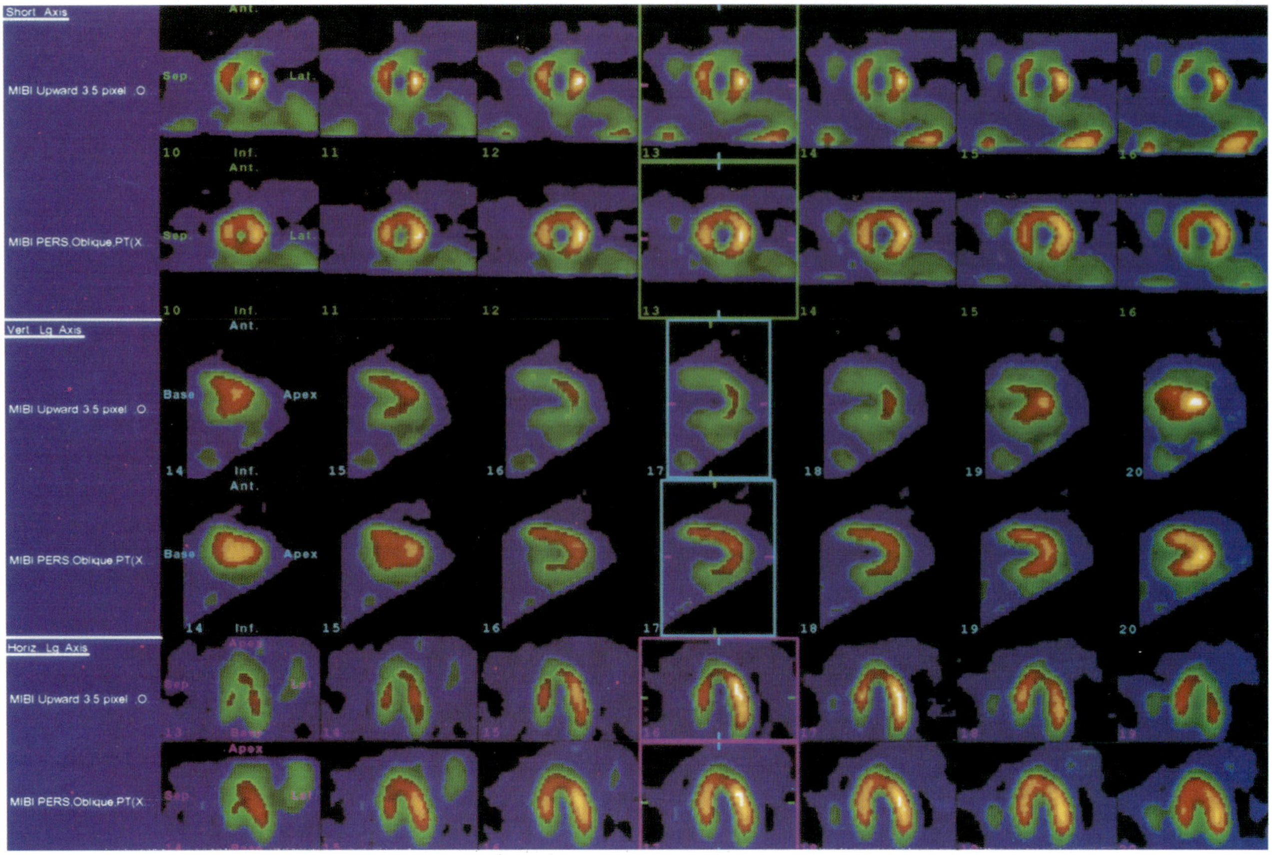

Figure 117

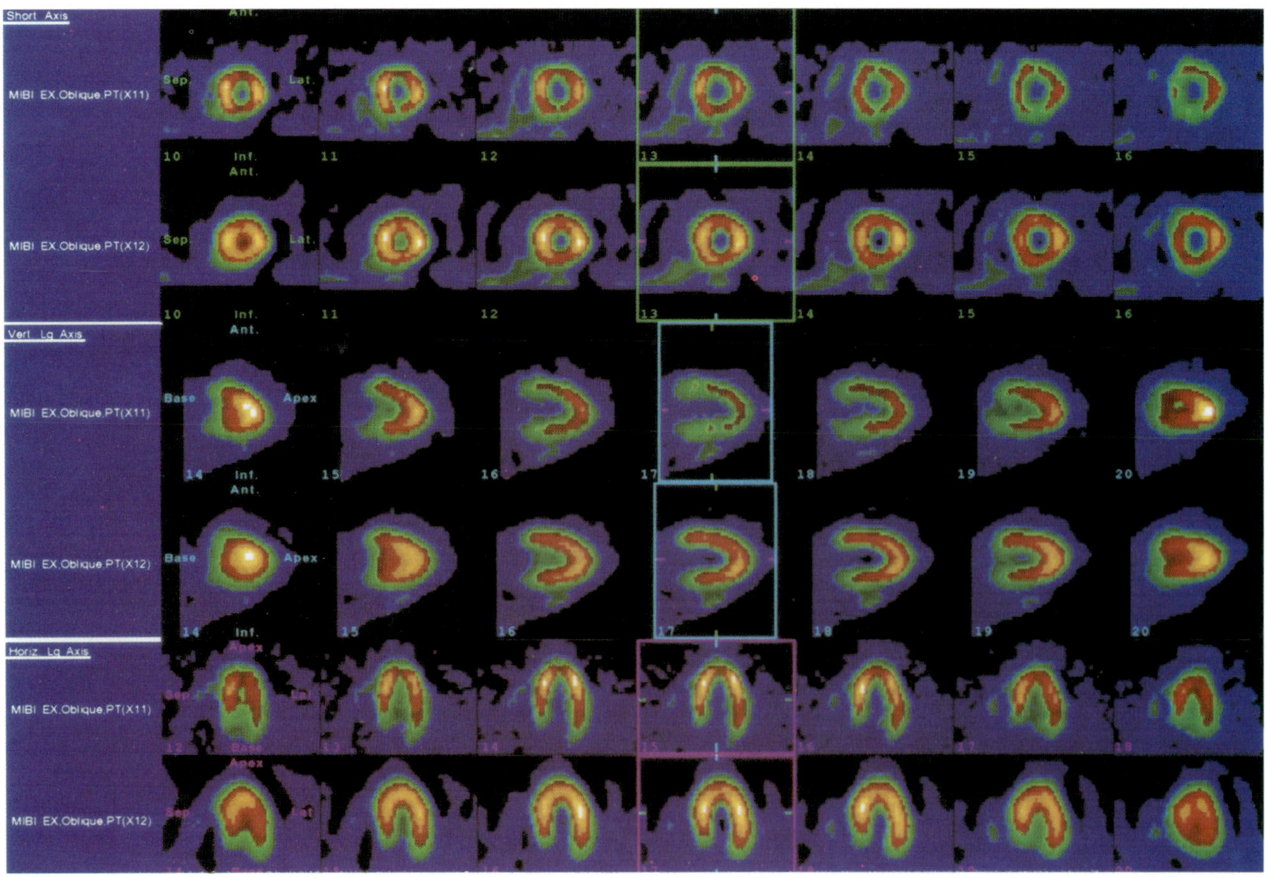

Figure 118

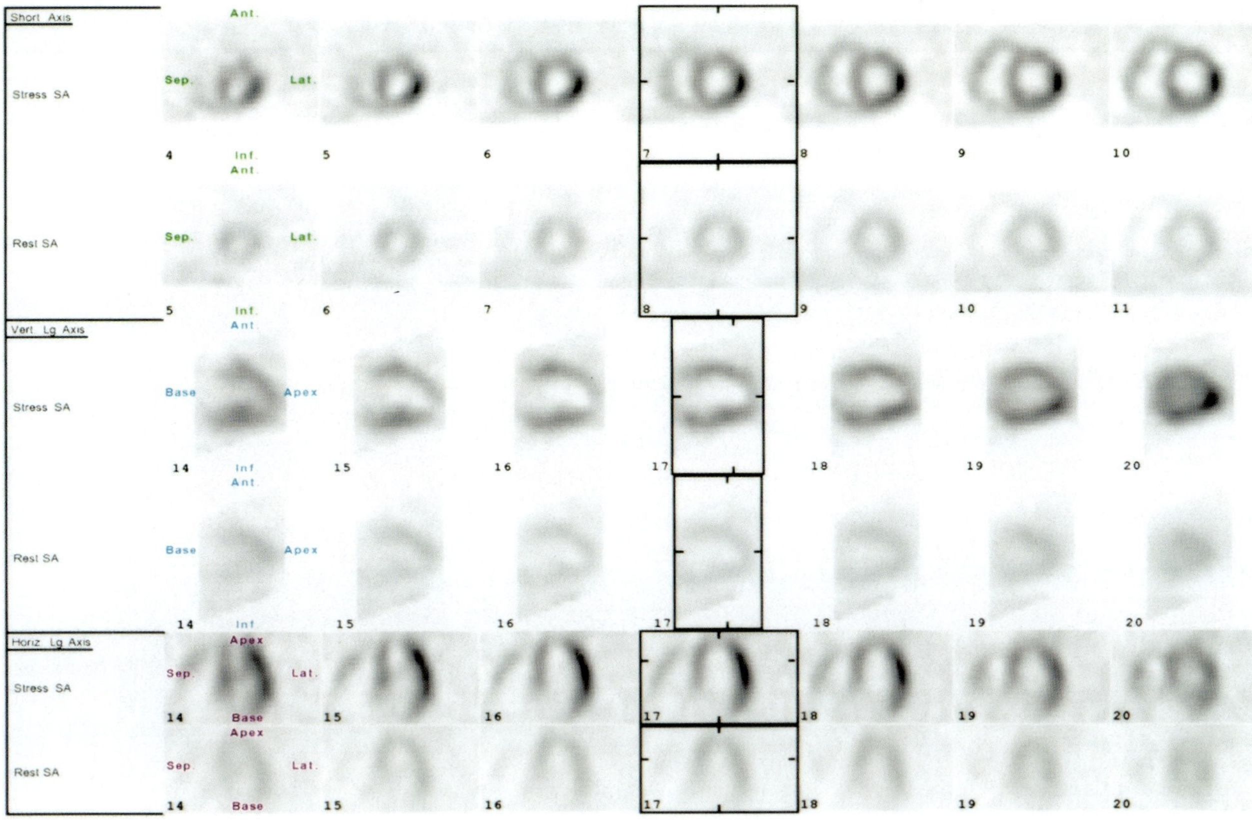

Figure 119

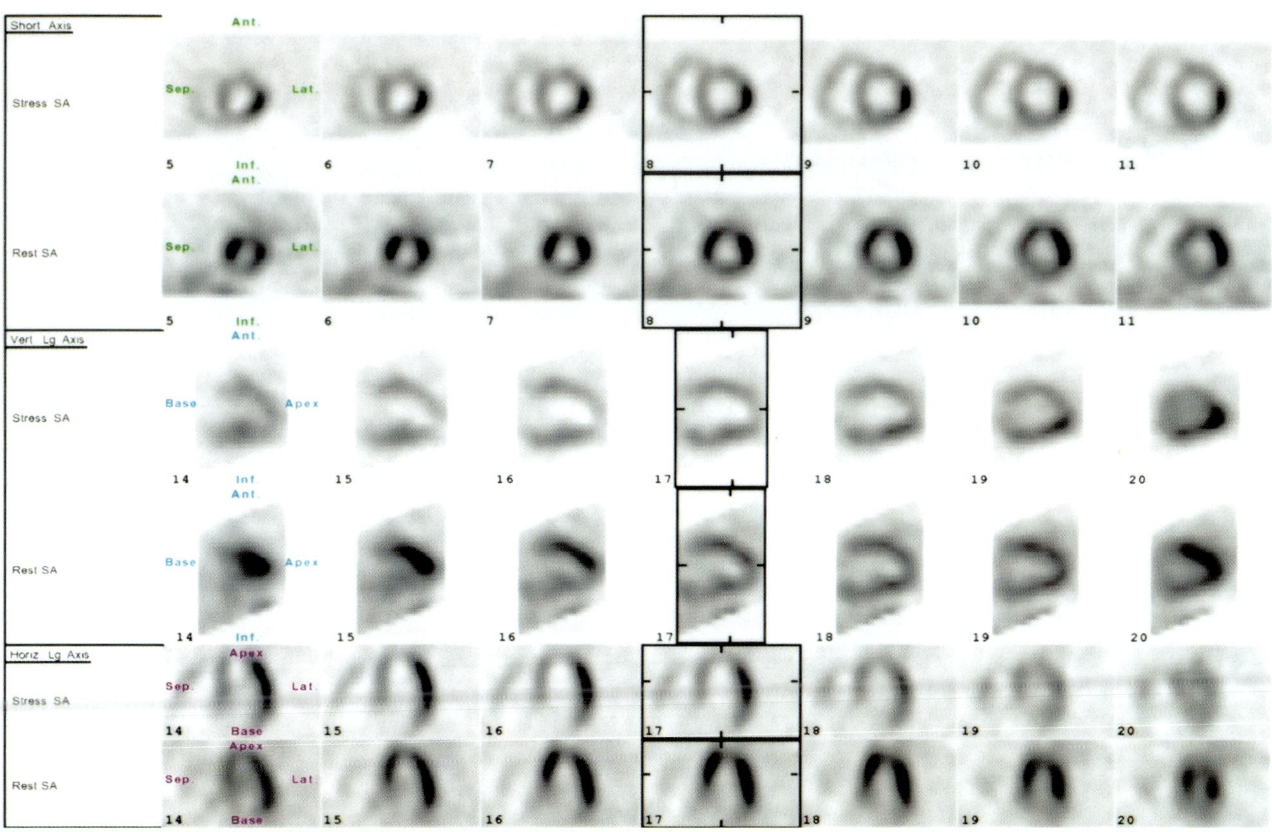

Figure 120

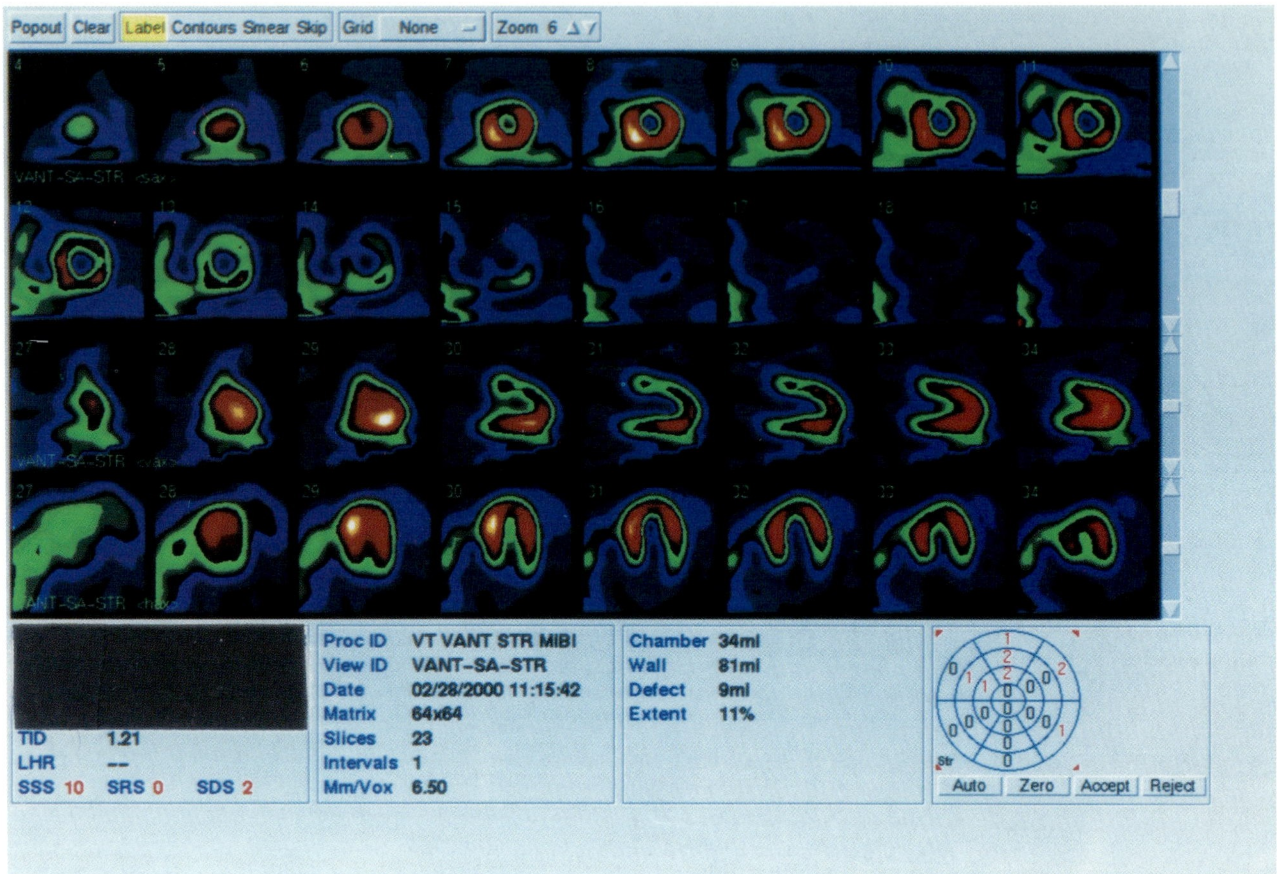
Popout
Clear
Label
Contours
Smear
Skip
Grid
None
Zoom 6
TID 1.21
LHR --
SSS 10
SRS 0
SDS 2
Proc ID VT VANT STR MIBI
View ID VANT-SA-STR
Date 02/28/2000 11:15:42
Matrix 64x64
Slices 23
Intervals 1
Mm/Vox 6.50
Chamber 34ml
Wall 81ml
Defect 9ml
Extent 11%
Auto
Zero
Accept
Reject

Figure 122

Answers and Critiques for Multiple Choice Questions

ITEM 1

Answer: a. The image itself is visually normal. Visual analysis should always corroborate the quantitative. There must be a compelling reason to call the study abnormal in the face of the visual impression. The counts-distribution profile suggests a minor deviation from the normal, in itself not compelling and probably within the range of statistical error. In addition, the basal location of the apparent anterior defect is not a typical coronary-related area. (Reprinted with permission from Wackers FJTh. Artifacts in planar and SPECT myocardial perfusion imaging. *Am J Cardiol Imaging* 1992;6:42–58.)

ITEM 2

Answer: a and c. A noncircular orbit may follow the body contour or conform to a simple ellipse. The type of orbit does not itself produce artifacts. Even a circular orbit rarely centers on the heart, because the heart is not centered in the body and the detector must clear the body over at least 180°. The loss of resolution with distance, as described previously, is always a factor in both types of acquisition. In fact, overall, better resolution is obtained by keeping the detector as close as possible to the patient. (Reprinted with permission from Maniawski PJ, Morgan HT, Wackers FJTh. Orbit-related variations in spatial resolution as a source of artifactual defects in Tl-201 SPECT. *J Nucl Med* 1991;32:871–875.). Figure 87 illustrates the effect of orbit configuration on reconstructed slices acquired in a healthy patient. In this case, varying distance from the heart and resolution related to the orbit that fits the body contour resulted in typical opposing defects. Attenuation and the likelihood of patient motion are not influenced by the camera orbit. (Reprinted with permission from Wackers FJTh. Artifacts in planar and SPECT myocardial perfusion imaging. *Am J Cardiol Imaging* 1992;6:42–58.)

ITEM 3

Answer: a, c, d and e. Acquisition at 180° relates to higher contrast and spatial resolution than 360° acquisition. Of course, this is also true for single-head cameras and relates to the greater degradation in posterior projections from attenuation, scatter and the detector response (*302,353–355*) included in the 360° data set. (Reprinted with permission from Eisner RL, Nowak DJ, Pettigrew RI, Fajman W. Fundamentals of 180° acquisition and reconstruction in SPECT imaging. *J Nucl Med* 1986;27:1717–1728.) Resolution degradation at depth, uncorrected by the backprojection algorithm, increases the incidence of artifacts in 180° orbits. This is particularly true of elliptical orbits, in which varying the distance of the camera from the target (heart) forces the detector to view the same structures at different distances and with varying resolution. (See Garcia EV. Quantitative myocardial perfusion single-photon emission computed tomographic imaging: quo vadis (where do we go from here)? *J Nucl Cardiol*

1994;1:83–93.) Elliptical 360° orbits are less problematic and relate to fewer artifacts than elliptical 180° orbits, because they always view an opposite projection and the far view balances out the close view, averaging out the differences in resolution. For all of these reasons, a 180° orbit is usually applied for SPECT perfusion acquisition, most often with a circular orbit or one that most closely parallels the body contour.

ITEM 4

Answer: f. A blown photomultiplier tube or dense attenuation would present a dense regional defect. Flood field heterogeneities would produce myocardial irregularities, whereas filter and cut-off variations relate to image processing, not acquisition, and do not explain image findings. The findings here relate to COR errors of 1 (upper right), 2 (lower left) and 3 (lower right) pixels that have been simulated. Created here are opposing anterior and inferior defects, as well as radioactivity "tails" that extend from the margins of the artifactual defects. (Reprinted with permission from DePuey GS. *Cardiac SPECT.* New York, NY: Raven Press; 1994.) The findings shown are similar to those described in relation to patient motion as a "hurricane sign," shown diagramatically in Figure 89. (Reprinted with permission from Sorrell V, Figueroa B, Hansen CL. The "hurricane sign": evidence of patient motion artifact on cardiac single-photon emission computed tomographic imaging. *J Nucl Cardiol* 1996;3:86–88.) In fact, the end result of a COR artifact is not dissimilar from patient motion.

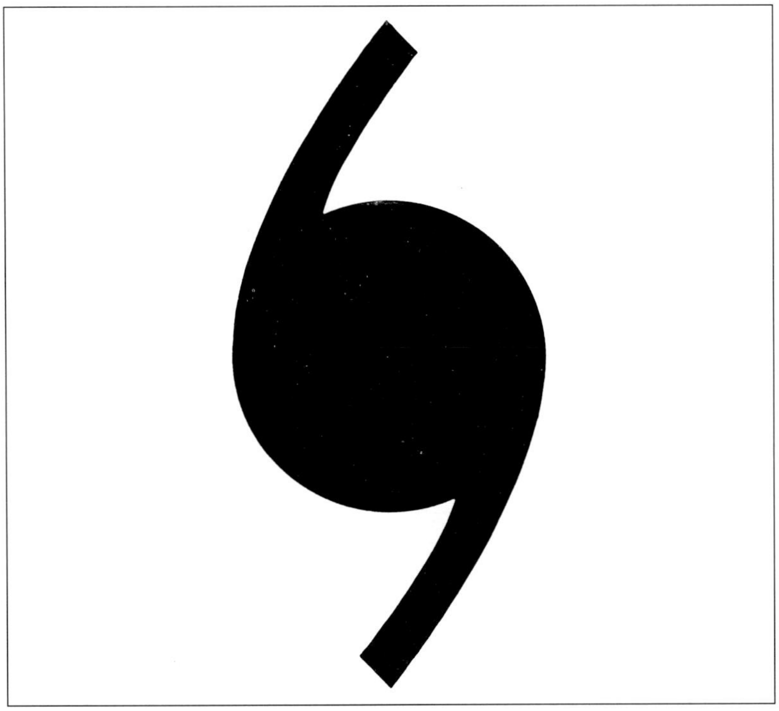

Figure 89

ITEM 5

Answer: d. The classic anterior defect, affecting the distal anterior–lateral wall but sparing the apex, is typical of breast artifact. This would be seen well in the projection images. The defect appears to worsen in some of the vertical long-axis redistribution images. Such "reverse redistribution" presents inconsistencies in defect localization and is caused by shifting soft tissue or nonreproducible soft tissue placement and gives further reassurance to the conclusion that the defect is based in artifact. (Reprinted with permission from DePuey EG. How to detect and avoid myocardial perfusion SPECT artifacts.*J Nucl Med* 1994;35: 699–702.)

ITEM 6

Answer: e. Shown is a ring artifact resulting from a defective photomultiplier tube in a region of the crystal adjacent to the left ventricle. This defect will be identified on the flood field, which should be tested for uniformity daily. The artifact results from the back-projection of flood field artifacts. For the same reason, ring artifacts also can occur in polar coordinate maps. (See Figure 66.) (Reprinted with permission from DePuey EG. How to detect and avoid myocardial perfusion SPECT artifacts. *J Nucl Med* 1994;35:699–702.)

ITEM 7

Answer:
a. Figures 60A and 60B
b. Figure 61
c. Figure 92
d. Figure 62 (see question 1)
e. Figure 59
f. Figure 93

ITEM 8

Answer: All are correct. As shown in Figure 44, wall motion and thickening are obvious aids. Prone imaging, usually by stabilizing the patient and altering breast position, provides a second look and often reduces attenuation effects. Projection data often will demonstrate the presence and extent of attenuation related to any given acquisition, and the dual-isotope protocol presents a unique comparison of relative regional activity with logical assumptions relevant to attenuation. Attenuation correction algorithms have not been proven in the clinical environment.

ITEM 9

Answer:
a. Figure 97A
b. Figure 97B
c. Figure 94
d. Figure 95
e. Figure 98
f. Figure 96
g. Figure 101
h. Figures 100A and B
i. Figure 99
j. Figure 102
k. Figure 104
l. Figure 103, the numerical designations indicate deviations from the COR.

ITEM 10

Answer: All are correct. The factors outlined are those that contribute to the drift in the COR. This makes for significant image defects. If a single hot point is seen to be 2 different points when viewed at a 180° angle, it will present 2 different points in the SPECT reconstruction. When identical regions or walls are seen to be different structures at different angles, major image discontinuities can appear. Figure 70 presents the same SPECT data processed in the 3 standard axes (short axis in 2 top panels, vertical long axis in 2 middle panels, and horizontal long axis in the 2 bottom panels) with a correct(top panel in each axis) and with an incorrect COR. Note the anterior apical defect created by processing with the abnormal COR correction. Figures 69, 103 and 104 also show the effects of COR artifacts. For this reason, COR evaluation must be done, assessed on the computer and the correction applied to subsequent image data. This is generally performed weekly with most SPECT cameras.

Such operational problems dealing with field regularity, as well errors in linearity, COR, energy resolution, sensitivity, magnification and other factors, should be checked routinely. A 2×10^6-count flood is performed daily to check uniformity and sensitivity. Cameras are peaked daily and with each new radionuclide imaged. Pixel size is measured daily until stable and then weekly in quantitative labs. Weekly checks of uniformity and sensitivity are performed with a 30×10^6-count cobalt flood acquisition. Resolution is checked with specifically designed linear phantoms.

This COR correction is then used to align the detector data with respect to the reconstruction matrix. Failure to correct for the COR, or the application of erroneous COR data, causes misregistration of pixels during the reconstruction process, which causes artifactual myocardial perfusion defects.

ITEM 11

Answer: a. Likely artifact. This defect is likely related to soft tissue attenuation from the left breast, with the anterior curvilinear area of reduced activity overlying the anterior aspect of the heart.

b. Likely artifact. Because of the classic distribution, sparing the apex and septum, and the findings on projection images, this, too, is probably related to soft tissue attenuation of the breast. Apparent reversibility relates to movement of the breast artifact on the redistribution study.

c. Likely perfusion defect. There is no evidence of attenuation artifact, and the distribution is classic for ischemia in the left anterior descending coronary distribution.

d. Ambiguous. The defect probably relates to the effects of the dense extracardiac activity, which could well result in an artifactual dense adjacent abnormality as a result of its interaction with the effects of attenuation and the back-projection algorithm. Delayed imaging of the ^{99m}Tc sestamibi stress study with prone imaging could be helpful.

e. Ambiguous. Here, the absence of a rest defect and apparent reversibility could relate to the effects of scatter of the dense extracardiac collection off the adjacent inferior wall. The extracardiac activity is not present at stress, which could well expose a true perfusion defect and result in the artifactual appearance of a reversible defect. The origin of the apparent stress defect must be determined and may be the result of scar or attenuation artifact. A delayed rest prone stress study could be helpful.

ITEM 12

Answer: a, b and d. Lung uptake, difficult to appreciate on SPECT images, is better seen on separate planar or projection images. The latter, however, are brief, data-poor images. Cavitary dilation may be more apparent than real if related to reduced uptake in a wall separating the camera from the blood pool. This transparent wall permits direct visualization of the cavity and the resultant appearance of dilation, often with accompanying photopenia. Washout cannot be evaluated well after reinjection or, of course, in relation to sestamibi or a dual-isotope protocol, but planar images can be so applied when acquired by the stress–redistribution protocol.

ITEM 13

Answer: a, b, c, e and g. Speed and efficiency are the main advantages. This permits its performance at all times of day. This then requires physician availability at different times through the day and may be difficult to support. It can be somewhat more expensive than other protocols. However, its efficiency brings greater logistic and clinical gains. Most of all, it remains accurate.

ITEM 14

Answer: All are correct. Practical advantages and maintained accuracy appear to be most important to the user, as the protocol is gaining in application. Nonetheless, interpretive methods must be adapted to imaging differences, such as the apparent larger cavity on the sestamibi image.

ITEM 15

Answer: b, c, d, and e. Proper circumferential profile analysis requires identification of the projection that looks up the ventricular long axis. This is generally identified by the symmetry of the related septal and lateral walls but could be problematic in the setting of infarction or ischemia.

ITEM 16

Answer: All are correct. The original studies by Bonow et al. (Bonow RO, Dilsizian V, Cuocolo A, et al. Identification of viable myocardium in patients with chronic coronary artery disease and left ventricular dysfunction: comparison of thallium scintigraphy with reinjection and PET imaging with ^{18}F-fluorodeoxyglucose. *Circulation* 1991;83:26–37, 1991) employed ^{201}Tl imaging poststress, after 4 hr and after reinjection. Some defects resolve after 4 hr, only to reappear after reinjection. These latter defects can resolve subsequently at 24-hr imaging. Although such redistribution can be impressive, it is a low-yield phenomenon.

ITEM 17

Answer: f. Images at 48-hr would be impractical because of their low-dose density. Sestamibi has no role in this situation. A higher dose may reduce imaging time but will not aid redistribution.

ITEM 18

Answer: b, c, d, e and f. We are learning that gallbladder radioactivity is not usually a problem and that earlier, rather than later, sestamibi imaging might aid the reduction of bowel background. Background-related artifactual defects may obscure adjacent perfusion defects or, alternatively, may sometimes produce a dense defect of an artifactual nature.

ITEM 19

Answer: a and d. Helpful is Table 1, in Self-Study Program III. *Nuclear Cardiology, Topic I: Physical and Technical Aspects of Nuclear Cardiology* (originally published in Faber TL. Multiheaded rotating gamma cameras in cardiac single-photon emission computed tomographic imaging. *J Nucl Cardiol* 1994;3: 292–303), which summarizes the relationships between acquisition times and sensitivities of multihead systems. Of course, a double-head camera with heads configured at 90° or 180° takes one-half the time to image a study acquired at 360°, when compared with a single-head camera. Although 3 heads sound plentiful, they cannot be as efficiently deployed over 180° as at 360°. Think about it!

ITEM 20

Answer: All are correct. Radionuclide at the left ventricular base, an area of sparse muscle mass, active motion and generally reduced relative radioactivity, is seen poststress but is not as evident in late images, in which the normal "horseshoe configuration" is restored. Lung uptake, cavitary dilation and basal uptake are the nonperfusion indicators of extensive coronary involvement and risk. Rarely seen in the absence of perfusion defects, they should cause added concern when applying the image results clinically.

ITEM 21

Answer: b, c, e and f. Currently, washout analysis is believed to add little in diagnostic sensitivity to SPECT analysis and is moot when using sestamibi or reinjection methods. The phenomenon illustrated here cannot be common. In the manuscript describing it and from which the example was extracted, diffuse washout abnormalities in the presence of normal planar images were seen in approximately 1% of patients with coronary disease. (Reprinted with permission from Abdulla A, Maddahi J, Garcia E, et al. Slow regional washout of myocardial thallium-201 in the absence of perfusion defects. Contribution to detection of individual coronary artery stenosis and mechanisms for occurence. *Circulation* 1985;71:72–81.) In addition, extensive work has documented an excellent prognosis in association with a normal planar perfusion image. The study by Kang et al. (Kang X, Berman DS, Kimchi EY, et. al. Prognostic value of a normal myocardial perfusion SPECT in patients undergoing coronary angiography [abstract]. *J Am Coll Cardiol* 1998;31:409A.) demonstrates an excellent prognosis in association with a normal image in patients without as well as those with coronary artery disease. However, discretion being the better part of valor, it may be worth having as a tool, provided data can be appropriately analyzed. If applying a ^{201}Tl protocol, the simple acquisition of a LAO planar image before reinjection will permit assessment of lung uptake, cavitary dilation and washout. Reinjection can then be performed, followed by SPECT acquisition, with little time lost.

ITEM 22

Answer: b, c and e. This example of dense, cavitary photopenia, or "the black hole sign," indicates dense hypoperfusion. (Reprinted with permission from Dae M, Canhasi B, Olvera S, et al. The etiology and implications of dense cavitary "photopenia" on myocardial perfusion scintigraphy. *Invest Radiol* 1985;20:388.) If induced by stress, it suggests a tight, high-risk lesion. It extends over the cavity, indicating its relationship as a property of the overlying wall. A similar phenomenon has been observed and described in relation to SPECT imaging and suggests the contribution of the perfusion of the overlying myocardial wall to the "cavity" in each slice. Because no more than 1%–2% of the injected dose is ever in the cavity after initial extraction, there is little radionuclide in the cavity to displace, even in the presence of a large thrombus. Therefore, this finding is not related to thrombus. However, when fixed, as is usually the case, it indicates the proper environment for thrombus formation.

ITEM 23A

Answer: b, c, d and e. In fact, the defect in the inferior wall proved to be an artifact related to high-intensity hepatic collection. Therefore, it was not a perfusion defect. The apparent counts reduction probably relates to the interaction of tissue attenuation and the backprojection method, in which the area of the inferior wall cannot be separated from the intense extracardiac collection, which latter contaminates or obscures inferior wall activity and prevents the identification of local counts. (Reprinted with permission from Nuyts J, Dupont P, Van den Maegdenbergh V, Vleugels S, Suetens P, Mortelmans L. A study of the liver-heart artifacts in emission tomography. *J Nucl Med* 1995;36:133–139.) The processing algorithm then erroneously concludes that the region must be void of activity.

An alternate explanation relates directly to the process of filtered back-projection as originally described by Shepp and Logan. (Shepp L, Logan B. The Fourier reconstruction of a head section. *IEEE Trans Nucl Sci* 1974; 21:21–43.) The method convolves the projection image data into a 3-dimensional SPECT image set using a negative filter function, which creates a band of reduced intensity (activity) around high-intensity objects (Sorenson J, Phelps M. *Physics in Nuclear Medicine,* 2nd ed. Orlando, FL: Grune and Stratton; 1987:394–401.) These "negative lobes" enhance contrast and eliminate otherwise evident "star artifacts."(See Germano G, Chua T, Areeda J, Kiat H, Berman D. Hepatic uptake creates artifactual defects in 99m-Tc myocardial SPECT images: a quantitative phantom analysis. *J Nucl Med* 1994;35: 356–359.)

ITEM 23B

Answers: b, c, d and e. The hepatic collection is mainly related to the biliary path of sestamibi excretion and the unfortunate acquisition during hepatic labeling. This usually can be avoided by employing ^{201}Tl, imaging sestamibi early, before or late after hepatic labeling, or using one of the newer ^{99m}Tc based, renal-excreted agents. Sometimes, similar problems may be encountered in relation to intense subdiaphragmatic localization of ^{201}Tl. Figure 106 demonstrates the original defect (left), as well as the restoration of inferior wall activity (right), after hepatic clearance on delayed imaging, 1 hr later (arrows). (Images reprinted with permission from Williams KA. Image of the month. *Am Soc Nucl Cardiol Newsletter* 1996;3:8.)

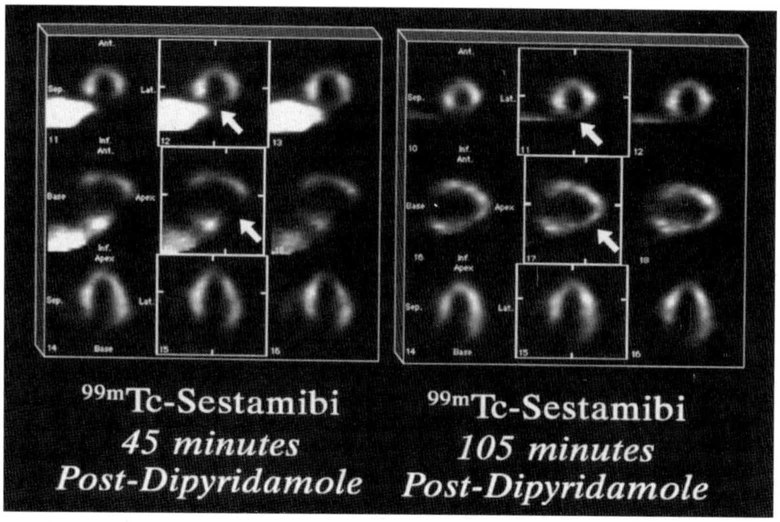

Figure 106

ITEM 24

Answer: f. Dilation seen here far exceeds that expected with ischemic dilation and in the absence of clear perfusion abnormalities. The study is said to have been "technically optimal," eliminating possibilities b and c. Volume depletion at rest is unlikely, because this generally occurs with longer fasting and the exertion of stress. Why would the patient be volume depleted at rest and not at stress? Stress-related tachycardia and reduced ventricular volume with heart rate would reduce the size of the heart in the stress study; the converse is seen here. In fact, the stress and rest studies were performed 1 mo apart. After the rest study was acquired, the patient was seen to be in a supraventricular tachycardia (SVT) at subsequent echocardiography. He returned for the stress study, which was said to show mild inferolateral ischemia. Volume differences at rest and with SVT explain the size changes. Yet, at the time of rest study acquisition, nobody knew of the rhythm! The study was not gated, an electrocardiogram was not made, a pulse was not felt and the patient was not even asked if he was experiencing palpitations. The physician in charge looked at the image but not the patient. This is a generic fault within the practice of nuclear medicine and must not be accepted in that field or the subspecialty of nuclear cardiology, especially because one advantage of the rest–stress protocol permits evaluation of the patient and his or her perfusion pattern at baseline before stressing the circulation. Such rate changes should be considered with different protocols in which stress-first ^{201}Tl protocols would place the patient under the camera early after exercise, sometimes for the first time. The lingering effects of exercise and the added effects of anxiety may influence apparent cavitary size. The rest study was repeated in sinus rhythm with normalization of ventricular and cavitary size (Figure 108). (Reprinted with permission from Wolinsky DG. Image of the month. *Am Soc Nucl Cardiol Newsletter* 1999;6:10.)

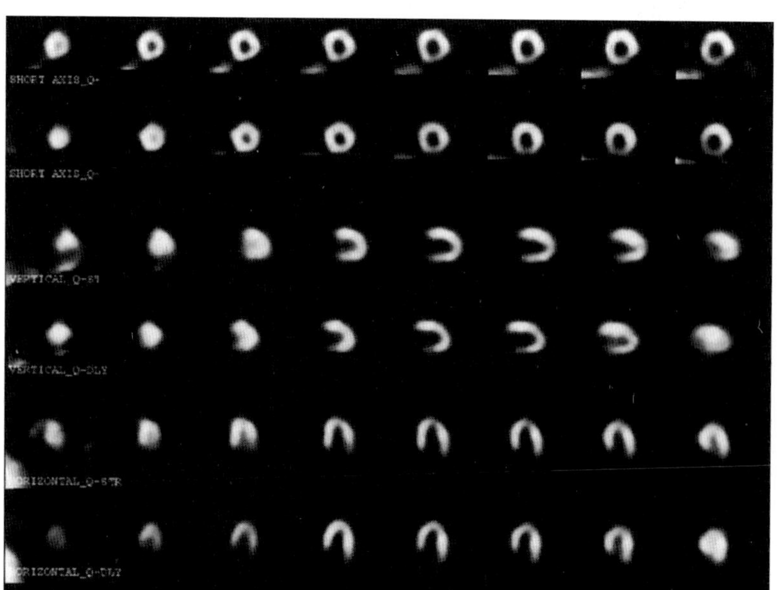

Figure 108

ITEM 25

Answer: c. Clearly, the ventricle is not dilated, and neither a small heart nor intracardiac shunts are indications for study. Although b may be accepted, this indication is not evident in the image, as is the vacant hepatic silhouette resulting from hepatic failure in this patient studied to exclude coronary disease before liver transplantation. Although exercise studies divert splanchnic activity to the exercising extremities, here the study was performed with sestamibi, with which hepatic transit is the main route of excretion. The gallbladder is seen as a punctate "hot spot" in the liver in the normal study. (Reprinted with permission from Cohen MC. Image of the month. *Am Soc Nucl Cardiol Newsletter* 1998;5:11.)

ITEM 26

Answer: false. Although Figure 110A suggested multivessel ischemia and was supported by the polar map findings, coronary angiography was normal, as was the image when reprocessed without motion correction, as shown in Figure 110B. In this case, with evidence of minor motion on the original projection set, the motion correction "cure" was more painful than the "disease." (Reprinted with permission from Williams KA. Image of the month. *Am Soc Nucl Cardiol Newsletter* 1999;6:10.)

ITEM 27

Answer: d. A comparison of the extracardiac deposits in stress and redistribution images shows them to be at different levels, in which the inferior hot spot at redistribution is nowhere evident at stress. This alone strongly suggests extracorporeal contamination, in this case on the patient's gown. With change of gown and reimaging (Figure 111C), these collections are gone! (Reprinted with permission from Iskandrian AS. Image of the month. *Am Soc Nucl Cardiol Newsletter* 1995;2:5.)

ITEM 28

Answer: All are correct. In this case (Figure 113), there was intense adherence of the radionuclide to the venous endothelium and not an infiltrated dose as occurred in another patient (Figure 114). In Figure 114, the intense "hot spot" marked the infiltrated dose, shown in the right arm, overlying the right side of the body, below and to the right of the myocardium, which is faint by comparison.

ITEM 29

Answer: a, b, d, e and f. Although c is usually true, in this setting in which continued poststress delivery of the radionucide is possible, the prone image, like the supine, could underestimate related ischemia. (See Figure 76.)

ITEM 30

Answer: a and e. Application of the bad flood (Figure 116) is the only possible process considered that could result in an extracardiac "hot spot." Of course, the distribution pattern in the upper panel of Figure 116 is not the one generally associated with breast attenuation. Opposing inferior and anterior

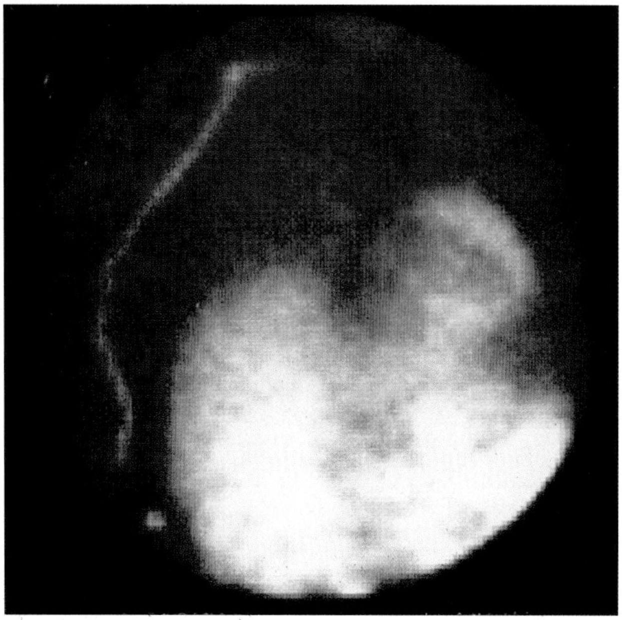

Figure 113

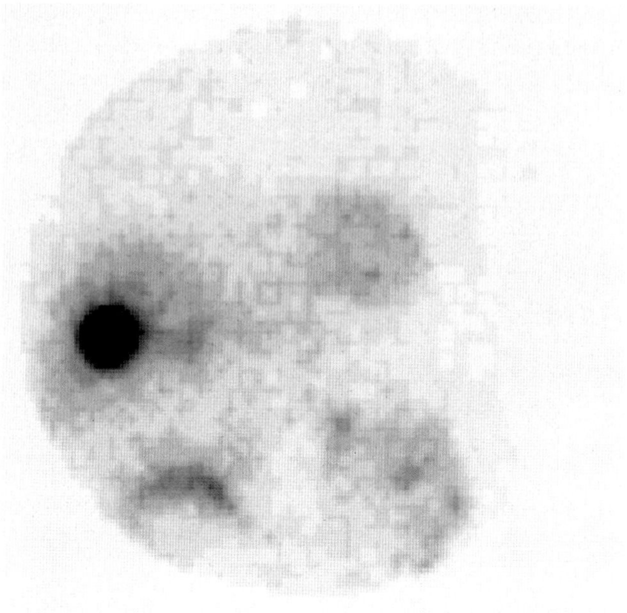

Figure 114

defects, as seen in Figure 117, are typical of vertical patient motion as "upward creep," a form of motion artifact more commonly seen with early poststress ^{201}Tl imaging. Figure 118 reveals relatively subtle differences in ventricular wall thickness, wall intensity and cavitary size, here influenced by the filter cut-off applied.

ITEM 31

Answer: true. Because of high background activity not evident in these slices, the intensity of the myocardium in the image is relatively reduced, compared with background and compared with the intensity of the myocardium in the stress image in Figure 119, in which intensities are spread out on a relative scale over the entire screen, that is, over both data sets. In Figure 120, each image set is normalized to the hottest myocardial pixel in each image set, making maximal myocardial intensity equal in both image sets.

It should be noted that although intensity differences exist, in Figure 119, the relative dilation of the stress image and its comparative heterogeneity are preserved. This becomes clearer in Figure 120, in which stress-related cavitary dilation and stress-induced anterior, apical and septal defects are evident. Demonstrating the identity of the relatives counts data content of the image sets in both figures, the polar map, shown in Figure 121, was identical when generated for both Figures 119 and 120.

ITEM 32

Answer: d and e. In fact, the supine poststress image, acquired and processed with the standard software without attenuation correction, was NORMAL! It is

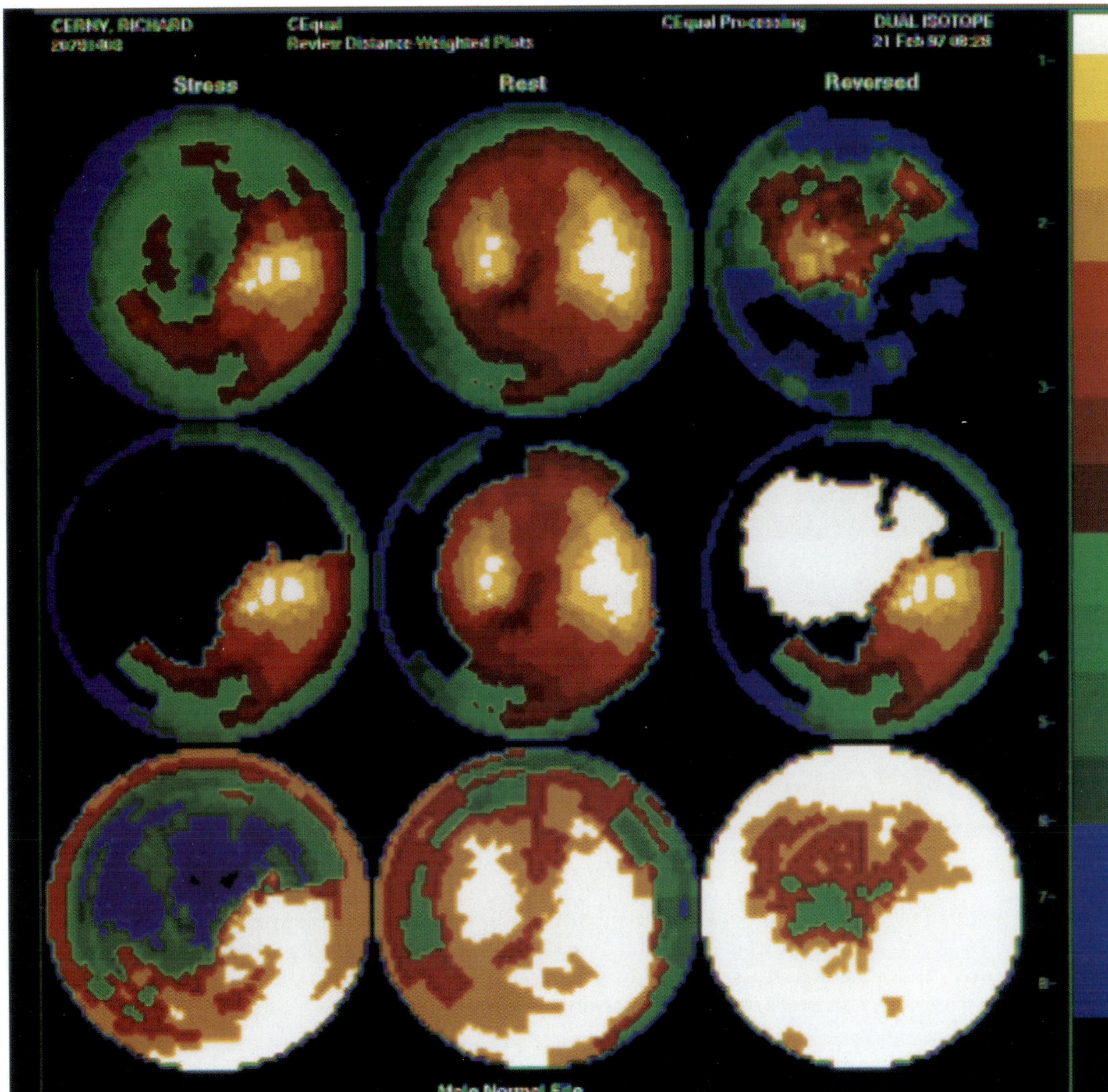

Figure 121

presented in Figure 123 in the same manner as the attenuation-corrected data discussed previously. In view of the clinical presentation, stress test results and many years of imaging experience with this method, it is likely a true reflection of the normal state of the coronary arteries. The attenuation correction method itself introduced anterior and lateral defects, suggesting multivessel coronary disease. Defects always may be artifactual in origin, and review of projection images is always wise. Perhaps this should be done before looking at the processed images and then reviewed afterwards. Answers b, c and f suggest that

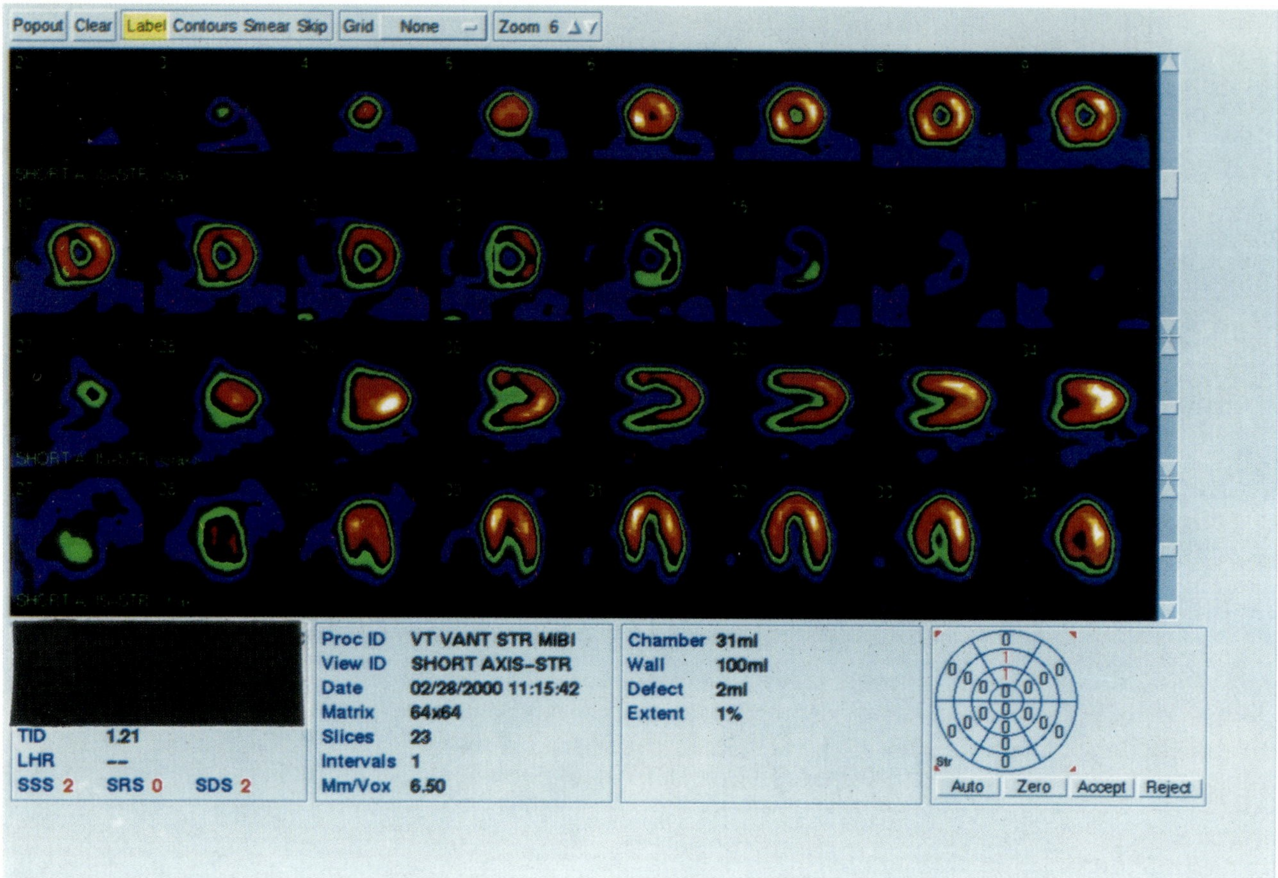

Figure 123

the defect is related to induced ischemia. Of course, this was not likely the case, and to proceed with any form of management based on this conclusion would be an error. Similarly, a rest study would only clarify whether the apparent defect in the stress study was fixed or reversible. It was, in fact, probably related to an error in the attenuation correction method.